WHAT WORKS, WHAT DOESN'T
The Guide to Alternative Healthcare

D0683106

WHAT WORKS, WHAT DOESN'T

The Guide to Alternative Healthcare

PAT THOMAS

Newleaf

Newleaf
an imprint of
Gill & Macmillan Ltd
Hume Avenue
Park West
Dublin 12
with associated companies throughout the world
www.gillmacmillan.ie
© Pat Thomas 2002
0 7171 3364 8
Index compiled by Cover To Cover
Design by Vermillion Design, Dublin
Typesetting by Carrigboy Typesetting Services, County Cork
Printed by the Woodprintcraft Group Ltd, Dublin

This book is typeset in 10pt Stone sans on 14pt.

*The paper used in this book comes from the wood pulp of managed forests.
For every tree felled, at least one tree is planted, thereby renewing
natural resources.*

A CIP catalogue record for this book is available from the British Library.

1 3 5 4 2

Contents

CONTENTS

PART III APPENDICES

Foreword

This is a book about how not to be disappointed with alternative healthcare.

Even now, putting the words 'disappointment' and 'alternative healthcare' together in the same sentence seems audacious. After all, everyone knows that alternative medicine is the kinder, gentler approach to healthcare. And yet as alternative medicine becomes more widely utilised and available the numbers of disappointments and failures are multiplying.

If you are interested in alternatives to conventional medicine you will no doubt be aware of the explosion of information on alternative healthcare over the last few years. If you are very observant you may also have noticed that two types of information prevail. First there is the unquestioning, laudatory type commonly found in the popular media that promotes the idea that alternative medicine can cure anything. Then there is the completely negative type that promotes the idea that alternative medicine is simply quackery and placebo.

Clearly the road less travelled in alternative medicine is the middle ground, from where it is possible to ask questions and observe and to see the all-important bigger picture of healthcare.

I believe completely in the philosophy of alternative healthcare. It is my first line of care for myself and my family and I have seen it work quickly and effectively over a wide range of conditions. I believe in the treatment of the whole person and not just the symptom and I have experienced in my own life how effective this approach can be in dealing with a whole range of health problems.

I believe in alternative medicine, but I also recognise its limitations and the existence of quacks and charlatans. I also recognise, as detailed early on in this book, that there is often a huge gap between the philosophy of alternative medicine and its everyday practice. For instance, when alternative medicine is practised in a conventional 'magic bullet' way – targeting symptoms with miracle cures – it ceases to be alternative medicine and becomes instead just another ineffective offshoot of the conventional system.

It is possible to believe in something wholeheartedly and still ask questions of it. In fact it sometimes takes greater faith to do so. Yet in alternative medicine opinions are increasingly becoming polarised into an 'anyone who isn't with us is against us' attitude which is antagonistic, unhelpful and unrealistic. I personally refuse to be pigeonholed into that position, and it is one reason why I wrote this book.

Although alternative medicine breaks many of convention's rules, one golden rule still applies: 'First do no harm.' If an alternative promises and then fails to work, if it makes the condition worse or produces new, more severe symptoms, it has broken the golden rule. What is more, this rule relates to more than just the physical body; it applies to the psyche as well. If a 'natural' remedy becomes just another emotional or psychological crutch, then a therapist has done just as much damage to the person in their care as if they had been given a synthetic drug.

The questions asked here are pretty basic. Does it work? Is it safe? Are there other options? To this end the information here is based on current research and is comprehensively referenced. However, I fully recognise the limitations of conventional thinking and research in helping us to understand how alternative medicine works and what it works best for. Those who clamour for more research into alternatives in order to make them more 'respectable' would do well to remember that very few conventional medicines and procedures have ever been 'scientifically' proven to work. In fact modern medicine is very unscientific. Tens of thousands of people experience a decline in their health status and even die as a direct result of conventional care every year. Our old ways of understanding the body – either as a simple machine or as an isolated biological battlefield under constant attack from invading germs – are breaking down. Nevertheless at the present time research data is one of the best tools we have for beginning to understand the benefits of the whole range of alternative medicines and therapies.

By using alternative therapies appropriately, and for conditions they have been proven to benefit, the disappointment factor can be minimised. Being aware of the strengths and weaknesses of each type of therapy can also give you a better picture of its real value. At the moment we have allowed the value of alternative healthcare to become bound up with the price tag it carries in the healthfood shop or the profit it can make for practitioners and manufacturers. And yet there is so much more to take into account when assessing the value of a thing. Let's open our eyes to all that alternative methods have to offer. Perhaps they cannot cure cancer; but if they can provide relaxation and a good night's sleep for a person suffering with cancer, without producing adverse side effects, that is a substantial step forward.

Another way to minimise disappointment is to look at our own expectations of therapy and the baggage we sometimes bring with us to alternative medicine. Alternative medicine is now a big consumer business and many people approach the selection of alternatives as they would any other shopping trip – with a big symbolic shopping trolley into which they collect all the latest therapies without giving much consideration as to how they work or what they are best used for.

You cannot be held responsible for the way in which some practitioners run their clinics or the aggressive and sometimes downright dishonest way in which some alternative remedies are marketed. But you can learn to think about healthcare as a consumer instead of as a patient. This means making yourself aware of the nature of illness and the total picture of health. It means acknowledging the parts our minds and emotions play in the way our physical bodies behave. It means being aware of (and fighting off) the very human tendency to want to switch off and leave it to the experts. It means choosing healthcare that suits your personality and your needs and saying no to those which don't (even if they come highly recommended by friends and relatives).

Becoming an intelligent consumer is one of the best ways to avoid disappointment with medicine of any kind and my hope is that this book will provide a springboard from which you can launch yourself on the road to confident and reasonable alternative choices in healthcare.

Acknowledgments

I had the ironic experience of writing a portion of this book while recovering from a disabling bout of pneumonia, so special thanks go out to my family, friends and colleagues who were so patient and supportive during and after this event. I am grateful as always to Lynne McTaggart and Bryan Hubbard at *What Doctors Don't Tell You* and *Proof!* for continuing to provide a platform for my writing, for being stimulating sounding boards against which to test theories and opinions and for providing such a valuable and necessary service to health consumers everywhere. Gratitude and love go to my agent Laura Longrigg – it's been a wild year. Thank you. I am also indebted to Eveleen Coyle and all at Gill & Macmillan who have been so supportive of me and have comprehensively restored my faith in book publishers. Finally to my son, Alexander, who has borne so much with admirable patience during this year: yes I am finished and, yes, let's break out the Scrabble board and plug in the Playstation.

Author's Note

This book focuses on the most common and widely available types of alternative healthcare. It also focuses on those for which there is some kind of research evidence.

There are many types of alternative healthcare available and more are being invented every day. While proponents claim major differences between therapies, a closer look reveals that very often they are merely variations on a theme (the many different types of massage are a testimony to this). Throughout this book where one therapy overlaps with another I have indicated this in bold italics. For example, if you are interested in homeopathy, you may also wish to read the information on other types of energy medicine such as *spiritual healing*. My hope is that this may help readers to understand more fully how and why certain types of therapies work and what they may be best used for, and also that it will assist individuals in finding the best alternative to suit their needs.

Certain practices which are no longer considered 'alternative', such as psychotherapy, have not been included. In addition, I have chosen not to include a separate section on 'nutritional therapy' as this rarely has anything to do with nutrition (which most practitioners, both conventional and alternative, would agree is the foundation of health) and instead is usually focused on the prescription of single supplements. While there is evidence that certain supplements can aid health under some circumstances, research into single supplements can be misleading suggesting that one nutrient is more important than others, and missing the synergistic actions of nutrients in the body entirely (and this, in turn, is a topic too big for a book of this type). Information on the importance of nutrition can be found in the introductory chapters as well as under *naturopathy*.

Part I

Getting Down
to Basics

Chapter 1

Santé

Achieving good health is now one of the single biggest preoccu-
pations in modern society. You may have bought this book
because you are interested in better health and feel that alternative
medicine may hold the key. Maybe it does. But there is something
else you may wish to consider first: what exactly is good health? In
typical Western fashion we appear to be pursuing something without
giving much thought to what it is, what it represents in our lives and
how it is best achieved.

In fairness, people have been struggling with this question since the
days of the earliest physicians. Clearly good health is more than just
the mere absence of illness or uncomfortable physical symptoms; for
if it was simply a matter of a well-behaved body how could it be that
some individuals, for instance those dying of cancer, often report
feeling a profound sense of well-being?

Fifty years ago scientists at the World Health Organization attempted
their own definition. Health, they said, was a 'state of complete
physical, mental and social well-being'. Given that this all encompassing state of wholeness is difficult to achieve, this definition met
with mixed reactions from health professionals. In fact, one physician
commented at the time that the only people he had known who
were in that state were either manic or about to have a heart attack!

Differences in the philosophical definition of health are not solely
what prevent us from seeing the bigger picture of health. Other
more pragmatic issues also cloud our vision. We are, for instance,

hampered by the way scientists study health and disease, reducing the body to a mechanistic series of causes and effects. We are also hampered by the fact that our doctors – the self-appointed guardians of public health – never study health in medical school. Instead they study disease, often in the way a general might study an enemy, continually looking for new strategies to eradicate it at all costs.

Conventional medicine has also gone down the road of specialisation; and while this has led to a better understanding of individual aspects of health and disease, it has also led to defining patients as collections of separate body parts and systems. Carving people up in this way means that the physician rarely sees his patients as whole individuals and is often oblivious to the continual interactions of the various body systems. For instance, the central nervous system is connected to the endocrine (hormonal) system and this in turn influences the emotional sites in the brain. The stomach and digestive tract are increasingly referred to as the 'second brain' and emerging research shows that this area of the body has a complex network of nerves, the enteric nervous system, similar to that of the central nervous system. These two nervous systems are constantly interacting, which may be one reason why, when your digestion isn't functioning well, your emotions may also be out of balance.

Modern medicine often congratulates itself on the fact that we are living longer than ever. But in celebrating the miracle of modern longevity we miss some crucial points about the nature of health and disease. It is not advances in medicine but in hygiene, housing and nutrition that have made the greatest impact on our longevity.

What is more, while we are living longer we are not living healthier or better. In spite of our increased longevity, a growing number of people in their prime report a lack of vitality and vague symptoms that they cannot pin down, symptoms such as insomnia, digestive problems, headaches, respiratory complaints, feeling run down, depressed and being susceptible to every 'bug' that is going around.

Such people are suffering from what US health expert Dr Jeffrey Bland calls 'vertical ill health'. They are not sick enough to take to their beds (and become horizontally ill), but they lack vitality. Worse, because so many of the people they know suffer from the same complaints, they consider these things part of the 'normal' human condition.

To combat this vague unwellness conventional medicine offers a variety of different drugs to help us stay vertical such as antide-pressants, decongestants, antacids and painkillers. In addition, many of us prop ourselves up with other things like alcohol, caffeine and nicotine and more recently 'energy' drinks (which are caffeine under another name) and herbal remedies such as guarana (also caffeine) and ginseng. But of course these things simply produce more adverse symptoms (which again most of us regard as 'normal').

Medic or physician?
Right up to the Renaissance the health profession was not called medicine. Instead it was called *physic* (from the Greek word *physis* or nature). Physicians were professors of physic and trained in the philosophy of nature. The word medicine is taken from the Latin *medico*, literally I drug. Treating disease with drugs was only a small part of the physician's work and the least-respected way of dealing with illness. Today drugs, along with enterprising new surgical techniques, are the main ways in which doctors 'care' for patients.

Enter alternative medicine
This book is, in part, about the way alternative medicine can be used to bring balance back to our view of health. Once considered a fringe interest, studies in both the UK and the US now show that more than 40 per cent of healthcare consumers will turn to alternative medicine before they will go to a conventional doctor. Visits to alternative practitioners have increased dramatically across the Western world.

Conventional medicine's failure to deliver 'good health' has moti-vated many individuals to take charge of their own health and has spawned an unprecedented interest in alternative healthcare.

Readers may be wondering at this point about the use of the term 'alternative' as opposed to 'complementary'. The choice is deliberate since the methods and goals of most holistic therapies are very different to those of conventional medicine.

For instance, alternative medicine is mostly aimed at self-healing and prevention rather than reacting to and suppressing symptoms as they arise. Similarly, alternative medicine believes in the innate ability of the body to heal itself; conventional medicine believes that only medicine or surgery can cure.

In alternative medicine there is a broader definition of good health that encompasses more than the mere absence of symptoms because, even in the absence of symptoms, a patient's essential vitality and ability to resist illness may be low. A competent therapist may be able to discern this and work with the patient to help strengthen and maintain a healthy immune system.

In contrast to conventional medicine, which is most at home treating acute diseases, alternative medicine has much to offer those who suffer from chronic complaints. And because many alternative therapies can be practised at home, they also place healthcare squarely in the context of the community rather than in isolated bureaucratic centres.

Because alternative therapies place no boundaries between physical, emotional and mental well-being, no aspect of the self is too trivial; posture, lifestyle, beliefs and values, energy and work and their impact on the total picture of a person's health are all relevant. Again this is in contrast to conventional ideas which look for single causes for single diseases.

The idea of partnership with the therapist is also in opposition to the dominant-subordinate relationships which many doctors and patients have. Because of this there is a certain amount of personal responsibility put upon the individual who seeks alternative forms of care. You must do what you can to help yourself whether it means changing your diet, taking the idea of relaxation seriously and integrating it into your life, or taking more exercise. It may also encompass more difficult tasks such as facing up to uncomfortable aspects of your emotional life, examining your own beliefs and behaviour and looking objectively at some of your relationships and priorities.

Perhaps most importantly most alternative therapies, when practised competently, are generally safe and medicines such as herbs and homeopathy are for the most part harmless and non-toxic. While any medicine – even the natural ones – can potentially produce adverse effects, these are still rare when compared to those of conventional medicine.

These distinctions will perhaps blur over time, but for now the most fundamental principles of holistic healthcare are so different from those of conventional medicine that they can only be regarded as an 'alternative'.

Does alternative mean better?

Although alternative medicine promotes a more holistic, patient-centred approach to health, proponents should not allow themselves to be too smug. One of the broader questions this book examines is whether alternative medicine is better than conventional medicine. In some cases there is evidence to show that it is. Some herbal remedies, for example, when tested against conventional medicines, have been shown to be more effective. But research into herbal medicine is still in its infancy; there is a great deal we do not know about the long-term consequences of using certain herbal products. Indeed, as the use of herbs becomes more common, the number of reported adverse effects increases exponentially (see Appendix 2).

As a philosophy alternative medicine is geared towards looking for the root of the problem and trying to see the bigger picture of health. But in practice many training in alternative medicine also focus on the process of disease to the detriment of understanding health and, for this and a variety of other reasons, not all practitioners of alternative medicine have a holistic outlook.

In addition, many alternative therapies and therapists ignore social issues that are continually working against the good health of the nation. These issues tend to cluster together, creating higher health risks in some groups. Poverty, for example, usually goes hand in hand with a poor living environment, an increased tendency to smoke, increased consumption of alcohol and low breastfeeding rates, all of which conspire to produce chronic poor health in a significant proportion of the population.

The risks such lifestyles bring with them are unlikely to be effectively addressed with aromatherapy, hypnotherapy or acupuncture. Addressing them with special diets may also be ineffective because many of the dietary requirements of alternative medicine (for instance organic foods) are either expensive or their ingredients are difficult to obtain in local shops. What is more, because most alternative therapies require a trip to a private practitioner, they are out of the reach of those who might benefit most from sound advice and achievable suggestions for a healthier lifestyle.

Health is as health does
The truth is that 'good health' is a very individual thing. It is the result of efforts in several directions at once; it's also more of a journey than a destination. Nobody feels whole and content every part of every day. Indeed, some would go so far as to say that without illness, and the impact that it can have on our lives, good health has no meaning at all.

At least 95 per cent of illnesses are self-limiting. In other words, they will heal by themselves and do not require any intervention. Of course prevention is an important part of healthcare, but just-in-case medicine – conventional or alternative – given without any real indication can make symptoms worse and produce a whole range of new and even more debilitating side effects.

For the majority of us good health remains, or returns, when we make the effort to create the conditions for it to exist. To this end it is generally accepted that healthy people behave in ways that are conducive to good health. These include:

Aiming for balanced nutrition The typical Western diet is a shambles of bingeing and/or denial. In search of the perfect diet (or more truthfully the perfect body) we slavishly follow trends initiated by 'experts' and celebrities. At any one time more than 50 per cent of women are on a diet and rates for male dieters are fast approaching the same levels. One week the trend is for high carbohydrate diets, the next high protein diets. Along the way there are diets that are high or low in fat, diets that don't mix proteins and carbohydrates, diets where all vegetables must be eaten raw, liquid diets, mono diets which only allow one type of food over the course of several days and, for some, the ultimate diet – fasting – which means no food at all.

When these diets fail to deliver permanent results most people revert to their old eating habits until yet another new fad catches their imagination and the cycle begins again. Balanced nutrition is about variety as well as moderation. It's also about balancing the need for convenience with the overwhelming benefits of fresh, unrefined foods. In a balanced diet no food is forbidden (unless you are intolerant or allergic). Everything from red meat to ice cream to cooked vegetables has its place (again in moderation); and because you are eating a wide variety of foods you will be getting a wide variety of nutrients, making it unlikely that you succumb to the overwhelming cravings that can lead to bingeing. Equally, in a balanced diet there is more to seasoning than salt. Using herbs and spices (herbal medicines at their most everyday level) liberally will bring out the best in your food, making eating a pleasure again.

Taking regular exercise An overwhelming amount of evidence shows that people who exercise regularly are less prone to disease (everything from heart disease to diabetes and cancer). They also feel better about themselves and even live longer. Your body can be a source of pleasure, strength and resilience and the importance of experiencing it as something other than a vehicle for carrying papers, briefcases, children and shopping cannot be over-emphasised. Your body really is the most remarkable thing you will ever own. Maintaining it by engaging in regular moderate activity once, or more often, each week is an investment in your future. Happily this need not entail structured exercise. Recent research suggests that finding 30 minutes a day to walk instead of using the car, to climb the stairs instead of using the lift, even window shopping while walking around a shopping mall, is just as effective as traditional forms of exercise.

Knowing when to take a break Healthy people are aware of the importance of getting enough sleep. They also understand the value of taking a break, not just yearly but daily and at weekends. They generally have hobbies and interests that absorb them fully and schedule time for these in their lives. They also have regular holidays and value, and actively pursue, time with family and friends. These individuals do for themselves what most 'stress management' experts make a lot of money teaching – they learn to spread the load, switch off and recharge their emotional batteries from time to time.

Not voluntarily poisoning the body The world is full of pollutants and toxins and we are powerless to avoid many of these. But we also have the power to say no to certain types of toxins. This can mean identifying allergies and avoiding those things that trigger them. It can mean not inhaling nicotine, or over-indulging in caffeine and alcohol. It can include avoiding toxic chemicals like fluoride and the volatile organic compounds found in most cleaning products, toiletries and perfumes. It can mean buying organic food, using natural wood in preference to plastic and seeking out paints and other types of home decoration that are low in toxins. Doing what you can to lower your exposure to toxins will have a greatly beneficial effect on your health in both the short and long term.

Pursuing spirituality Spirituality is a part of all of us whether we engage in the rituals of an organised religion or not. We are all divine. We all have the capacity to experience things outside our usual realm of imagination and our usual frames of reference. People who devote time and energy to their spirituality are exercising the muscles of humility, empathy, belief, hope, forgiveness and love. Such things are medicine for the soul and a healthy soul can act as a barrier to illness or, should illness arise, make it much easier to bear.

Paying attention to and taking responsibility for our feelings and actions Feelings are facts. They are relevant to our lives and to the way we interact with others. They are also relevant to our level of health. Healthy people acknowledge the full range of human emotions – not just the nice ones. They do not blame others (parents, employers etc.) for their lives or their actions and are mature enough to understand that not all feelings need to be acted upon. For instance, anger, fear, bitterness and resentment can be expressed without turning them into actions that hurt others.

Because this is a difficult concept to take on board, many 'bad' feelings simply get stored away in the dark recesses of our psyches where they can generate disease just as easily as germs can. Anything that eats away at the psyche can eventually eat away at the body. For example, psychologists have found that there may be such a thing as a 'cancer personality'. Two major theories about this predominate: one says that people who deny or repress emotions or are too focused on conforming to social norms are more vulnerable; the other suggests that personalities dominated by sadness, depression and unmet emotional needs seem more prone to developing cancer than others.

Building and maintaining strong social support Those who would like to live longer and healthier would do well to pay heed to the abundance of research showing that loneliness is the most powerful and destructive disease of all. People with strong social support networks, those who are fully engaged in their community, are inevitably the healthiest individuals. In contrast, people who are lonely have more depression and even more heart disease and cancer.

To fit all these healthy behaviours into one lifetime sounds like a vast prescription to take on board, but no law says we have to do it all at once. Good health does not have to be an all-or-nothing proposition. In fact, all too often the all-or-nothing approach is simply an excuse to do nothing. By taking on board what you can, you can make beneficial changes in your level of health. Even if you don't stop smoking, by taking time to relax and meditate you may stimulate bodily repair mechanisms that help you limit some of the damage caused by cigarettes. You may not have time to exercise three times a week, but taking the stairs instead of the lift or walking to the next bus stop each day can have a gradual knock-on effect, improving your circulation and stamina.

Disembodied medicine

Finally, while most discussions of health and illness suggest that illness is the result of a disease process in the body, nothing could be further from the truth. Physicians in every culture except our own have understood things in a different way. They knew that the symptoms we associate with illness are really the body's attempts to get well and to regain a state of homeostasis or balance.

Good examples of this process abound in our experience of common conditions such as fever, coughs and inflammation. For example, fever is uncomfortable, but it is not a disease process; it is the body's attempt to kill off invading bacteria and viruses. Coughing is not a disease process; it is the body's attempt to get rid of excess mucous. Inflammation in a joint or elsewhere is the body's way of protecting that area while the process of repair takes place. Likewise, a skin rash is not a disease process but often the body's way of ridding itself of toxins (the skin is the major excretory organ in the body).

Over the years medicine has turned its back on the idea that symptoms such as these are signs of a strong body trying to get well. To the modern specialist the symptom *is* the disease – something to be attacked and suppressed at all costs. Such a view is reinforced by our tendency to define health as the absence of symptoms – a body that doesn't trouble us in any way with niggles, gurgles, aches or pains. This, however, is a kind of disembodied medicine and with such miserly expectations the body inevitably becomes the enemy and its owner a prime target for profit-hungry magic bullet salesmen (again, conventional *and* alternative).

To free ourselves from our troublesome bodies we wage war, buying more and more stuff to try and quiet the body and make it behave. And yet to really be healthy we need to do the opposite, to make friends with our bodies. To many this sounds like a lot of new age rhetoric, rather like hugging trees and practising unconditional positive regard for others. But the fact is you must live in your body. If you are at war with it your life will always be a struggle, no matter what kind of medicine you use.

Chapter 2

Becoming Your Own Health Expert

In this country most people get their information about health matters via the media, and the media has a lot to answer for in terms of the way we look at our own levels of health expertise. First of all, our media suffer from an almost incurable disease itself – *expert-itis*. Whether writing about conventional medicine or alternatives, the media tendency is to ignore context and uncritically reproduce everything that any so-called health expert has to say. This can often lead to the passing on of incomplete, contradictory or simply wrong information. It can also reinforce the idea that others know more about your health than you do.

The conventional approach to healing also encourages the patient to switch off and leave everything to the experts, and of course many people take this attitude with them when they make the shift to using alternative medicine. Unfortunately, it is very difficult to make sensible choices about healthcare when you are 'switched off'.

The first thing that health consumers need to do in order to begin to make sensible healthcare choices is to cure themselves of expert-itis. Often this requires a substantial leap of faith and a belief in the miracle of your own body. You don't need a PhD or a degree of any kind to understand your body – you live in it. Absolutely nobody knows better than you about your life. Nobody has a more intimate knowledge of what you eat, how you sleep, what your emotional state is. No amount of careful history-taking can ever reveal every relevant detail about your relationships and life experiences. All these things combine to paint a picture of who you are, what your individual vulnerabilities are, and where you are likely to need a little extra support in order to stay healthy.

The seven principles of good health

Nevertheless, if you are still finding it hard to break free from the grip of expert-itis, it may be because you need more practical information and support. Generally speaking there are seven guiding principles that can help most health consumers make informed choices about their care. Bear these in mind and you can avoid being fooled into believing that your continued health depends on someone else's expertise. You may even be able to negotiate the minefield of modern healthcare with greater confidence. As you will see, these principles, while primarily aimed at conventional attitudes, also apply to alternative medicine.

Principle 1: Diagnosis is an imperfect science.

Today our doctors have an impressive collection of instruments that can allow them to measure and monitor virtually every part of our bodies. At the last count there were more than 1,400 different gadgets ranging from simple blood pressure cuffs to the most sophisticated computerised nuclear magnetic imaging devices.

There are some who hold up this kind of gee-whiz technology as evidence of how far medicine has come. Sadly, it also shows just how far we have slipped backwards. Many of our doctors have become deskilled – they have literally lost the ability to make a diagnosis based on their own judgment and on taking a good look at the person sitting in front of them.

What's more, in order to use machinery to assess human conditions, one must also accept at some level that people are like machines – that they are all made to the same specifications, that they all respond in the same way to the same drugs and that their bodily levels of fluid, hormones, chemicals, microbes and anything else you can name remain static from day to day, week to week, year to year.

Clearly this is nonsense. But for a doctor who has become deskilled there is only one thing left – a total belief in the infallibility of the machines at his disposal. Instinctively we know that machines and the people who use them are fallible, and the medical evidence bears this out.

One of the most common tests performed in doctors' surgeries is the measurement of blood pressure. High blood pressure can indicate a risk of heart and kidney problems. Yet an individual's blood pressure can vary by as much as 30 points over the course of a day, and white coat hypertension, that is hypertension caused by the anxiety of having one's blood pressure measured, is a recognised medical phenomenon. Also interesting is the fact that not only can blood pressure vary during the course of the day, it can vary between an individual's arms at the same sitting!

There are no controls over the use of some of this technology and often the accuracy of a diagnosis depends on operator skill. Prenatal ultrasound screening is a good case in point. Anyone can buy and use an ultrasound machine, even someone who has never had any better training than watching his colleagues until he feels confident enough to 'have a go'. But not long ago a major British study showed that one in 200 babies aborted because ultrasound detected abnormalities were perfectly normal. The same study found that ultrasound fails to pick up significant handicaps in one out of every 100 cases. Soon after that a major study in Oxford concluded that ultrasounds were wrong in one-third of all cases.

Laboratory tests for blood and urine are also far from infallible. In America in 1989 the prestigious Center for Disease Control and Prevention studied a representative sampling of laboratories and found that about a quarter of all test results were incorrect. The telling commentary in the medical journal the *Lancet* concluded that many routine laboratory diagnostic tests are a waste of time and money.

Of course alternative medicine makes less use of gadgetry than conventional medicine but blood tests are a common phenomenon for those trying to identify things like allergies and the presence of parasites or toxins. More and more machines, such as Vega machines, are used to provide a diagnosis – without a shred of evidence that they actually work. Also in alternative medicine the pendulum seems to have swung too far in the other direction. Understanding that an illness is more than just a collection of symptoms squeezed into a convenient pigeon-hole is important. But some practitioners take this philosophy too far, refusing to make diagnoses at all or if they do they give their clients vague mumblings about being 'out of balance'.

This is partly a problem of language – at the moment in the West unless we define disease by its conventional name we have no real language to describe it. Of course a Chinese medicine practitioner may describe a specific condition as being a disease of 'damp cold', but this is not meaningful to the majority of Western patients. It is also a problem of power – by not giving a patient a clear explanation of what may be wrong, the practitioner reinforces his or her position of power over the patient. It is up to alternative practitioners to fashion a language that is informative and accurate and does not exclude the patient, but they have thus far failed to do so.

Principle 2: It doesn't pay to be a guinea pig.

Although we tend to think of medicine as a science, in reality it's no such thing. We naturally want to trust our doctors. We want to assume that no one would subject us to drugs or procedures which are untested, unsafe or ineffective. We also want to trust that our practitioners have already done some of the donkey work for us, that is, that they have satisfied in their learned minds the difference between the value of a thing (its immediate social and medical impact) and its evaluation (monitoring its effects over the longer term).

But the fact is that over 80 per cent of medical procedures are untested. Remember your health is big business. By the time a drug is ready to be tested on humans, it may have been researched for more than a decade and developed at a cost of more than £150 million. Because of this, the temptation to cut corners, to shorten the lag-time between prototype and marketable commodity is considerable. In the

US the Food and Drug Administration has found what they call 'serious deficiencies' in 11 per cent of clinical drug trials.

Equally, a 1994 review in *Science* magazine found that the conclusions reached by medical research are often flawed by the most basic errors in design and analysis – either the trials weren't randomised properly or the researchers divided their results into smaller and smaller subgroups, or simply removed specific data from the analysis in order to make their study prove a predetermined conclusion, usually that a drug or procedure is safe and effective.

Even when properly executed, clinical trials of drugs can only ever give us a picture of their short-term benefits and risks. It is only when a drug is on the market that we can begin to see how many adverse effects emerge. Of course a drug can be studied once it is on the market, though quite often it is not until it is linked with a serious or fatal reaction.

The same problems plague new surgical techniques and technology. Keyhole surgery is a good example. One in five of all abdominal operations are performed with this method; unfortunately, many surgeons have begun to use this technique without adequate training. Fads in medicine change rapidly and as one doctor wrote in the *Lancet*: 'It was merely the surgeons' enthusiasm for something new, and the worry of being left behind if they did not master the technique, that led to the explosion in popularity of this minimally invasive surgery.'

So how minimally invasive is it? Studies show that serious complications arise in 15 out of every 1,000 procedures. One survey of more than 77,000 keyhole operations concluded that over half of the deaths after the surgery were attributed to complications of the technique. Researchers now believe that there are flaws inherent in the procedure itself and even if our doctors do boost their level of skill, it won't make much of a dent in the reports of adverse reactions. Nevertheless, it is estimated that very soon 70 per cent of all operations will be performed by this method.

In utilising alternative medicine consumers are often unwitting guinea pigs too. As is the case with conventional drugs, it's only when an alternative such as a herbal supplement becomes widely used that we begin to see some of the potential pitfalls of its use. St John's wort is a good example. Unlike many herbs on the market, it had enough reasonable research to show it benefited mild to moderate depression to warrant wider use. However, with wider use came adverse effects such as gastrointestinal irritation, allergic reactions, fatigue, and restlessness as well as interactions with a range of conventional drugs including heart drugs, antidepressants, anti-seizure drugs, cancer drugs, anti-transplant rejection drugs and birth control drugs.

Many other popular herbal supplements have no particular research behind them. And because nobody is looking, we have no idea how they really behave in the body over the long term and how they may combine synergistically with other supplements and drugs for ill or good.

Similar problems are being found in aromatherapy. Allergies to lavender, once rare, are becoming more common because of the increasingly widespread use of lavender essential oils and scented products.

Principle 3: There is no such thing as a magic bullet.

No single drug will work to cure all types of disease and the same drug can react very differently in different people. The assumption that all patients will respond in the same way to a particular drug is, in part, reinforced by the way they are studied. Scientists will, for instance, select groups of people who are as alike as they can be in order to eliminate any variable that might interfere with their research. But once a drug is out in the real world, it is no longer in a controlled environment. Anyone and everyone could be taking it and reacting to it in a variety of ways. Many of today's magic bullets offer patients nothing more than the opportunity to trade off one set of debilitating symptoms for another. In the most extreme cases a magic bullet may cause the death of someone whose symptoms could have been managed more effectively by less drastic measures.

For instance, heart patients are often given beta-blockers to regulate the heartbeat and to lower blood pressure. But in 1996 a clinical trial was stopped early because patients were dropping dead from sudden irregular heartbeats caused by beta-blockers. Exercise and the consumption of 'good fats' such as can be found in nuts are often just as effective as beta-blockers in improving heart health.

One of the saddest examples of the failure of magic bullet ideology is antibiotics. Today the vast majority of antibiotics are prescribed on a just-in-case basis, or for viral ear, nose and throat infections. But as any medical student can or should be able to tell you, viral infections do not respond to antibiotics.

Sixty years ago antibiotics were the miracle drugs of the century. They carried with them the promise that we would no longer be at the mercy of harmful microbes. Now they have been so over-prescribed and so inappropriately prescribed, that they have caused the emergence of antibiotic-resistant super bugs. As a result, what was once a genuine lifesaver is in many cases ineffective. What is more, antibiotic over-use has been implicated in a number of unrelated diseases and disease-like states – not just fatigue and tummy upsets, but allergies, seizures, psychosis, kidney and liver damage and even autism.

Alternative medicine is not averse to promoting magic bullets; some practitioners and supplement manufacturers positively embrace the idea. Indeed all the unnecessary products and paraphernalia that are sold over the counter at healthfood shops are as focused on useless 'magic bullet' promises of good health as the Prozac and paracetamol we pick up at the chemist.

Aided by the media many consumers now believe that echinacea will kill all germs; that plant estrogens will 'cure' menopause; that because sharks 'don't get cancer' consuming shark cartilage will prevent humans from getting it; that silver, which is poisonous when ingested in any other form, is actually beneficial when taken in a 'colloidal' form; and that drinking a tea made from a rotting Kombucha mushroom or taking a supplement made from the velvet harvested from wild elk antlers can keep us young for ever. In alternative medicine as in conventional medicine one principle is always consistently true – if it sounds too good to be true, it is.

What does it all mean?

Many alternative medicines and therapies are accompanied by claims which can sound impressive, but which on closer inspection are almost meaningless. These include:

Traditional

This claim is a double-edged sword. It usually implies that the product or therapy has been used for hundreds, even thousands of years. This kind of pedigree is often taken as an endorsement of the quality or effectiveness of the therapy. Traditional is also applied to products in the US that were in use before 1938. With one stroke of a bureaucratic pen these substances, too numerous to test in our lifetime, were deemed to be generally safe and so do not require testing. Since most supplement manufacturers are loath to test their products because of the cost involved, the traditional tag is used to suggest efficacy that may not be there. Colloidal silver is a good example of a product that was in use before 1938 and which has been sold without any published data on its safety or efficacy as a cure for a wide variety of conditions. However recently the FDA declared it misbranded (for being dispensed with misleading information) and restrictions have finally been placed on what manufacturers can and cannot claim about it.

Natural

There is no real definition of natural. It is usually taken to mean something that is harmless and beneficial and which comes from a natural rather than a laboratory source. However, it would be naive to assume that all natural substances are harmless. What is more, many alternative therapies involve some very unnatural practices such as sticking needles into the skin, enforced fasting and/or vomiting, or injecting mistletoe into a tumour.

Holistic

Holism relates to the outlook of the practitioner (and patient) and their ability to see the bigger picture of health. Some conventional practitioners do practise in a holistic way and some alternative practitioners practise magic bullet medicine – seeking to repress symptoms rather than seek out causes of illness.

No side effects

All remedies and therapies have side effects. Getting better is a side effect. So is getting worse. What the claim is really trying to say is no adverse effects. But once again few therapies can claim to be 100 per cent free of adverse effects. Aromatherapy, for example, can cause allergic reactions – not life threatening but certainly an adverse effect. And hypnotherapy, while genuinely useful, can sometimes leave patients feeling profoundly disoriented – also an adverse effect.

Proven in clinical trials

Most drugs and procedures used in healthcare are not well proven. In alternative medicine the claim for proof is a moving feast. Usually it does not refer to clinical trials published in respectable medical journals. Instead, it often refers to uncontrolled and unscientific observations carried out in the inventor's clinic or practice. Sometimes it refers to customer feedback, but anecdote, however useful, is not the same as evidence. Other claims of proof refer to unpublished research emanating from a university or hospital, which while useful is not considered definitive.

Principle 4: It's different for girls.

Sometimes the most obvious truths are the hardest to grasp. Females are not males. They have a different physiology, lead different lives and have different needs. But in medicine, different is bad. Different is scary and unpredictable and needs controlling.

As a general rule good health, like so much else in our society, is defined by what is appropriate and normal for a fit, young male. But females, because of their ability to conceive and bear children, have a rather more complex biology than men. Medicine has long wrestled with the 'problem' of female biology and the way that, for instance, women tend to react differently to certain drugs and surgical procedures. Indeed, women are often excluded from drug trials on the basis that their physiology complicates things. This results in two things. First of all we are in the dark about what kinds of different reactions women might experience when taking drugs which have been tested primarily on men. Secondly, it reinforces the idea that there is something inherently wrong with the way women's bodies function. Few women today do not perceive their bodies, at some level and for a variety of reasons, to be a 'problem'. This makes them very vulnerable to the idea that they need to be fixed.

Doctors often perceive women as being at the mercy of their hormones. The belief that women need to be hormonally 'normalised' is behind many of the 'cures' offered to them today. At one end of her life a woman's fertility gets 'normalised' with the birth control pill, at the other with hormone-replacement therapy. A woman who has been 'fixed' in this way, of course, has an increased risk of stroke and estrogen-dependent cancers of the breast and endometrium, and far from being protective HRT does not prevent memory loss and can actually increase the risk of heart disease and osteoporosis.

One of the greatest failures of alternative medicine is the way it has taken the raging hormone ethos of conventional medicine on board. Given that women are the major users of alternative medicine this is potentially a very serious thing. Today nearly every herbal remedy for women is based on so-called 'natural' plant estrogens. Alternative doctors, it seems, are as willing as their conventional counterparts to muck around with women's bodies and the inadequacies, even dangers, of this approach are fast becoming apparent. Plant estrogens, far from being natural and mild, can be very potent and cause many of the same problems that synthetic ones do. Indeed they can combine in the body with synthetic estrogens and become stronger still. As long as women continue to accept that their bodies are a problem to be managed, such outrageous practices will continue.

Principle 5: Your body speaks your mind.
No discussion of health could be complete without examining the relevance of illness. Today we believe that good health is our 'right', something which should be bestowed upon us (by governments, doctors and so on) rather than something which is acquired through our own actions. But perhaps the idea of perfect health and well-being is just a cultural myth. Perhaps holding on to the ideas of the

'rightness' of health and the 'wrongness' of illness can prevent us from understanding that health and illness can be part of the same normal, healthy process. What we call illness, apart from being part of a larger health process, can also be profoundly meaningful on other levels.

Many bodily symptoms are the result of, or can be worsened by, a poor emotional state. When exploring the mind-body connection, it's all too easy to focus on the effects of stress. However it's not just a question of stress, but of the whole panoply of human experiences and emotions which influence our levels of health.

For example, medicine has yet to convincingly answer the question of what causes heart failure. The risk factors that are commonly highlighted, such as smoking, obesity, a sedentary lifestyle and a high fat diet account for only half of all heart disease. To find the other half we must look to sociology and psychology. Large studies over a number of years, in both San Francisco and eastern Finland, have observed that those who are lonely and socially isolated are two to three times more likely to die from heart disease (and other causes) than those who feel connected to others. The inference is profound – some heart attack victims may, quite literally, be dying of a broken heart.

In the search for good health, it behoves us to ponder what might happen if we allowed similar metaphors to influence our diagnosis and treatment of illness. What changes might occur if, for instance, we asked ourselves what emotional mechanism prompts the body to attack its own tissues, as in auto-immune diseases. Or what kind of mental or emotional inflexibility might facilitate crippling disorders such as arthritis.

In his ground-breaking book, *The Healing Power of Illness*, Thorwald Dethlefsen offers a radically different perspective on everyday symptoms that most of us take for granted. Rashes, he says, always indicate that something which has hitherto been held back (repressed) is trying to break through the repression in order to come to the light (consciousness) allowing something that was previously invisible to show itself.

He also reminds us how often a person with a cold says something like 'stay away from me'. Initially it seems like a protective gesture aimed at those around us, but keeping people away may well have an emotionally protective effect for the sufferer as well.

Taking ideas such as this on board can take a great deal of courage, as it can change your view of yourself and the world dramatically. But it may also provide the one thing that always seems to be missing from medical diagnosis – insight into why we sometimes get ill. At the same time it paves the way towards acceptance of the mounting evidence of the effectiveness of mind/body therapies. For example, there are more than 500 studies attesting to the healing contribution of transcendental meditation over a wide range of disorders.

Happily many alternative practitioners do recognise the body/mind connection. However, like conventional doctors, few are trained in counselling or psychotherapy and as a result they don't always know how best to support a person whose psyche is strongly influencing the course of their illness. Acknowledging the psyche's part in illness is only the first step. Practitioners must be skilled enough to either work effectively with the psyche or well connected enough to refer a client on to someone who can.

Principle 6: It might not be a bug.
In principle 4 it was mooted that the emotions and psyche have the power to make us ill. But illness can also speak to us about the state of both our internal and external environments. While conventional medics still look for germs, injury and genetics as the main causes of illness, increasingly it seems that environment plays a large but unrecognised role. For example, increasing numbers of people are being affected by chronic complaints such as headaches, skin rashes, catarrh and breathing difficulties. Environmental doctors would say that many of these individuals are quite literally 'allergic' to the 21st century. We are all being bombarded with chemicals and toxins throughout the day. Children in particular can suffer more because their immune systems are still developing and because they are smaller and thus are taking in more toxins per pound of body weight

than adults. It's hardly surprising then that conditions like asthma and allergies are on the rise among young people.

Again alternative medicine has led the way in this wider understanding of the causes of illness. But because we live in a society where things must be either black or white there is a tendency among some alternative practitioners to believe that all symptoms are emotional in origin or that all diseases have their roots in a toxic environment. This can cause complications in some patients' conditions. For instance, emerging evidence suggests that diabetes can be linked to exposure to pesticides. But if a diabetic patient is encouraged to fast and reduce the amount of insulin they take without full consideration of their condition, the result can be a substantial worsening of their health and in rare circumstances death.

Principle 7: There is still so much we don't know.

With advances in medical science coming at us thick and fast every day, it can be hard to grasp the idea that we actually know very little about how the body functions and what effect the drugs and chemicals we are exposed to either directly or indirectly may be having on our health. Conventional medicine often has very little to offer people suffering from conditions such as chronic fatigue, allergies and auto-immune diseases, because these diseases are not well understood. Often in treating chronic conditions a doctor may prescribe a medication based on habit or an educated guess. If the symptoms disappear in the short term, the treatment is deemed a 'success'. But because we are so focused on the short term, if more worrisome symptoms emerge at a later date, the doctor may see this as an entirely unrelated event and not as a result of the drug regime.

Alternative therapists can be just as dogmatic and lacking in insight as their conventional counterparts. Each type of healthcare has a tendency to believe that their techniques have the capacity to address nearly all health problems. And each type of healthcare is wrong. In reality the practice of both conventional and alternative medicine is made up mostly of partial triumphs and outright failures broken by occasional spectacular successes. The arrogant idea that proponents of alternative healthcare have a better handle on health matters than others obscures the fact that we still know very little about the way our bodies function and that their systems of care cannot yet explain everything there is to explain about the intricate workings of the body. Alternative practitioners may be on the right track, but they have not yet arrived at the destination.

Part II

The Alternatives

Chapter 3

Avoiding Disappointment

The idea that anybody using alternative healthcare could be disappointed with the experience is not one that is usually given much space. So much has been written about how you can find true good health through practices such as herbalism, homeopathy, aromatherapy and massage that the idea of such therapies failing to deliver seems almost unthinkable. Yet alternative medicine often does fail, in many ways.

The most obvious way in which alternative therapies can fail us is that they don't work. A person may take up a therapy that has been recommended to them by a friend or buy a supplement they have read about somewhere and in spite of high hopes may find that it does not produce the hoped for outcome. Equally, therapists may make recommendations, insinuations or outright promises about what they can achieve and then fail to live up to their word. In addition, much of the way we use alternative medicine today is inappropriate. Lacking in basic information, or seduced by so many promises of the safety and efficacy of alternative healthcare, many people self-treat with the wrong medicines, in the wrong dose, for the wrong disease.

The consequences of such failures may not seem so great at first. Yes, some people will become disillusioned. In some instances, if high expectations of one therapy don't pan out, a person may in their frustration begin to believe that all alternative medicine is ineffective.

However, if such frustrations go on long enough and are experienced by a wide enough group of people, a second problem arises because all these disappointments and avoidable failures are chipping away at the respectability and, if we are not cautious, the availability of alternative medicine.

There are any number of regulatory organisations just waiting in the wings for enough people to be disappointed with alternative medicine so that they can legitimately swoop in, regulate it, restrict its use and take control of it (and ultimately make a profit from that control). The bottom line with alternative medicine is – if we abuse it, we will lose it.

A substantial step on the road to legitimising alternative medicine would be to stop randomly throwing 'natural' alternatives at every disease that comes along and start using them with a bit of restraint and common sense. To this end there has been an interest in what is being called integrative medicine – a melding of conventional and alternative practices as and when it is appropriate to the patient's condition. While relatively new in the West, practitioners of traditional Ayurveda, who are often medical doctors, have long moved effortlessly between conventional and more alternative practices. This paradigm, however, has not been widely accepted in the West where issues of who 'controls' this new type of medicine are still yet to be resolved. At the moment the power rests solely with conventional medicine and practitioners of alternative medicine (probably quite legitimately) fear that without an equal voice in the process, integration will be just another form of suppression.

The troubling issue of proof

Another way of trying to legitimise alternative healthcare has been to subject it to scientific scrutiny. Most of us would like to know that the healthcare we choose has been proven to be effective through good quality research. As we have already seen, this is not the case with a great deal of conventional medicine. It is likewise not the case with alternatives. Several things stand in the way of producing good quality research into alternative medicine including:

Lack of funding Those who fund medical research are often reluctant to give money to those researching alternative medicine.

28

Because many products such as herbs cannot be patented, pharma-ceutical companies have no interest in funding such studies since they cannot make a profit from them. Just to put things into per-spective, in 1995 only 0.08 per cent of NHS research funds were spent on complementary medicine.

Poor research skills Many alternative practitioners have never had any training in practical research skills or in evaluating existing data. They may have no access to library facilities, supervision or other resources. Most training in alternative therapies does not emphasise the value of good quality research.

Small study sizes Often studies into alternative medicine involve very small numbers of people. Only with large numbers of partici-pants can a study claim to have the 'power' to prove anything. Large numbers allow researchers to confirm efficacy but also give them the opportunity to detect adverse effects more accurately. To get around this, many researchers use what is called a meta-analysis – pooling the results of several similar small studies in order to boost the power of the findings. This works to some degree but is hampered by the fact that many studies into alternative medicine are of poor or uneven quality – making it difficult (sometimes impossible) to compare like with like. Meta-analysis also suffers from its own limitations. By its nature it looks for the places where all the studies agree. The places where they differ, however, may also be highly significant.

In alternative medicine there is the added difficulty of testing alternative therapies and procedures using conventional methods. The gold standard of scientific testing is the randomised, double-blind placebo-controlled trial. In this type of trial the experimental substance or procedure is tested against a placebo (something with no known therapeutic value). In order to eliminate bias, neither the testers nor the participants know which group is receiving which. However, the randomised, double-blind placebo-controlled trial is not infallible and may even produce misleading results since it can only be used to test the most mechanical of biophysical responses. Current methods of research which rely on easily measurable outcomes do not adequately address issues such as psychological outcomes, the nuances of relationship and the emotional needs of those being studied, even though these are deeply relevant.

Also, as our knowledge of the complexity of the body expands, it is becoming increasingly important to widen our definitions of 'treatment' and 'health'. While nobody would dispute the validity of evidence-based medicine, it is likely that to better understand health, 'evidence' from a variety of sources must be considered.

Because they function largely outside the healthcare system, alternative practitioners are in a good position to see the bigger picture and to pick up on trends and the changing needs of healthcare consumers long before those working inside the system can perceive them. They are in a position to construct a new kind of science – one which uses a combination of observation, anecdote, dialogue, complaints, and human input as well as available scientific, sociological and psycho-logical evidence to reach its conclusions about appropriate care, and to identify problems and opportunities for change.

But in reality most practitioners haven't done much more than complain about the unfairness of their situation. They recognise the limitations of modern medical research but have done little to address it. While it can sometimes be satisfying to cry 'not fair' and play the victim, such reluctance to play the game and get their heads around designing trials that would reflect their multifaceted approach to healthcare may eventually be alternative medicine's undoing.

The problems of researching alternative medicine are a classic catch-22. Without funding research is not forthcoming. Without experience of performing research, alternative practitioners are unlikely to hone their research skills and become more proficient at designing studies and interpreting data. Without proof many useful and efficacious alternative therapies will continue to be considered poor cousins of 'real' medicine.

Hidden agendas

When alternative medicine is put to the test, the problems of apply-ing conventional methods to research alternatives, and conventional attitudes to analyse that research, soon become apparent, as do the problems of hidden agendas. This problem of using conventional methods to assess alternative therapies was eloquently illustrated in a recent study of breast cancer and alternatives published in the *New England Journal of Medicine* in 1999.

The study, conducted at the Dana-Farber Cancer Institute in Boston, followed 480 women who had been newly diagnosed with either early or more advanced breast cancer. All were receiving standard care, but more than 28 per cent reported using at least one form of alternative care after initial surgery. About 70 per cent of these women had never considered alternative therapy before surgery. Using standard psychological measurements, the authors concluded that the women who used alternative therapies tended to be more depressed and anxious.

This study in itself was pretty depressing since, in analysing the data on the women's depression, the researchers drew a largely unfounded line connecting the use of alternative therapies to emotional instability. The fact that women who had chemotherapy were most likely to seek alternatives was not explored in great depth. Yet, chemotherapy is widely known to have a pronounced depressive effect on cancer patients. Women seeking alternatives at this stage of the disease may already be hopeless and depressed. Also, women who choose to pursue both conventional and alternative therapies in tandem may be left trying to reconcile, often without support, two entirely different patterns of care.

Many conventional studies into alternative therapies have a hidden agenda and are designed to put alternative therapy in a poor light. It is hardly surprising then that this breast cancer study concluded that it was the alternative therapies that caused the depression instead of the aggressive chemotherapy.

In contrast, a smaller study, conducted at the same time, of 39 patients (22 males and 17 females, with an average age of 63.5 years) showed good results on many levels. Using a patient question-naire called the SF 36 – which contains 36 questions covering eight categories of health – the researchers aimed to gain a picture of the patient's total health when using an alternative therapy. The SF 36 has been, used to study conventional care and the credibility of this method is now backed up by at least 250 quality studies. This was, however, the first time this method had been used to study alternative care.

Using this method researchers were able to demonstrate across the board improvement in chronic diseases which ranged from hypertension, diabetes type II, kidney cancer and immune disorder when treated with a wide range of therapies including chelation, stress reduction, vitamins and minerals, allergen avoidance and herbs.

Making choices

If you are new to the use of alternative therapies (and even if you are not) there are some sensible guidelines to consider which may help you make sense of whether a particular therapy (or a therapist) is the right choice for you.

First consider your practitioner. The best practitioners are those who see themselves as facilitators. In other words, they seek not to conquer disease but to help the body achieve wellness. Some would say the difference is small, but it is not. With one the body is the enemy, it is out of control and needs mastering; with the other the body is fully capable of healing itself and maintaining balance, given optimum conditions.

To some extent your choice of therapist is led by your choice of therapy, and your choice of therapy will be led by what you feel is wrong with you. Nearly all therapies can claim some success with a bafflingly wide range of conditions, but some are more effective than others for specific problems. Thus if you are experiencing joint or muscle pain or recurrent headaches, then one of the manipulative therapies such as osteopathy, chiropractic, reflexology, shiatsu and various other forms of massage are a good place to start.

If you need help with the effects of stress, the psychological therapies including classic psychotherapy, meditation, yoga, tai chi and hypnotherapy should be your first consideration. And if your problem is biochemical, then nutritional, homeopathic or herbal therapy including Ayurveda are the logical place to start. Consider also the following advice:

Contact professional organisations Many of the professional organisations listed in this book keep a register of therapists. They will be able to supply you with a list of qualified therapists in your area. It is then up to you to contact them and discuss your requirements and see if these fit with the type of therapy that is being offered.

Get personal You have the right to know how long a particular therapist has been practising, what type of treatments they offer and if they are fully insured. If you have a specific condition which needs treating, ask what experience the therapist has in treating this condition, what his or her success rate is and how long it can take to effect a cure. Ask what you can expect during the first and subsequent sessions and, of course, what the cost of first and subsequent visits is.

Which therapy
The choice of a therapy or remedy is often highly individual, so don't simply rely on claims and recommendations. Try to make an informed decision. Try also to resist all the media hype that promotes the idea that all therapies are good therapies. In addition, consider the following guidelines.

Be informed Getting information on your choices is important. This book provides background information to all the most common alternative therapies and highlights areas where research has shown the therapy to be effective. However, you may wish to consult other books or phone the organisations connected with particular therapies to obtain more information. Many organisations produce leaflets illustrating their specialities.

Consider more than one approach You may also wish to consider a combination of approaches. For instance, massage therapy such as shiatsu can greatly enhance the balancing effects of nutritional or other biochemical therapies.

Ask what's in it Refuse to be passive about the 'stuff' which you are being offered. Always ask what's in a particular remedy, tincture or pill. Check which oils your aromatherapist is using. These are not trade secrets and should not be treated as such. Ask also what each of the ingredients does and what you can expect from a particular remedy. Any therapist who is reluctant to answer such basic questions should be regarded with suspicion.

Give it time Alternative therapies do not work in the same way as conventional therapies. Whatever form of therapy you choose, and provided you do not actually feel worse, give it time. Conventional medicine works, in the main, by suppressing symptoms. Alternative therapies work by addressing the cause and healing the whole body. This process can take time. Bouncing from one practitioner or therapy to another because things aren't moving fast enough is likely to be counter-productive.

Less is more With all alternative remedies, take a 'less is more' approach. Generally speaking you should only take a remedy up to the point where you begin to feel better. The aim of alternative medicine is to support the body's own ability to heal and change, not to undermine it or do all the work for it. Studies into some herbs, for instance, have shown that taking larger amounts does not always produce better or faster results than taking small regular doses. The same is true for homeopathy, and a good osteopath or reflexologist will know when 'hands off' is better than 'hands on'.

It shouldn't hurt This sounds obvious but it is amazing what some people will put up with! Massage, chiropractic or osteopathy should *never* hurt. If it does, inform your practitioner. If he or she does not listen, change your practitioner. Homeopathy, herbs and even massage can sometimes produce unexpected side effects. These should not be severe and should not last a long time. Some therapists are very enthusiastic about these reactions and encourage their patients to put up with all manner of adverse effects. However, if you are unhappy with the effect of a particular therapy and your practitioner doesn't acknowledge and act upon your feelings, change your practitioner. This advice also applies to GPs, consultants and other medical professionals. You always have the right to switch to someone new if you are unhappy with your care.

Work with your body Have some faith that your body can do what it is supposed to. It can tell you what is wrong both physically and emotionally if you learn to listen to it. It can get better. Before you go running to any practitioner, conventional or alternative, spend a few days trying to 'tune in' to your real needs.

Get plenty of rest, eat good food, accept help from others and pay attention to any feelings and intuitions you have. Ask yourself whether your body is talking to you in metaphor. So, is your backache telling you to stop carrying so much? Are your chronic headaches a sign to 'get out of your head' and pay closer attention to the demands of your body? Are you nauseous because you just can't stomach something any more? If things improve after a few days, then you have found a solution, or a beginning of one. If you still feel you would like extra help, then choose a therapy that you feel comfortable with.

Chapter 4

Acupuncture

Commonly used for

Pain Relief • Digestive Disturbances •
Allergies and Respiratory Problems • Insomnia
• Headaches/Migraine • Nausea •
Musculoskeletal Complaints • Osteoarthritis
• Heart Conditions • Stroke • Neuralgia
• Addiction • Pregnancy and Birth

• *Requires a professional therapist*

Acupuncture has been an important part of ***traditional Chinese medicine*** for more than 2,500 years. Like many great discoveries, it evolved through a mixture of serendipity and science. In China, thousands of years ago, a strange wartime phenomenon was observed: soldiers whose bodies were pierced by arrows sometimes recovered from illnesses which had plagued them for many years. Eventually the idea evolved that by penetrating the skin at certain points diseases could be cured.

The first recorded use of acupuncture in the West was in Paris in 1810 when a doctor named Berlioz used it to treat symptoms of abdominal pain in a young female patient. Dr Berlioz, who was ridiculed by his colleagues and roundly criticised for his recklessness, nevertheless claimed the treatment was a success and continued to use acupuncture in his practice. Shortly afterwards, a handful of British doctors also began to experiment with acupuncture and the use of this ancient therapy was, amazingly, mentioned in the very first edition of the prestigious British medical journal, the *Lancet*, in 1823.

The first Western scientific studies into acupuncture were published in 1827 when the therapy was judged to be an acceptable and effective method for treating rheumatism. But it is only over the last 20 years or so that it has come to be more widely researched and accepted by healthcare practitioners and the general public in the West. In that time acupuncture has repeatedly demonstrated its ability to gently nudge the body back into harmony and relieve niggling discomforts without appearing to cause major or unnecessary changes in body chemistry. Indeed, the World Health Organization (WHO) has gone so far as to state that there is now sufficient medical evidence in support of acupuncture for it to be considered an important part of everyday healthcare.

According to the WHO there are 104 different conditions that acupuncture treatment may benefit including migraines, sinusitis, colds, asthma, addictions, myopia, ulcers and other gastrointestinal problems, nerve pain, ringing in the ears, paralysis and loss of speech from stroke or other brain damage, sciatica and osteoarthritis. On this basis it has recommended that acupuncture should be fully integrated into conventional medicine.

In the US in 1997 the National Institutes of Health recognised that acupuncture was an effective treatment for post-operative pain, pain from dental procedures and nausea and vomiting due to a range of conditions from pregnancy to chemotherapy. It also noted that acupuncture can be effective for tennis elbow, muscle pain and menstrual cramps.

In the UK, in response to mounting research into the success of acupuncture in easing such a wide range of conditions, the British Medical Association (BMA) has recommended that access to acupuncture for NHS patients should be widened.

The recommendation came on the heels of a two-year study published in 1995 and carried out by the BMA into patient access to acupuncture and other complementary and alternative therapies via general practitioners. In it, a survey of GPs revealed that 58 per cent had arranged complementary or alternative therapies including acupuncture for their patients. Among GPs surveyed, acupuncture – which was usually performed in GP surgeries, pain clinics or physiotherapy departments – was the most common form of alternative therapy referral, with **osteopathy** and **homeopathy** also proving popular.

How does it work?

In the West we don't appear to have a vocabulary to adequately explain how acupuncture works. According to the Chinese, the life energy that surrounds us and flows through us is called *qi* (pronounced chee). Many things, including illness, environmental factors and emotional states can disturb the flow of qi. When this energy is disturbed, either because it is blocked or because it is moving too slowly or too fast, imbalance and eventually illness will result. The ultimate aim of Chinese medicine is to restore health by bringing a person's qi back into balance. Acupuncture is one of several methods a practitioner of **traditional Chinese medicine** may employ to bring about this beneficial change.

There are over 2,000 acupuncture points on the body, though in everyday practice only about 200 are commonly used. These run along 12 pathways or energy channels known as meridians. Each meridian is linked to a particular organ in the body, thus each organ can be treated by stimulating the relevant meridian. Using needles as fine as a human hair, an acupuncturist aims to activate and/or unblock the body's energy channels, treat disease, boost immunity, harness the body's natural healing powers and alleviate fatigue.

In addition to the 12 main meridians, there are eight others, many of which are specific to women's physiology and childbirth. Of particular interest are the *ren* and *chong* channels. The ren channel, for example, controls conception and nourishment of the foetus and, according to the Chinese philosophy, a woman can only conceive when the ren and chong channels are functioning well.

In Chinese medicine, harmony and balance are dependent on the smooth, uninterrupted flow of qi. According to this philosophy the qi is responsible for the proper function of all spiritual, emotional, mental and physical processes. Although the use of needles is most commonly associated with the practice of acupuncture, a therapist may also bring elements of **massage** (or *tui na*, a form tissue stimulation similar to that used in **osteopathy**), **herbal medicine**, dietary advice and recommendations for therapeutic exercise such as *qi gong* into his or her practice in order to restore a patient's health.

Although it may seem on the surface of things a rather simple therapy, acupuncture involves the knowledge of a complex system of health. A therapist will be applying aspects of **traditional Chinese medicine** that include, for example, balancing yin (dark, female energy) and yang (light, male energy) in the body. He or she will also be balancing other opposing forces which form part of the philosophy of yin and yang, such as heat and cold, internal and external, deficiency and excess, as well as assessing and responding to the cyclical effect of the five elements – water, wood, fire, earth and metal – the influence of which can be felt at different times of the year in your body.

There is probably no reason why you should concern yourself too deeply with the philosophy behind the practice if you do not want to. However, since some of these principles encompass what you eat (for instance, some foods are considered yin and others yang, and an imbalance in these foods can lead to disharmony in the body) and other aspects of your lifestyle, it may be worthwhile to go into greater depth about your treatment with your practitioner.

There are many approaches to acupuncture. In the West six common types of acupuncture have been identified. These are:

- **Traditional Chinese acupuncture** The most common type of acupuncture, and the one which most of us will encounter, uses a wide range of techniques to make a diagnosis, including an examination of the whole body and its different pulses. From this examination a practitioner will make a decision about which points on the appropriate meridians to treat.

- *Auricular or ear acupuncture* Where the needles are inserted exclusively into one of the hundreds of acupoints believed to exist on the ear.

- *Korean hand acupuncture* Based on the principle that all energy circulating in the body originates in the hands and feet (similar to the principles of *reflexology*). Practitioners will needle specific points on the hands or feet to treat illness.

- *Myofascially based acupuncture* Assesses the meridians for tender points that may suggest a blockage in the flow of qi which, in turn, is contributing to the patient's complaints. Needles are then inserted in those points to correct the energy flow.

- *Five element theory* An esoteric form of acupuncture that recognises that the cause of illness is not simply physical in nature. The philosophy of the five elements is one of the basic philosophies that underpins Chinese medicine. It assigns all living and inanimate objects one of five qualities – wood, fire, earth, water or metal. In the body these elements are linked in a specific sequence of circulating energy pathways. These pathways can be disrupted by, among other things, our emotional responses – anger, joy, sympathy, grief and fear – to outside events. Using an understanding of this sequence and its relationship with the five elements, a practitioner makes a diagnosis and chooses which points to use as a treatment.

- *French energetics* Based on the principles of bioenergetics which believes that positive energy (cosmic energy, the life force and so on) can be channelled from the universe and directed within the body to remove any pain and bad energy which may be affecting the patient. In principle, if not in practice, this therapy is similar to a type of Western *spiritual healing* known as *therapeutic touch*.

In addition, some practitioners may use electro-acupuncture, where needles are stimulated with a mild electric current to enhance their effectiveness.

Technique, technique, technique

Even among therapists practising the same type of acupuncture, no two will work exactly alike, as was evidenced by a small study of 'technique' published in the US in 2001. When seven acupuncturists practising traditional Chinese medicine were asked to evaluate a single patient suffering from chronic back pain, most agreed on the diagnosis, but there were wide variations in the treatment recommendations, with individual practitioners using anywhere from 5 to 28 needles. Of the 28 acupuncture points selected, only four were used by two or more of the therapists.

Should prospective patients be worried by this variation in technique? No, because the nature of acupuncture is for treatments to vary. Through experience different practitioners will try or use different acupoints to stimulate the flow of energy through the body.

What the research says

Acupuncture is one of the most thoroughly researched and documented of all alternative therapies. As such you can choose it with confidence to treat a variety of conditions. In addition to addressing specific problems, acupuncture is believed to have a general strengthening effect on the immune system, to improve circulation, blood pressure, the rhythm of the heart, digestion, and the production of red and white blood cells. It may also stimulate a variety of hormones which help the body respond more efficiently to injury and stress.

When acupuncture is studied, it is usually compared to what is known as sham acupuncture. In sham or fake acupuncture needles are inserted into places that do not lie along any known meridians and which have no known therapeutic effects.

Pain relief

No one knows why acupuncture works to relieve pain. One theory is that the pain-relieving effects of acupuncture may be related to endorphins – natural narcotic-like substances produced by the brain. When we are injured, the body steps up the production of endorphins which, when released into the bloodstream, have the effect of numbing the receptors in the central nervous system, suppressing pain and inducing an overall sense of calm, relaxation and well-being. Sticking a needle into the body may be perceived by the system as a mild injury and so may boost endorphin production, but this has never really been proven.

Pain and its relief are notoriously difficult to study because the experience of being in pain is a subjective one. Trials into the pain-relieving effect of therapies like acupuncture, *massage, chiropractic* and *osteopathy*, as well as those using conventional methods and drugs, regularly show mixed results because of the subjective nature of pain.

Nevertheless, several scientific reviews have analysed the now considerable data on acupuncture and pain relief and found that overall acupuncture does show a measurable effect in relieving pain from a variety of conditions, though some have argued that the evidence is not as strong as practitioners claim.

Systematic reviews (where the results of many studies are pooled together) of the evidence for acupuncture in treating low back pain, for instance, do not endorse its use and one review of 12 trials into backache has argued that the effect, while positive, is not significantly more than placebo treatment or simply doing nothing.

But individual trials sometimes show benefit. For instance, an early trial in the *American Journal of Chinese Medicine* in 1980, involving 50 people with chronic low back pain, divided participants into two groups. One received acupuncture immediately; in the other, treatment was delayed and individuals put on a waiting list. More than 80 per cent of those who received immediate treatment experienced a reduction in pain of almost 50 per cent. In the delayed treatment group, a third got better and 25 per cent got worse before they eventually received acupuncture. But when the delayed treatment group did finally have acupuncture treatment, 75 per cent of them also improved. Four weeks later 58 per cent of all those who had received acupuncture continued to show improvement.

Two years later, in another study of people with neck pain, one half received acupuncture and the other half didn't. Eighty per cent of those treated with acupuncture showed improvement three months later, with a 40 per cent reduction in pain, a 68 per cent reduction of hours of pain each day and a 32 per cent improvement in activity level. In the no-treatment group 60 per cent got worse and around 13 per cent improved. In a more recent study published in the *British Medical Journal* in June 2001, acupuncture was found to be more effective than massage for treating chronic neck pain, but only in the short term.

Similarly confused results have been found for arthritic pain. In one study of patients awaiting knee surgery for arthritis, acupuncture provided significant improvement in pain and range of motion and significant reductions in the use of painkillers. Nearly a quarter of those treated with acupuncture felt so much better that they opted out of surgery altogether. But, again, other studies have shown less benefit.

Total anaesthesia?

In 1979 a 58-year-old man in China with a brain tumour located near his pituitary gland underwent surgery using electro-acupuncture as anaesthesia. The patient received only a mild preoperative sedative, and the four-hour operation included removal of a portion of the skull as well as the tumour. The patient remained fully conscious, alert and relaxed. Five needles attached to a low voltage battery provided his pain relief. The patient was able to walk out of the operating room without assistance after the operation.

Headache

One area of acupuncture pain relief where there are probably more positive studies than negative ones is headache. A study of over 20,000 people at the University of California found that acupuncture reduced both the frequency and severity of muscle tension headaches and migraines. More recently a review of well-designed trials into acupuncture for the relief of headache pain concluded (somewhat grudgingly) that the ancient Chinese therapy had value in the treatment of this type of pain.

The researchers identified 22 trials involving a total of 1,042 people and found that though the studies were small, the trend suggested that acupuncture provided significant pain relief and that true acupuncture was shown to be on average one and a half times more effective than fake or sham acupuncture.

Acupuncture can also work for migraine – sometimes. In one 1989 trial, comparing real and sham acupuncture in 30 individuals with chronic migraine, real acupuncture was much more effective in reducing pain and medication use than sham acupuncture, and this effect persisted for a year. Other studies of migraine, however, have found less benefit.

Where acupuncture seems to be least effective is in treating stress-related headaches. Several studies comparing real to sham acupuncture found little difference between the two – interestingly both treatments were somewhat helpful. Another study comparing acupuncture to physiotherapy (in this case defined as exercise, massage and relaxation) found that acupuncture was the least effective method for relieving stress-related headaches.

Nausea
Most studies in this area centre around the use of anti-nausea *acupressure* bands that, when worn correctly, put pressure on a therapeutic point known as P6. A 1996 review analysed several trials of acupuncture or acupressure and found that in 27 out of 29 trials acupuncture/acupressure was successful for treating nausea associated with a variety of experiences including chemotherapy, travel and also pregnancy.

Acupuncture is already widely used to prevent dental pain. But holistic dentists have found that ear acupuncture may also be useful in helping those who are normally unable to undergo treatment because of an exaggerated gagging reaction. Scientists theorise that by stimulating the correct nerve in the ear, chemicals are released that influence the functioning of the vagus nerve – the nerve that controls gagging and the swallowing reflex.

Addiction

Several studies have looked into the efficacy of acupuncture as a way of addressing addictions. In 1989 the *Lancet* published a study showing that when alcoholics already on a treatment programme had acupuncture included as a therapy, it significantly increased the number who completed the programme, reduced their need for alcohol and led to fewer relapses and readmissions to the detox centre. Other studies have found it effective in helping to reduce addiction to opium and heroin. Used with pregnant women addicted to crack cocaine, acupuncture alongside a detox programme improved the birthweights of their babies.

Acupuncture has not however been found useful for treating addiction to cigarettes or for eating disorders.

Stroke

Although sometimes promoted as a cure, opinions are mixed as to whether acupuncture can aid recovery for the majority of stroke patients. Two trials, in 1993 and 1996, found that stroke patients benefited from a better quality of life after receiving acupuncture.

But in 1998 Swedish researchers found that acupuncture was no better than sham treatments at improving the neurological function of stroke patients. Researchers divided 104 stroke patients into three groups: deep acupuncture, superficial acupuncture or a sham treatment. All the individuals were over 40 years old and all had such severe damage to their neurologic systems that they could not walk without support and/or could not eat and/or dress without assistance.

Why did this trial find less benefit than the previous trials? It is possible that acupuncture, like all stroke treatments, is more effective in younger patients and when applied very early after a stroke. Equally, like conventional interventions, it may not be as effective in those with severe neurological damage.

Musculoskeletal complaints

Small studies generally confirm that conditions such as fibromyalgia, carpal tunnel syndrome and wrist pain appear to respond well to acupuncture treatment.

A large review in the *Journal of the American Medical Association* in November 1998 confirmed this finding, suggesting that musculo-skeletal conditions such as fibromyalgia, myofascial pain and tennis elbow were conditions that might respond especially well to acupuncture. The reviewers went even further by acknowledging that the conventional treatment of these conditions – usually involving anti-inflammatory medicine such as aspirin, paracetamol or steroid injections – have very little in the way of scientific evidence to show that they work and often have many more adverse effects.

Fertility and pregnancy

There is some evidence that acupuncture can help women with painful periods and Swedish researchers have also reported that some women with polycystic ovary syndrome (PCOS) may benefit from treatment by electro-acupuncture. In a Swedish study in 2000, 38 per cent of the women receiving acupuncture experienced a return of regular ovulation, though the treatment was most effective in women who were not obese and who had less evidence of severe hormonal disruption.

Because it has no known side effects for mother or baby, some women (even those who feel a little nervous about the idea of needles) turn to acupuncture to help facilitate a healthy pregnancy.

While it is often promoted as a way to induce labour, no firm evidence exists to show whether it really works or not. One small trial involving 120 women found that acupuncture appeared to soften the cervix and so make labour shorter and easier. In this trial the average length of the first stage of labour was three hours in the acupuncture group compared to $5^{1}/_{2}$ in the conventional care group. Women receiving acupuncture also had fewer inductions.

Some evidence exists to show that acupuncture can be used to turn a breech baby and thus facilitate an easier birth. The majority of breeches turn spontaneously before term. However, a few persist to term.

In one careful study first-time mothers with breech babies in their 33rd week of an otherwise normal pregnancy received either moxibustion or no intervention for two weeks. At the end of this period 75 per cent of the babies in the moxibustion group had turned, compared to 47 per cent in the control group. Moxibustion involves the use of heat to stimulate an acupuncture point – in this case a point on the little toe known as BL 67, or *zhiyin*. The authors suggest that this ancient Chinese technique may help to turn a breech by increasing foetal activity.

Other conditions

Acupuncture is also used to treat heart and respiratory conditions, though the evidence is less abundant for these situations. Animal experiments have shown that acupuncture can lower blood pressure, but people studies are not conclusive.

Acupuncture may also be useful in promoting sleep. A study of 40 people with difficulties in either falling asleep or remaining asleep were diagnosed according to traditional Chinese medicine. The groups then had either true or sham acupuncture several times a week. Those receiving true acupuncture slept significantly better than those who did not.

Cautions

Acupuncture, while largely safe, has been associated with occasional complications. In one Australian study, fainting was the most common adverse effect followed by increased pain and nausea/ vomiting. More serious complications such as pneumothorax (puncturing the chest cavity) and convulsions were very rare.

Complications of acupuncture, particularly the more serious ones, need to be seen in the context of the widespread use of acupuncture throughout the world. For example, in one Japanese study that reviewed the outcomes of 55,291 acupuncture treatments, there were only 64 adverse events – the most frequent of which was the failure to remove a needle after treatment. This represents an adverse reaction rate of approximately 0.001 per cent, or one in every 1,000 treatments.

Compared to the adverse events associated with conventional procedures this is very low and as a major review published in the *British Medical Journal* in 2001 concluded, the risk of complications can be greatly reduced by making sure that you are treated by an experienced practitioner. Looking at over 60,000 acupuncture treatments the reviewers found that with experienced practitioners the adverse event rate was less than one in 10,000 procedures.

If you are pregnant you should seek a therapist who is experienced in working with pregnant women as there are certain acupuncture points which should not be stimulated during pregnancy. Again, serious complications are rare, but a good acupuncturist will usually be cautious about over-stimulating the body during pregnancy and will generally opt for gently strengthening the body and giving advice on diet and lifestyle.

What to expect

Acupuncture cannot completely heal conditions where there is a permanent structural injury (for instance spinal injury) or where the internal organs are scarred or damaged in some way, though it may help to relieve certain symptoms. Other than this you can consult an acupuncturist for just about anything about which you would normally consult your GP.

In acupuncture, diagnosis is a blend of intuition and science that some Westerners, who are new to the concept, may find difficult to grasp. Yet, it's not very different from the way the average general practitioner works – making a diagnosis on the basis of an educated guess or a 'hunch'. The critical difference is that your acupuncturist will be trying to identify a whole pattern of disturbance rather than just targeting single symptoms.

The number of consultations you will require will vary enormously according to what condition is being treated. The average appointment lasts anywhere from 30 minutes to an hour. However, your first appointment will need to be longer because of the time needed to take a comprehensive case history. Your acupuncturist will need detailed information about your lifestyle, diet, work, medical history and emotional state. A diagnosis will be made on the basis of this information as well as from examination of your pulses (in Chinese medicine there is more than one) and your tongue.

Some people feel apprehensive that the needles will hurt – in fact, acupuncture is a virtually painless process. The needles are very fine and usually only penetrate the superficial layers of the skin. Because your practitioner is working with energy channels, the places where the needles are inserted may not correspond to where you are experiencing pain. Once inserted you may feel a mild tingling sensation, but as the energy flow improves you should also feel a growing sense of well-being. The needles may be removed after a minute or two or left in for up to 30 minutes. There is no pain on removal.

Your therapist may use a variety of techniques to stimulate acupuncture points, including finger pressure (**acupressure**), massage, electricity and even heat, known as moxibustion. In moxibustion, a cigar-shaped bundle of herbs known as *moxa* (the Chinese word for mugwort) is lit and held a short distance from the skin in order to heat either the needle or the acupoint. This should not produce any burning, though you will sometimes feel intense heat.

Because acupuncture is a gentle therapy, it is rare to have any negative reactions to it. Although most people leave the treatment room feeling relaxed, occasionally some may experience a less pleasant reaction. If you have been suffering from a chronic condition or if energy has been stagnant in a particular area of your body for a long time, moving that energy may release accumulated toxins into the body. As your body tries to rid itself of these toxins, you may experience a wide range of physical symptoms such as headaches, nausea, sweating or skin rashes, as well as emotional ones such as melancholy and fatigue. These symptoms should not last more than a few days. If you are at all worried by your reaction, always phone your practitioner.

Some GPs and other practitioners such as midwives are also trained in acupuncture and may offer this as a treatment on the NHS. However, most people still have to seek out private practitioners. If you wish to investigate acupuncture further, you can get a list of qualified acupuncturists in your area from the British Acupuncture Council or the British Medical Acupuncture Society. Practitioners belonging to the latter group are also conventionally trained doctors of medicine.

Acupressure

If you are drawn to the philosophy of acupuncture but dislike needles, you may find that acupressure suits your needs just as well. Acupressure originates from Japan and is a less invasive form of acupuncture which uses the same meridians and vital points. It is similar to the practice of **reflexology** and also the basis of **shiatsu** massage. In order to help the body balance its energies, the acupressure therapist will use finger pressure, heat or cold to stimulate acupuncture points, or *tsubos*, on the body.

Tsubos are different from other areas on the body in that they have more neuroreceptors and conduct more electricity. Oriental practitioners would say that these are the points on the body where the *ki* (as it is called in Japan) flows very near to the surface of the body. A sensitive practitioner will be able to feel this flow of energy at each tsubo. Firm pressure and non-damaging heat and cold applied to a tsubo can change the energy which flows from that point through the spinal cord and into the brain.

Acupressure can be done through most types of clothing, but for most acupressure techniques it is best to work directly on clean, dry skin. It can be a part of regular, formal therapy or you can learn to use it as a self-help measure. Because it requires no special equipment apart from a clean pair of hands, it is a very portable therapy and an effective form of first aid.

How does it work?

Because it involves the stimulation of acupuncture points as well as touch, it is likely that the benefits of acupressure are in line with those of both **acupuncture** and **massage**. However, acupressure has not been subjected to the same degree of scientific scrutiny as acupuncture. Nevertheless, there is evidence to suggest that gentle pressure on the tsubos stimulates the body, in the same way that it does with acupuncture, to release pain-relieving, mood-enhancing endorphins.

Acupressure is not really a diagnostic tool, although to some extent an experienced practitioner will be able to 'feel' where there is an imbalance in your body. Most people consult an acupressure therapist to deal with existing problems such as backache. Acupressure may also be useful for relieving headache pain, neck and upper back stiffness, lower back pain and, of course, labour pains. Contact the Shiatsu Society for a list of registered practitioners in your area.

Cautions

Acupressure, like **massage**, should not be applied in the following states:

- at a place on the body where there is an open wound, infection or swelling

- on any area of the skin which is red, inflamed or broken or where there is scar tissue, rash, blisters or varicose veins

- over the site of a broken bone or injured nerve or organ.

Pregnant women should also take care. To avoid the risk of inducing premature labour, acupressure should not be applied to the following sites in a woman who is less than 38 weeks pregnant:

- the abdomen

- small toe, including the toenail

- the back or inside of the lower legs, beginning at the knees

- the web of tissue between the thumb and forefinger, referred to as the *hoku*.

What to expect

Your therapist will want to know a bit about your medical history, and you should in particular inform him or her of any medications you are taking. History-taking in acupressure is not as important as it is in many other alternative therapies. Nevertheless, your practitioner should always take the time to listen to what is ailing you.

Treatment usually takes place on the floor. You may be asked to lie on a *futon*, a thin mattress, or simply on a folded blanket or towel. Some points on your body will feel more tender than others and this is usually interpreted as a sign of imbalance. Gentle initial massage will help relieve that tender feeling. An acupressure session will usually last half an hour to an hour and you should be given a short time to rest and allow your body to integrate the subtle changes in its energy after each session.

Like acupuncture, most people leave acupressure sessions feeling relaxed and calm. However, if you experience any adverse symptoms which last more than a day or two, always phone your practitioner for advice.

Chapter 5

Aromatherapy

Commonly used for

Fatigue • Insomnia • Nausea • Fluid Retention
• Respiratory Problems • Headache
• Pregnancy and Postnatal • High Blood Pressure
• Infections • Pain Relief

• *Requires a professional therapist* • *Suitable for self-help*

Smell is the most ancient of all the human senses. It affects our lives and emotions in ways which scientists have not even begun to explore.

Throughout history highly concentrated oils extracted from flowers, herbs and animal sources have been used to calm or stimulate the emotions and enhance well-being. The use of balms, ointments and scented oils is even documented in the Bible. Scent has historically been thought to have the power to heal and repel evil and as such has played a part in religious rituals across many cultures. For the Egyptians, it was part of the burial ritual and a symbol of status. The Greeks believed fragrance connected them to the gods. The Romans used perfumes for seduction and herbs as aphrodisiacs, whereas in the Middle Ages perfume was used mainly to cover up the stench of disease.

The modern use of essential oils as a therapy, however, began in the 1930s when the French chemist René Maurice Gattefosse coined the term 'aromatherapy'. Fascinated by the benefits of lavender oil in healing his burned hand without leaving any scars, he started to investigate the healing potential of other essential oils.

During the Second World War, a French army surgeon, Dr Jean Valnet, successfully used essential oils to treat wounded soldiers and patients in a psychiatric hospital. Not long afterwards, Marguerite Maury, an Austrian beauty therapist and biochemist, elevated aromatherapy to a holistic therapy when she began prescribing essential oils as a remedy for her clients. She is also credited with the modern practice of using essential oils in massage.

Today aromatherapy is something of a catch-all phrase for a wide range of healing techniques – from **massage** to hydrotherapy to creating a pleasing ambience in a room – that involve the use of highly concentrated oils derived from plants and flowers.

How does it work?
Essential oils are thought to affect the body in two ways. The first and most obvious is through their aroma. Humans have the ability to distinguish between more than 10,000 different smells. But smell is a complex sense that involves much more than the detection of odour. When we breathe in an odour we are taking in a mixture of chemicals and in recent years it has become apparent that these chemicals can affect us in many ways.

The ability to perceive odour is so connected to our well-being that it hardly seems surprising that people who have lost their sense of smell often suffer from a high incidence of psychiatric problems such as depression and anxiety.

Exactly how odour is perceived and processed in the brain is not well understood since it involves complicated physical and psychological pathways that can be impossible to separate. We do know that, of all the senses, smell has the most direct connection to the mind and emotions. All fragrances, natural and synthetic, are able to breach the blood brain barrier (the protective membrane that surrounds the brain) and gain direct access to the limbic system – the emotional switchboard of the brain. Studies have shown that inhaling fragrances can cause changes in both the circulation and electrical activity in the brain.

Apart from their direct effect on the brain, aromatherapy oils can also enter the blood system through the skin (for instance when used in massage), through the lining of the lungs (when they are inhaled) and, more rarely, when taken orally (this is not a method which is advised unless under competent professional supervision). Once absorbed into the bloodstream, the medicinal properties of the oils – whether they are antifungal, antibacterial, antiviral or antiparasitic – can begin to have an effect.

External use only

Essential oils should never be taken orally except under professional supervision. Tea tree oil and eucalyptus have been associated with childhood poisonings and ingestion of pennyroyal has also been found to be fatal.

Nevertheless, some oils can be beneficial when taken orally. When a plant oil is taken internally (for instance, peppermint oil to relieve symptoms of IBS), it can also be considered a form of *herbal medicine*.

What all this means is that aromatherapy probably works on the mind and body at the same time. In therapeutic use there are about 150 essential oils distilled from plants, flowers, trees, bark, grasses and seeds. Each has a distinctive chemical make-up and a unique therapeutic, psychological and physiological effect. Some are antiseptic, others are antiviral, anti-inflammatory, pain relieving, antidepressant and expect-orant. They can be used, among other things, to stimulate, relax, improve digestion and eliminate excess water.

Some sceptics put the benefits of aromatherapy down to the effect of the *massage*, rather than the oil. This may not necessarily be correct. When studies were conducted using both plain vegetable oils on their own and with essential oils mixed in, those receiving the essential oils usually experienced more improvement. For instance, in one study cancer patients were given either a massage with plain almond oil or almond oil mixed with roman camomile. Those in the camomile group experienced fewer symptoms, less anxiety and noted that their quality of life improved. Similarly, recent Japanese data has shown that a footbath with lavender oil produced greater biochemical changes associated with relaxation than did a plain foot bath.

A single essential oil can contain as many as 100 different chemical components. The predominance of one type of chemical component over the others determines how an oil will act on the brain and body. Essential oil chemistry is complex, but the main components of essential oils generally include alcohols, esters, ketones, aldehydes and terpines. Their effects are summarised opposite.

What the research says
What all this means is that we know a lot about the composition of plant oils and we have a lot of theories about how their application might be beneficial. But actual research is almost non-existent because so many serious scientists dismiss the idea that essential oils on their own could be of value. From a scientific standpoint, the therapeutic benefits of aromatherapy are widely thought to be on a par with comfort eating and retail therapy. Because of this, funding for large-scale aromatherapy research is not forthcoming. Therefore we have to rely on mostly anecdote and the subjective experience of aromatherapists and patients.

Antimicrobial action
One area that has received some attention, however, is the powerful antibacterial, antiviral and antifungal qualities of essential oils when applied topically, and this may be one area where the use of essential oils can be said to be truly effective.

Many essential oils including lavender, geranium, peppermint, eucalyptus, lemon grass, orange, clove and thyme have been found to exert an antimicrobial action. Among the most thoroughly studied of all is tea tree oil which has shown great benefit in the treatment of fungal infections such as athlete's foot. In one study it was as effective as the drug tolnaftate in improving symptoms of athlete's foot. It has also been shown to be as effective as the drug clotrimazole in treating fungal nail infections. Tea tree has also been

Essential oil chemistry

Chemical	Properties	Commonly found in
Alcohols	Bactericidal (kills bacteria), stimulant, energising, vitalising, antiviral, diuretic	Rose, pettigrain, rosewood, geranium, peppermint, myrtle, tea tree, sandalwood, patchouli, ginger
Aldehydes	Anti-inflammatory, calming, sedative and antiviral	Oils with a lemon-like smell including lemon balm, lemon grass, citronella, eucalyptus, sandalwood, anise
Esters	Antifungal, sedative, calming, antispasmodic, anti-inflammatory	Roman camomile, lavender, clary sage, pettigrain, bergamot, geranium, palmarosa
Ethers	Calms the nervous system, antiseptic, stimulant, expectorant, spasmolytic, diuretic	Cinnamon, clove, anise, basil, tarragon, parsley, sassafras
Ketones	Wound healing, mucolytic (eases the secretion of mucous), stimulates new cell growth	Camphor, rosemary, sage, eucalyptus, hyssop, geranium, peppermint, rose
Lactones (part of the ester group)	Anti-inflammatory, mucolytic	Arnica, elecampane
Phenols*	Bactericidal, tonic, immune stimulating, invigorating, warming	Clove, cinnamon, thyme, oregano, savory, cumin
Sequiterpines	Antiphlogistic (moves fluids), anti-inflammatory, sedative, antiviral, anti-carcinogenic, bacteriostatic and immune stimulant	Blue or German camomile, lavender, clary sage, pettigrain, bergamot, sandalwood, eucalyptus, clove
Terpines	Very stimulating, potential skin irritants, antiviral	Lemon, orange, bergamot, black pepper, pine oils, nutmeg, angelica, marjoram, frankincense

* Can be liver toxic if used in large amounts over extended period of time.

shown, in laboratory tests, to kill antibiotic resistant *Staphylococcus aureus* bacteria. Whether it can do the same in humans remains to be seen.

Future cancer treatment?

The essential oil of lavender contains a monoterpine compound called perillyl that has been found to have an inhibiting effect on cancer cells. In laboratory studies it has been found to inhibit the rapid growth of early cancer cells by 70 to 99 per cent. It is too early to say what this might mean in terms of healthcare, but studies are currently ongoing to see if capsules of this compound given to those suffering from breast, prostate and ovarian cancer are a viable alternative to the antiestrogen drug tamoxifen, a side effect of which is an increase in the risk of uterine cancer.

Stress

Essential oil massage has been found effective in improving the well-being of cancer patients and other people in hospital. In one study 122 individuals who were in an intensive care unit reported feeling much better when a massage with lavender oil was administered, compared to when they were simply given a massage or allowed to rest. No changes in blood pressure, respiration or heart rates were noted, suggesting that the effects of massage were very gentle.

In another study conducted by researchers at the University of Vienna, orange oil was diffused in the waiting room of a dental office via an electrical dispenser. The patients who were exposed to the room odour were then compared to a group who were not for signs of anxiety, alertness and calmness. Those exposed to the odour were significantly more relaxed and the effect was most pronounced on women.

Similarly, studies with students have revealed greater alertness, better moods and enhanced brainwave activity and ability to do maths problems when exposed to the aroma of either rosemary or lavender essential oil. What has yet to be determined is whether this effect is physiological or psychological (though some would argue that it really doesn't matter as long as it works).

Insomnia

Because essential oils can be used to aid relaxation, they may also be useful in aiding sleep. In 1991 British researchers at the University of Leicester, measuring sleep patterns in the elderly over a six-week period, also found that being in a scented room was as effective as sedative drugs. Another small but often quoted study reported in the *Lancet* in 1995 showed that elderly people 'slept like babies' when a lavender aroma was pumped into their bedrooms at night. These people had all had difficulty falling asleep and normally had to take sleeping pills to get to sleep prior to the aromatherapy.

Headache

Tiger Balm, that pungent red ointment infused with essential oils of menthol, camphor, clove and peppermint, was found in a 1996 Australian study to be as effective as the pain reliever acetaminophen in relieving tension headaches. It was also found to work faster. In another study in 1995 at the Neurological Clinic of the University of Kiel, Germany, the use of a combination of peppermint oil with just a trace of eucalyptus proved to be particularly effective in relieving tension headaches. The combination is thought to have a powerful analgesic effect. Adding more than a trace of eucalyptus to the mix did not alter the pain, but was effective in relieving muscle tension.

Pregnancy and postnatal

Essential oils are often recommended as a way of aiding relaxation during pregnancy and labour and, when used externally, as a way of healing cuts and tears after birth.

Studies on the use of lavender oil for healing perineal trauma after birth show mixed results. But a unique eight-year study in Oxford involving more than 8,000 mothers has shown that aromatherapy is an effective way for women to manage labour pains.

The study was conducted by Oxford Brookes University between 1990 and 1998 and found that the use of essential oils can reduce maternal anxiety and fear as well as inducing a sense of well-being. The findings are important because fear and anxiety can slow a labour down and make the mother feel unable to cope with the pain.

As if to underscore this point, this particular study showed a considerable drop in the use of opiate pain relief by the women who used aromatherapy. In comparable teaching hospitals the rate of opiate use for pain relief is around 30 per cent; in the Oxford study it was around 0.4 per cent.

The oils used in the research included lavender, frankincense, camomile, rose, jasmine, eucalyptus, peppermint, lemon, mandarin and clary sage. They were administered in a variety of ways including massage, in a warm bath, a footbath, and as drops on the forehead or palm.

Jasmine flowers are sometimes used in India as a way of suppressing lactation. Traditionally, they are taped to the breast of the mother to stop her producing milk. In one interesting study jasmine flowers taped to the breasts was compared to the conventional drug bromocriptine. The flowers worked as well as the drug. This effect has also been confirmed in animal studies where the cages of mice either had jasmine scent in them or were lined with flowers which came into contact with their mammary glands when they walked. Those animals whose mammary glands came into contact with the flowers produced even less milk than those inhaling the fragrance.

Insect repellent
Many texts on aromatherapy recommend that essential oils, particularly citronella, can be used to stop pesky mosquitoes biting. Today some natural insect repellents contain quantities of citronella and chemists may also sell citronella candles to burn out of doors to keep the bugs away. Citronella, alone or mixed with other oils such as geranium and palmarosa, is claimed to be very effective at repelling insects and such studies as exist seem to confirm this. One from the University of Guelph in Ontario, Canada, in 1996, comparing the use of citronella candles and incense to plain candles or no candles, found that the reduction in bites with the candles and incense was 42.3 and 24.2 per cent respectively. Another study in Thailand in 2001 found that several essential oils including citronella, turmeric and basil (especially with the addition of 5 per cent vannillin, derived from vanilla) repelled three different species of

mosquito (both day-biting and night-biting) for eight hours – making them as effective as conventional repellents made with the insecticide deet.

> **You get what you pay for**
> Oils from readily available sources that are easy to extract the oil from, such as oranges, are relatively cheap. But oils from rare sources or those where the process of extracting oil is difficult, such as jasmine and rose, will always be expensive. Cheaper oils are either synthetic or cut with other less expensive oils. Jasmine, for instance, may be mixed with ylang ylang and rose may be mixed with geranium, bois de rose or palmarosa. Adulterated oils will not have the same therapeutic effect as pure oils.

Other uses

In a recent small trial a mixture of thyme, rosemary, lavender and cedarwood in a base made from jojoba and grapeseed improved signs of hair loss in men. The men in the study massaged the oils into their scalps daily and results were compared to a group of men who only used the base oil mixture for massage. In seven months the essential oil group showed a small but significant improvement. These findings, however, have not been corroborated by other studies.

In another interesting study inhaling vapour from black pepper extract helped to reduce craving for cigarettes. A group of 48 cigarette smokers were deprived of cigarettes overnight and then divided into three groups and given devices to puff on for three hours. One group's device delivered the smell of black pepper, in another the smell of mint and in the third just plain air. Subjects were assessed for mood and craving. Both black pepper and mint subjects felt more satisfied with their device. But only black pepper decreased significantly the craving for cigarettes. Other evidence suggests that exposure to a variety of odours can help to reduce the craving for cigarettes.

Using essential oils

Essential oils are a fairly pleasant, versatile and portable way of taking care of yourself. The way an oil is used will enhance its effect on the body. For instance, massage without essential oil has long been known to improve emotional states such as anxiety and depression as well as reducing levels of pain. Combined with correctly selected therapeutic oils, which can be inhaled and absorbed through the skin, its effect can be even more profound.

Only a very few essential oils are safe to use neat on the skin. The best way to use most oils is to mix them in a base, or carrier oil. Simple sunflower oil from your kitchen cupboard is as good a choice as any other. Other good choices include sweet almond, apricot kernel, grapeseed, safflower and hazelnut oils. To enrich a base oil, try adding heavier oils such as carrot, borage seed, avocado, evening primrose oil, jojoba, wheatgerm or sesame oils. Because they are so rich and heavy, these oils should account for not more than 10 per cent of any base mixture.

When mixing oils in a base, there is a general rule that says you should use no more than one drop of essential oil to one millilitre of base oil. For example, a tablespoon of oil equals about 15 ml – thus you could use up to 15 drops. Mixtures intended for babies and children should be very diluted – 2–3 drops per 15 ml. There are many ways of using them, the most common of which are:

In the bath Mix your choice of essential oil or oils in a light base oil, such as apricot kernel oil, or in a neutral, water-dispersing oil which you can purchase at some health food shops and natural toiletry stores. Alternatively, mix it into a small amount of whole milk. Pour this mixture into the bath. If possible, aim to relax in the bath for at least 15 minutes.

For massage A good way of addressing skin problems, aching muscles and joints and fluid retention. Always use essential oils diluted in a light base oil.

As a compress This method is good for bruises, headaches, varicose veins, burns and scalds. Add between eight and ten drops of essential oil to half a cup of water. Disperse well. Soak a face cloth in the mixture and apply to the relevant part of the body.

An inhalation A particularly good choice if you have a cold, cough or any other breathing difficulty. A simple and portable way to make an inhalation is to put a few drops of your chosen oil on a hankie. Wrap this in a plastic bag and carry it with you to use as and when you need to. At home, you can make a steam inhalation using a bowl of hot water and five to ten drops of essential oil. Lean over the bowl with a towel over your head and breathe deeply. Alternatively, you can now buy hand-held inhalers which are small plastic containers, not unlike coffee mugs, with a special mask that attaches to the top.

Foot baths Fill a basin large enough to take both feet with hand-hot water. Then add 8–10 drops of your favourite oil. This is a good way to soothe feet after a long day. If your ankles are swollen, try following the hot bath with a cool one to improve circulation. You can do the same thing for sore, swollen hands.

Room scents You can spread the scent of an essential oil throughout a room using an oil burner, or by placing one or two drops on a cool light bulb before turning the light on. If you heat your home with radiators, place five drops of essential oil in a bowl containing a little water and place this on top of the radiator.

Is it natural?

Today, everybody is jumping on the aromatherapy bandwagon. But while there are a number of 'aromatherapy' products available in supermarkets and chemists, many of the fragrances used in them are synthetic. Artificial fragrances can be found in bath oils, shampoos, lip balms and body rubs. They are also becoming more common in dish detergent, fabric softeners and other household cleaners. They are also used in foods where they are called flavours or aromas.

The cosmetic industry long ago abandoned the use of genuinely natural ingredients. Today it bases its products on fragrances derived from petrochemicals. Synthetic oils, however, do not work in the same way as natural ones and may produce a range of undesired effects.

Studies have shown, for example, that inhaling synthetic fragrance chemicals can cause negative circulatory changes in the brain. Subtle negative changes in brainwave activity can also occur with exposure to petrochemical fragrances. Perhaps not surprisingly, these types of fragrances are a frequent trigger of migraine headaches.

To produce the desired results, essential oils should always be from natural sources. When you are buying any essential oil or fragranced product, to assure yourself that it is from a natural source, always look for the Latin name of the flower or herb on the label. Otherwise you could be buying a synthetic oil or an adulterated mixture derived from petrochemicals.

Cautions

There are few contraindications for the use of aromatherapy, but a few points are worth bearing in mind. Skin irritations are not uncommon and the longer you use an oil without a break, the more likely it is that such reactions will occur. Reactions to lavender, once uncommon, are becoming increasingly common, probably because of the much wider use of the oil and the herb in the home. If you are allergic to chrysthanthemums, asters, marigold, goldenrod or ragweed, you may also be allergic to camomile. People who suffer from hay fever may also be sensitive to these extracts.

Tea tree oil, which is being used more and more widely now, is also a significant source of allergic reactions. In one study of sensitive individuals 59 per cent experienced an allergic reaction to plant extracts with the most common allergens being tea tree oil, dandelion, feverfew and members of the *Compositae* species (relatives of the daisy which include camomile and yarrow); and 34 per cent reacted to balsam of Peru.

If you have an allergy to nuts, you may experience a skin reaction to some base oils such as almond or peanut oil. If you have very sensitive skin, do a patch test first. Mix two or three drops of essential oil in a tablespoon of base oil. Put some of this mixture on to a fabric plaster and leave this on the inside of your arm for 24 hours or until any irritation occurs (whichever is sooner).

Similarly, bergamot and other citrus oils can increase the photo-sensitivity of the skin and should not be used if your skin is going to be directly exposed to the sun. Perhaps more importantly, certain oils can have an effect on blood pressure which for some individuals (those with a heart condition or pregnant women) may not be entirely therapeutic. Oils such as rosemary, sage, hyssop and black pepper can raise blood pressure, while others such as lavender, clary sage and ylang ylang can lower it dramatically. If such reactions are relevant to your health, make sure you double check which oil your therapist is using.

Watch out also for types of 'aromatherapy' that don't use essential oils. Aromatherapy candles and incense can release toxic chemicals into the environment as they burn. For example, in 2001 researchers in Taiwan have found that the smoke produced by burning incense is laden with cancer-causing PAHs or polycyclic aromatic hydrocarbons – highly carcinogenic chemicals that are released when certain substances are burned. And according to the researchers who measured levels in a temple in Taiwan, levels of PAHs were 40 times higher in a poorly ventilated temple than in houses where people smoke tobacco, 19 times higher than those measured outdoors, and even slightly higher than those measured on a busy street corner.

While most of us do not burn incense to the degree that it is burned in temples, the fact that we live in homes sealed against the elements may mean that with regular incense or candle use levels of toxic PAHs can also build up in the average home. In addition:

- Don't administer any oil for more than three weeks without a break. The olfactory receptors can literally become exhausted, at which point the therapeutic value of the oil is lost. Depending on how often and how strongly you use them, this rule can also apply to room scents.

- When combining oils, take a less is more approach – no more than five different oils in a single mixture. Study into the synergistic effects of different oils is lacking. What there is suggests that some combinations may be beneficial, for instance, improving the germ-fighting ability of oils with low to medium antimicrobial action. But others such as an oil's influence on the

WHAT WORKS, WHAT DOESN'T

way muscles relax and contract or the potential allergenic action of the oils may raise the risk of producing undesired effects in some – for example, pregnant women and those with asthma.

Aromatherapy in pregnancy

There is ongoing disagreement, even among professional aromatherapists, concerning which oils are safe during pregnancy and which ones are not. Research has done little to clarify this matter. In everyday use, most essential oils are used in such small quantities by women that the risks are little more than theoretical. Such cautions may be most relevant for women who have trouble conceiving or who have a history of miscarriage. Even so, some may reason that it is better to err on the side of caution with the following oils: basil, camphor, clary sage,* cypress, juniper, jasmine,* hyssop, lavender*, lemon balm, majoram, myrrh, mugwort, nutmeg, pennyroyal, peppermint,* plecanthrus, rose,* rosemary, rue, sage, savin, tansy, thuja and wormwood.

Most women can use these oils during pregnancy without any problems. However, those who are prone to miscarriage should exercise caution and wait until the second trimester before using them. Side effects are unlikely, but if any should occur, discontinue use.

What to expect

The best advice is not to have unrealistic expectations about essential oils. While aromatherapists may claim that essential oils can be used to treat just about anything, this is not strictly true. Essential oils are a therapy only in the loosest sense. On their own they have only been proven to address a handful of complaints – usually related to stress. However, you may find that using essential oils is a good adjunct to other therapies.

Like any other competent therapist, your aromatherapist should take a complete case history at your first session. The therapist will choose a mixture of oils specifically for you, depending on what was uncovered during the history-taking. Most aromatherapists use **massage** to enhance the effect of the essential oil, so you may be asked to undress and lie down, covered with a warm towel or sheet, on the massage floor, mattress, couch or table. Your therapist may employ a number of different massage techniques including **shiatsu** or **reflexology**. The depth of the massage and the parts of the body massaged will be chosen to suit your needs and comfort. An aromatherapy massage should never hurt.

Your aromatherapist should be qualified to treat a wide range of health conditions. Make sure you are not going to someone who is simply trained to use aromatherapy as a beauty treatment or for general relaxation. Such therapists generally have only completed short courses in aromatherapy and may not have the training necessary to practise therapeutic aromatherpy. If you are unsure about your therapist's credentials, ask.

To find a qualified aromatherapist, contact the International Federation of Aromatherapists or the International Society of Professional Aromatherapists (ISPA).

Essential Oils for Common Complaints

A basic selection of oils to ease a wide range of conditions

Essential oil	How does it work?	Most useful for	Try blending with
Chamomile *Matricaria chamomilla* (German) *Anthemis nobilis* (Roman)	Anti-inflammatory, antiseptic, digestive, tonic	Skin problems, wound healing, heartburn, indigestion, headache, cystitis, fluid retention, nausea, back pain, constipation, soothing and calming	Almost any other oil but particularly lavender, geranium, jasmine, bergamot, rose, neroli, clary sage, sandalwood, mandarin
Clary Sage* *Salva sclarea*	Hypotensive, aphrodisiac, digestive, antiseptic, anti-depressant, sedative, tonic	Anxiety, stress, improving circulation, relieves pain and cramp, enhances contractions	Orange, grapefruit, mandarin, geranium, sandalwood, lavender
Eucalyptus *Eucalyptus globulus*	Diuretic, expectorant, analgesic, antiseptic, stimulant	Headaches, colds and flu, cystitis, diarrhoea, muscle aches, respiratory conditions	Lavender, chamomile, mandarin, tea tree, lemon
Geranium *Pelargonium odorantissimum*	Antiseptic, astringent, diuretic, refreshing, toning, hypotensive	Fluid retention, anxiety, high blood pressure, diarrhoea, tension, depression, skin conditions, cramp, varicose veins	Bergamot, clary sage, orange, rose, lavender, jasmine and sandalwood
Grapefruit *Citrus grandis*	Uplifting, tonifying	Stress, exhaustion, skin conditions, constipation	Bergamot, neroli, tea tree, clary sage, sandalwood, mandarin and other citrus oils, geranium, lavender
Jasmine *Jasminum officinale*	Antidepressant, stimulant	Painful periods, muscle tension, anxiety, respiratory problems	Rose, sandalwood, neroli, geranium and mandarin and other citrus oils, chamomile, lavender

Essential oil	How does it work?	Most useful for	Try blending with
Lavender *Lavandula augustifolia* *Lavandula officinalis*	Antibacterial, decongestant, anti-depressant, aids sleep, reduces pain	Skin complaints, insomnia, colds and flu, burns and scalds, anxiety and depression, cramp, muscle aches, stretch marks, back pain, heals wounds, lowers blood pressure, eases headache	Most oils but in particular geranium, jasmine, chamomile, mandarin
Mandarin (tangerine) *Citrus reticulata*	Refreshing, uplifting, antiseptic, antispasmodic, sedative, digestive and tonic	Depression, cramp, anxiety, heartburn, constipation, nausea, stretch marks	Particularly lavender and neroli but also sandalwood, geranium, jasmine, chamomile
Neroli (orange blossom) *Citrus bigaradia* *Citrus aurantium*	Antidepressant, sedative, antibacterial, digestive, tonic, aids circulation	Constipation, flatulence, diarrhoea, oedema, insomnia, stress, skin conditions, stretch marks, eases breathing during labour	Geranium, grapefruit, mandarin, lemon, sandalwood, clary sage, ylang ylang, chamomile, rose
Rose *Rosa damascena*	Antidepressant, sedative, antiseptic, diuretic, laxative, uterine tonic	Depression, anxiety, loss of interest in sex, dry skin	Mandarin, sandalwood, neroli, chamomile, jasmine, lavender, clary sage, geranium, ylang ylang
Sandalwood *Santalum album*	Antiseptic, aphrodisiac, digestive, diuretic, expectorant, sedative and tonic	Respiratory infections, skin conditions, anxiety, fluid retention, lack of energy, heartburn, varicose veins, soothes and refreshes	Ylang ylang, rose, neroli, jasmine, lavender and geranium, bergamot, tea tree
Tea Tree *Melaleuca alternifolia*	Antiseptic, antifungal, anti-inflammatory, stimulates the immune system	Cystitis, skin conditions, respiratory problems	Lavender, geranium, mandarin, lemon and grapefruit will all mask its rather medicinal smell

* *Not recommended for use in early pregnancy, but can be safely used in late pregnancy and during labour.*

Chapter 6

Ayurveda

Commonly used for

Fatigue • Immune Function • Skin Conditions • Digestive
Disorders • Migraine • Hypertension • Musculoskeletal Disorders
• Menstrual and Menopausal Problems • Beauty Treatment

• Seek advice from a qualified practitioner

Without knowing it you may already have dabbled in some form of Ayurvedic medicine. Also known as traditional Indian medicine or Vedic medicine, individual components of Ayurvedic medicine such as **yoga, fasting/detox, meditation, urine therapy** and a range of **herbal remedies** have become increasingly popular ways of maintaining health during the last several decades.

The word 'Ayurveda' has two roots: *ayur* meaning 'life' and *veda* meaning 'knowledge' or 'science'. Thus Ayurveda is the science of life. While used for thousands of years in India as a legitimate and holistic therapeutic system, today when Ayurveda is mentioned it is most likely to be in the context of a celebrity who is using it to maintain their beauty and youthfulness.

This narrow idea that Ayurveda is some kind of way to beat gravity and the grim reaper has been largely aided by media-friendly new age mystics such as Deepak Chopra whose own Ayurvedic centre in California offers a way for the very wealthy to indulge in Ayurvedic facials, massage and other luxury treatments.

In truth, there is a great deal we do not know about the true nature of Ayurveda and what it can or cannot achieve in the realm of human health. Despite 6,000 years of traditional use, volumes of Ayurvedic knowledge have yet to be translated from their original Sanskrit. Some modern proponents invest Ayurveda with a mystical aspect, promoting the idea that Vedic medicine is a traditional spiritual discipline. However, others believe that there is little spiritualism in the ancient practice of Ayurveda and – as is typical when an Eastern tradition is adopted by the West – certainly not much of the traditional to be found in its modern practice.

As a system of healthcare Ayurveda works along similar lines as **traditional Chinese medicine** and many other ethnic healthcare systems. It is also just as intricate. Based on a system that distinguishes between individual bodily 'humours' or constitutional types, Ayurveda is primarily a system of healthcare and prevention rather than a way of curing disease. It sees the body as a whole and uses a variety of approaches to maintain a state of balance physically, emotionally, mentally and spiritually. It is believed that in this state of balance disease is much less likely to take hold of the individual. In Ayurveda the life force – the divine energy that flows through the body maintaining balance, and the equivalent of the Chinese *qi* – is called *prana*. Prana, like qi, flows along invisible channels, or *nadis*, and poor health is the result of blockages in these channels.

Stripped to its bare bones much of what is involved in the Ayurvedic system of medicine will be familiar to many Westerners. Where Ayurveda uses herbs, astrology, meditation, yoga and dietary advice to achieve this balance, the closest Western equivalent, **naturopathy**, would use aromatherapy, relaxation, massage, herbal medicine, diet, exercise and prayer.

An interpretation of the symbolism of Ayurveda would suggest that traditional Ayurvedic beliefs are, in fact, firmly grounded in the physical, not spiritual world. For instance, Ayurvedic philosophy teaches that all things on earth are made from the same five – largely earthbound – elements (or *bhutas*): earth, water, air, fire and space (or ether). Each bhuta has specific individual qualities.

Al things in nature are a combination of all the bhutas, but in each of us one will usually predominate. In Ayurvedic philosophy different bhutas can predominate in different parts of the body, thus those places which are watery (blood, bile mucous, sweat, urine) are predominantly water, whereas places which are more solid (bones, nails, teeth) are predominantly earth. Where transformation occurs, such as in metabolism or the digestive tract, fire predominates, and so on.

Within each individual the bhutas combine to make a predominant energy – the controlling force, or *dosha* – which maintains the dynamic balance within the body. The three doshas are:

- *Vata* – a combination of air and ether

- *Kapha* – a combination of water and earth

- *Pitta* – a combination of fire and water

In Ayurveda human constitution is usually determined by a combination of two of the doshas (though in some only one predominates). Thus a person could be a vata-pitta type or a pitta-kapha type. Under this system there are eight basic combinations:

- *Vata*

- *Pitta*

- *Kapha*

- *Vata-Pitta*

- *Pitta-Kapha*

- *Kapha-Vata*

- *Vata-Pitta-Kapha* (unbalanced)

- *Vata-Pitta-Kapha* (balanced)

This way of classifying or 'typing' individuals is common in both traditional and modern alternative systems (see also **homeopathy**) and has both advantages (ease of diagnosis and prescription for the practitioner) and disadvantages (the patient can so easily become a 'type' and not an individual).

How does it work?

The whole aim of Ayurveda is to restore and maintain good health. This it does by what could simply be described as a prescription for 'clean living'. While it is acknowledged that the causes of disease are often bacteria and viruses, the Ayurvedic practitioner is also looking for what has made the body particularly susceptible to these things which are, after all, on us and around us all the time.

In Ayurveda a person becomes susceptible to illness when the doshas are not in harmony. Disharmony can be caused by almost any kind of disturbance – for instance, weather changes, planetary influences, emotional upsets, how you were treated as a child, smoking, alcohol, drugs, environmental pollution or infection. When there is disharmony, the body releases toxins or *ama* that restrict the natural flow of energy and interfere with the body's natural organisation and intelligence. In Ayurvedic medicine it is ama that is the root of all disease and it is eliminated by the application, *panchkarma*, the process of cleansing the body.

What the research says

There have been no studies into the effectiveness of Ayurveda as a system of care. Over the years, some of the components of Ayurveda such as **yoga, meditation, fasting/detox** have been studied separately and found to be effective for certain conditions. In contrast, only a handful of the 800 or so herbs used in traditional Ayurvedic treatment have ever been studied (in a conventional sense) at all, though some of these have shown promise.

The type of Ayurvedic herbal medicine we know in the West is largely influenced by Maharishi Mahesi Yogi – the same Indian swami who introduced yoga to the wider world. His particular brand of Ayurveda is known as Maharishi Ayur-Veda and it belongs to the same well-funded movement as Transcendental Meditation. Maharishi-Ayur-Veda runs its own health centres and also markets its own exclusive line of products.

Potential but little proof

Many studies into Ayurvedic herbs use Maharishi brand herbs. For instance, a preparation called Maharishi Amrit Kalash-4 (MAK-4) – a paste which consists of raw sugar, ghee (clarified butter), Indian gallnut, Indian gooseberry, dried catkins, Indian pennywort, honey, nutgrass, white sandalwood, butterfly pea, shoeflower, aloeweed, liquorice, cardamom, cinnamon, Indian cypress and turmeric – was found to reduce the incidence of breast cancer in rats. Interesting but not necessarily relevant to humans.

Another remedy MAK-5 – a mixture of *Gymnema aurantiacum*, *Hypoxis orchioides, Tinospora cordifolia, Sphaeranthus indicus, Lettsomia nervosa*, butterfly pea, liquorice, *Vanda spatulatum* and Indian wild pepper – was shown in a laboratory test to thin the blood. Again interesting but difficult to show how it might work in humans.

Laboratory investigations have further shown that both MAK-4 and MAK-5 are rich in antioxidants such as vitamins A, C and E, bioflavonoids, catechin, polyphenols, tannic acid and riboflavin.

One very small human study found that both MAK-4 and MAK-5 could inhibit cholesterol and so may be useful in the prevention of atherosclerosis. In this study, 10 people with high cholesterol levels were treated with both preparations – MAK-4, 10 g twice daily and MAK-5, 500 mg twice daily on an empty stomach – over an 18-week period. Blood tests showed that total cholesterol, other fats and LDL ('bad') cholesterol were all reduced; HDL ('good') cholesterol levels remained stable. Unfortunately the study was too small from which to draw universal conclusions.

Another mixture (not a Maharishi herb) has shown interesting potential. Sixty people were given an Ayurvedic remedy called HP 200, which is made from the anti-Parkinsonian components of several plants – anticholingerics in *Datura stramonium*, levodopa in *Mucuna pruriens* and *Vicia faba*, dopamine agonists in *Claviceps purpurea* and MAO inhibitors in *Banisteria caapi*. The HP 200 powder was mixed with water and given orally for 12 weeks. At the end of the study, those taking the herb showed a statistically significant reduction in symptoms. Adverse reactions were rare but included gastrointestinal upsets.

The herb *Phyllanthus amarus* (a herb used in Ayurveda but also in many other ethnic practices) was shown in one study to kill the hepatitis B virus, but several other studies have failed to duplicate these results and the herb's potential remains uncertain.

Tonic mixtures

Among the most promising traditional Ayurvedic herbals are the *rasayanas* – powerful tonic herbs and mixtures reputed to strengthen the 'primordial tissue' that nourishes the rest of the body. Rasayanas are purported to enhance longevity, youthfulness, memory, intellect, the immune system and physical endurance.

Based on traditional uses for rasayanas, US researchers in 1997 concluded that many rasayanas work by acting on components of the immune system, which in turn have broad effects on the entire body.

To reach this conclusion they studied the accumulated evidence for six traditional rasayanas – *Emblica officinalis, Tinospora cordifolia, Asparagus racemosus* (now *Protasparagus racemosus*), *Withania somnifera, Terminalia chebula* and *Piper longum* – on animals.

In laboratory studies using both normal and immuno-suppressed animals, pretreatment with all six rasayanas protected animals from infection, shortened recovery time and lowered the death rate. The plants produced a stronger healing effect when combined with antibiotics. Important immune functions, such as the body's ability to identify and destroy foreign substances, also increased in treated animals as compared to control groups.

The researchers also found evidence to support the view that the traditional use of specific rasayanas strengthened individual tissues or organs, for example, *Emblica officinalis* for the pancreas; *Asparagus racemosus* for the stomach; *Piper longum* for the lungs and *Tinospora cordifolia* for the liver. However, because their findings were based on animal data no direct conclusions can be drawn regarding potential benefits for humans.

The liver-protective effect of *Tinospora cordifolia* has been found, however, in human studies. In one involving 30 patients with obstructive jaundice (when the bile ducts are blocked by stones or tumours, preventing the normal excretion of bile into the intestine), researchers found that *T. cordifolia* combined with conventional therapy reduced mortality to 6.25 per cent, compared to 39 per cent in the placebo group. Those taking *T. cordifolia* also reported feeling better and had an improved 'quality of life'.

In another study of 50 tuberculosis patients, *T. cordifolia* in combination with conventional therapy produced fewer side effects than when conventional therapy was combined with a placebo. A third study of 40 women with breast cancer showed that white blood cell counts remained higher and general well-being improved in subjects given the herb as a complement to cancer chemotherapy.

Another rasayana, *Withania somnifera* (more commonly known as *ashwagandha*), is sometimes called Indian ginseng in reference to its rejuvenative and tonic effects on the nervous system. In fact, numerous studies show ashwagandha to be comparable to **Panax ginseng** in its activity.

Traditionally, all parts of the plant were used as medicine, but the root, which has a sort of damp-horse smell, is most commonly used today. Ashwagandha contains at least 26 active components and this complex chemistry may explain its broad range of therapeutic properties including its ability to fight fatigue, reduce inflammation, calm, improve breathing and act as a general tonic.

Studies on humans are limited, but in one study involving mice, ashwagandha prevented stress-related gastrointestinal ulcers, increased physical endurance and prevented the depletion of vitamin C and cortisol (a normally protective hormone though high levels, often brought on by stress, as well as low levels can cause health problems) in animals that were stressed with a swimming exercise.

In another double-blind study, 101 healthy men ranging in age from 50 to 59 took either ashwagandha or a placebo for one year. Signs of ageing such as greying hair and calcium levels significantly improved in the herb group compared to those taking a placebo. Up to 70 per cent of those using ashwagandha also noticed increased libido and improved sexual function.

Cautions

The greatest risk most of us are likely to encounter in Ayurveda comes from the use of herbal remedies that, like those used in **traditional Chinese medicine**, occasionally contain heavy metals such as lead and mercury as well as toxins such as arsenic. These can reach dangerous levels and consumers are well advised not to buy herbs from questionable sources. Mixtures used as tonics and aphrodisiacs appear to be particularly risky.

When the Medical Toxicology Unit (MTU) at Guy's and St Thomas's Hospitals in London surveyed adverse reactions caused by herbs and dietary supplements, Ayurvedic medicines came high on their list of potentially dangerous substances.

The researchers noted at least nine reported adverse reactions among people who had used Ayurvedic herbs between 1991 and 1995. This however must be seen in context. It is a very small number and a closer look at the data revealed that most cases of adverse effects were in people who were self-treating with poor quality herbs.

In addition to potential toxins or contaminants, some Ayurvedic remedies and practices can have a profound effect on the system. For example, people who are very weak or whose energy is very depleted should not undertake rigorous fasting and detox as it may further complicate their condition.

What to expect

Ayurvedic treatment aims to restore an individual's unique consti-tutional balance and is probably most effective in individuals who are feeling 'run down' or 'not quite right'. There is little evidence that Ayurveda on its own can cure disease. In India practitioners move easily between Ayurvedic and conventional treatment according to what the patient's condition requires. Here this type of integration is rare.

A consultation with a traditional Ayurvedic practitioner is usually very thorough. Your practitioner will ask you questions about your health and lifestyle, may wish to observe how you stand and walk and may palpate different parts of your body.

Having determined your constitutional type, your practitioner will advise you on ways to help rebalance your doshas. To this end several different types of therapy aimed at the physical, emotional and spiritual levels may be used. In traditional Ayurveda these include:

Palliation In addition to a specific diet appropriate for a person's constitution and condition, the use of warming herbs such as ginger, cinnamon, black pepper, *Piper longum* or chitrak may be recommended to kindle digestive fire and burn toxins out of the body.

Snehana Oil massage to aid the movement of toxins from deep tissues to the gastrointestinal tract.

Swedana Sweat therapy, usually directly after snehana to further aid toxin release.

Panchkarma Usually follows the above three treatments and traditionally involves any or all of five separate actions: *vamana* (therapeutic vomiting), *virechana* (purgatives and laxatives), *basti* (therapeutic enema), *nasya* (nasal administration of medication) and *rakta moksha* (purification of the blood, blood letting – rare in the West).

Rasayana and **vajikarana** Types of rejuvenation therapy, usually using herbs appropriate to the person's condition or constitutional type.

Chromotherapy Different doshas resonate with different colours and this therapy involves the use of specific coloured lights beamed directly on various parts of the body, or water placed in the sunlight with specific coloured cellophane attached to the jar, or simply wearing specific colours of clothing.

Practitioners also give complex dietary advice based on a wide range of different tastes – bitter, sweet, strong and so on – and types of food much more wide ranging than is usually suggested by a Western nutritionist. In Ayurveda no foods are forbidden and for some types a diet heavy in meat, for example, may be prescribed as the most appropriate one. In addition, your practitioner may use *marma* – the Ayurvedic version of **acupressure** to help move toxins through the body and may recommend **yoga** and the use of mantra and breathing exercises.

The physical examination

In traditional Ayurveda a full physical examination has several components to it. These include:

Akruti – a general physical examination of the entire body

Nadi – examination of the pulse

Jihva – observation of the tongue

Shabda – listening to a person's speech and voice

Druga – examination of the eyes

Sprasa – tactile examination by palpation.

In some cases it may also involve:

Mutra – examination of the urine

Mala – examination of the stools.

Modern Ayurvedic practitioners can be very eclectic in the way they practise, however, and not everyone consulting a Western Ayurvedic practitioner will be given this full range of examinations.

Training as an Ayurvedic practitioner is rigorous – six years at a university in India or Sri Lanka – so you can be assured of your practitioner's skill. There are fewer than 40 fully qualified Ayurvedic practitioners in the UK. To find one, contact the Ayurvedic Medical Association UK. Anyone not on their list is not a fully qualified Ayurvedic practitioner and may only have undergone a short course. There are also several Maharishi Ayur-Veda health centres throughout the UK that can offer treatment, though this can be expensive.

What's in a name?

In Ayurvedic herbal medicine herbs are rarely used singly. Mixtures of herbs and spices are chosen for their tastes – sweet, sour, salty, pungent, bitter and astringent. Each tonic is balanced to produce the desired effect. Nevertheless, many of us use Ayurvedic herbs singly without knowing it. A look at the chart below shows that some of the most commonly used Vedic remedies can easily be found in the herbs and spices section of the local supermarket and can be used in a health-promoting way in everyday life.

What's in a name?

Ayurvedic name	Western name	Commonly used for
Dungri	Onion *Allium cepa*	Colds, parasites, bronchial disorders, joint stiffness, skin disorders, fluid retention, eliminates toxins
Kumari	Aloe *Aloe vera*	*Externally*: Inflammation, wounds, burns and scrapes, skin problems, muscle spasms and cramp *Internally*: as a purgative and tonic
Ajwan	Celery seed *Apium graveolens*	Colds, coughs, sinus congestion, digestive problems, high blood pressure, menstrual irregularities
Lashuna	Garlic *Allium sativum*	Tonic, colds and flu, parasites, skin problems, stiff joints, fluid retention, eliminates toxins
Choraka	Angelica *Angelica sinensis*	Menstrual problems, anaemia, poor circulation, digestive disorders, colds and flu, joint pain
Rai	Mustard *Brassica nigra*	Coughs and cold, backache, joint pain, constipation, digestive troubles
Merchi	Cayenne pepper *Capsicum annum*	Gastrointestinal and bowel problems, poor digestion, arthritis and muscle cramp
Sushavi	Caraway *Carum carvi*	Digestion, flatulence and colic, parasites, constipation
Brahmi	Gotu Kola *Centella asiatica*	Fatigue, depression, low libido, hypertension, insomnia, stress
Taj	Cinnamon *Cinamomum zeylancium*	Respiratory ailments, colds, indigestion, intestinal infections, poor appetite, anaemia, parasites
Bola	Myrrh *Commiphora myrrha*	Menstrual disorders, ulcerated skin, gum disease, haemorrhoids, mouth ulcers, canker sores

Ayurvedic name	Western name	Commonly used for
Dhania	Coriander *Coriandrum sativum*	Allergies, hay fever, liver support, arthritis and joint pain, parasites
Jeera	Cumin *Cuminum cyminum*	Digestive disorders, flatulence, migraine, allergies, exhaustion
Haldi	Turmeric *Curcuma longa*	Poor circulation, indigestion, anaemia, diabetes, poor immunity, wounds and bruises
Elaichi	Cardomom *Elettaria cardomomum*	Fatigue, respiratory problems, laryngitis, poor digestion, nausea
Lavanga	Cloves *Eugenia caryophylatta*	Colds, coughs, respiratory problems, indigestion, hiccups, low blood pressure, toothache
Mulathi	Liquorice *Glycyrrhiza glabra*	*Internally*: Poor memory, respiratory problems, fatigue, digestive disorders, constipation, ulcers, gastritis. *Externally*: herpes, cold sores
Pippali	Long pepper *Piper longum*	*Internally*: Asthma, bronchitis, sore throat, digestive disorders. *Externally*: arthritis , joint pain
Tulsi	Basil *Ocymum basilicum*	Parasites, coughs, respiratory problems, headaches, fevers, joint pain
Mari	Black pepper *Piper nigrum*	Indigestion, sinus congestion, poor circulation, removes toxins
Jaipala	Nutmeg *Myristica fragrans*	Stress, insomnia, diarrhoea, vomiting, poor appetite, flatulence
Methica	Fenugreek *Trigonella foenum-graecum*	Constipation, fever, sore throat, boils, rashes, digestive disorders, diabetes, high cholesterol
Ardraka	Ginger *Zingiber officinalis*	Nausea, vomiting, colds, flu, coughs, belching, motion sickness, laryngitis, headache, low libido, diarrhoea

Chapter 7

Biofeedback

Commonly used for

Headache • Urinary and Faecal Incontinence
• Constipation • Circulatory Problems
• Stroke Rehabilitation • Anxiety • Insomnia
• Irritable Bowel Syndrome • Migraine • Asthma
• Mild Hypertension • Post-traumatic Stress Syndrome

• Requires professional instruction

For many years the prevailing view of the human body was that it is a system that could not be controlled – that it breathes, blushes, belches, pumps blood and adrenaline, and sometimes relieves itself without any conscious input from its owner. And yet you can't tickle yourself. If you try to, your mind will block or control both the physical sensations and the impulse to laugh. Concepts like this suggest that while many of the body's functions and responses seem to be involuntary, they can with practice be controlled by the conscious mind.

Biofeedback is a 20th-century therapy but nevertheless has connections with ancient practices such as ***meditation***, mindfulness and progressive relaxation practised for centuries by yogis. It is also a behavioural therapy with connections with the practice of counselling and psychotherapy. Although it initially involves the use of a machine, biofeedback is also a do-it-yourself therapy – true to the spirit of self-responsibility that pervades alternative medicine.

While mindfulness and the control of certain bodily functions has been practised for many years in the East, the idea that a person can learn how to modify his or her own bodily processes is a relatively new concept in the West. Before the 1960s scientists believed that autonomic functions such as heart rate, pulse, digestion, blood pressure, brainwave activity and muscle behaviour could not be voluntarily controlled.

But today we know that many of these functions can be to some extent determined by the mind. This process is officially called **psychophysiological self-regulation** and biofeedback is one method that can help individuals become proficient at it. With biofeedback a person can consciously alter brainwave activity when at rest and regulate several autonomic functions such as breathing, heart rate and blood pressure in order to improve their overall health.

The concept of using machines to provide feedback for biological processes was pioneered in the 1930s by O. Hobart Mawrer, who used an alarm system triggered by urine to stop children wetting the bed. But it was not until the 1960s that US scientists began to use biofeedback to monitor the altered states and the ability to self-regulate of yogis. Eventually biofeedback began to attract the attention of physicians, some of whom used the concept of biofeedback to teach subjects to relax or 'mellow out' and to achieve a drugless high. By the early 1980s many different medical disciplines including primary care, psychology, general practice, neurology, alcohol and drug rehabilitation, dentistry and pain management had begun to incorporate biofeedback into their practice.

Today biofeedback is used as a therapy in its own right as well as an adjunct to other therapies, both conventional and alternative.

How does it work?
Biofeedback is a general term for any process that measures and reports back immediate information about the way the body is functioning. As the machine feeds back this information to the person being monitored, he or she can learn to actively regulate body functions. The type of machine used can vary and the machinery can

83

Type of biofeedback	Measures	Electrode placement	Conditions benefited
EEG (Electroencephalo-graph)	Brainwave activity	Scalp	Addiction, epilepsy, brain damage, hyperactivity, insomnia
EMG (Electromyograph)	Muscle tension and spasms	Various muscles	Muscle pain, teeth grinding, stress, asthma, physical rehabilitation, tension headaches, menstrual symptoms, arthritis
EDR (Electrodermal response)	Sweat gland activity	Fingers	Anxiety, overactive sweat glands
Thermal	Blood flow monitored as skin temperature changes (the more blood the warmer the skin temperature)	Fingers and elsewhere	Migraine, Raynaud's disease, hypertension, anxiety, asthma
Perieometer	Muscle contraction	Anal sphincter and pelvic floor muscles	Faecal and urinary incontinence
Breath	Breath rate, rhythm, volume, location	Chest, abdomen, mouth and nose	Anxiety, asthma, hyperventilation

be as elaborate as a specially programmed computer system or as simple as a thermometer taped to a finger (see chart above). Because of the diversity of the machines involved and the sometimes individual approaches to therapy, biofeedback is really a collection of different therapies rather than one distinct entity.

During a session electronic sensors are attached to various parts of the body – forehead, neck, fingers, toes, back muscles and anywhere else that normal function has been disrupted, and a patient may receive feedback from two or three of these instruments, depending on the disorder being treated. The sensors measure brainwaves, electrical signals to muscles, skin temperature, pulse and other seemingly autonomous functions.

These measurements 'feed back' in a variety of ways, including visual displays and auditory tones, offering a constant stream of physiological data. With the help of the therapist the person learns to interpret this data (for instance, an increase in finger skin temperature is thought to correspond to the person feeling more relaxed) and relate it back to his or her physical condition and eventually control whatever process is being monitored.

While biofeedback requires special equipment initially, once the technique is mastered individuals can use it any time or place to achieve the desired results. The machinery is just a catalyst for the individual to learn more about their internal states, how they affect the body and how they can be controlled to bring about favourable changes and a sense of control.

What the research says
Biofeedback has benefited from a great deal of research over the years and has been shown to be useful for a range of conditions. Many of the conditions that respond to biofeedback training are stress related, such as headaches, insomnia, asthma, gastrointestinal disorders, mild hypertension and muscular problems.

Headaches
Headaches ranging from the mild to the severe appear to improve with biofeedback. While most treatments are geared towards controlling pain by relieving stress, there is some evidence that when migraine is caused by dilated blood vessels in the head, biofeedback can be used effectively to reduce the pain and severity of attacks. What is more, biofeedback can sometimes be effective against even the most stubborn muscle tension headaches, succeeding where

other treatments have failed. Though numbers in the study groups are invariably small, the results are remarkably consistent.

For example, in a study of 31 headache sufferers, electromyographic (EMG) biofeedback was compared with a sham treatment that gave no instruction on how to control EMG activity and another group where symptoms were only monitored. Only the biofeedback group showed changes in EMG activity and significant improvement in symptoms.

Biofeedback has also been tested against drug therapy and shown to both enhance the effectiveness of medication and in some cases produce better results. Research has demonstrated, for example, that biofeedback is at least as effective as the beta-blocker/antihypertensive propranolol. In one study in 1995, relaxation/thermal biofeedback was shown to enhance the effectiveness of propranolol therapy. Although the combined therapy was very effective, it had more side effects than relaxation/biofeedback on its own.

This is an important point because, while drug therapy can be effective for migraine, the side effects it produces can mean that sufferers don't stick with their therapy over time. In a three-year study comparing use of the anti-migraine drug ergotamine and biofeedback, drug users were less likely than those who used biofeedback to stick with their regime.

Many headaches can be made worse by stress and often biofeedback combined with relaxation can be particularly effective in relieving headaches caused by muscle tension. With an improvement rate of 44 to 65 per cent, it is often more successful than using drugs. In one 1997 study, 44 people with chronic tension headaches were assigned to either six sessions of relaxation and EMG biofeedback or to a control group that received no treatment. More than half the relaxation/biofeedback group reported a 50 per cent reduction in headache activity following treatment.

In another trial comparing relaxation technique with EMG biofeedback, the relaxation group fared better when it came to the relief of migraine or muscle tension headaches, but not so well with mixed headache. In addition, when 23 migraine sufferers were assigned either to biofeedback-assisted relaxation or to a group who relaxed on their own, the biofeedback group reported a greater decrease in pain and need for medication.

There are notes of caution, though. In one study, while both relaxation and biofeedback worked equally well, the relaxation technique was more effective in reducing medication consumption at one-year follow-up. Also, according to one of the largest studies conducted in 1989 and involving 793 people, biofeedback, singly and in combined therapy, may be most effective when given over a longer number of sessions (at least 15) and when the symptoms have been present for two years or less.

Incontinence

Although it affects both sexes, women seem to suffer from incontinence somewhat more than men. Indeed, it is a genuine problem for as many as 38 per cent of the female population over 60. Often there is nothing mechanically wrong, but the fear of losing control can become an unbearable burden and a self-fulfilling prophecy.

Biofeedback can also be used to help women identify their pelvic muscles and learn to contract and relax them at will. With this method people report 54–95 per cent improvement of incontinence with the use of biofeedback in combination with other behavioural treatment.

For instance, in a recent trial published in the *Journal of the American Medical Association* in 1997, women with urge incontinence were divided into three groups that received either biofeedback treatment or the drug oxybutynin hydrochloride (Ditropan), 2–5 mg three times daily, or were left untreated for eight weeks.

Biofeedback patients had four sessions in which they learnt progressively to identify, relax and control pelvic muscles while keeping abdominal muscles relaxed; how to respond to urgent signals to urinate; and how to contract muscles to ensure complete voiding. No patient required more than two biofeedback sessions to correct the problem and at the end of the treatment period incontinent accidents per week fell by 81 per cent in the biofeedback group to 2.8 per cent. This compared very favourably to 5.7 per cent for the drug group and 8.2 per cent for controls. The study also acknowledged the depressing fact that although behavioural modifications are the best cure for incontinence, they are seldom recommended by physicians due to lack of physician expertise in this area.

In another study in 1996, biofeedback proved a better method than physiotherapy in pelvic floor rehabilitation after trauma. In this study, 40 women with genuine urinary stress incontinence used either a biofeedback system, comprised of a surface electrode inserted into the vagina and a catheter in the rectum, or physiotherapy to help retrain the pelvic floor muscles. Among the 34 women who completed the full treatment, there was a statistically significant improvement in the biofeedback group, which seemed to last over the longer term. The women in the biofeedback group were also better motivated to continue training afterwards.

Biofeedback has also been used to repair the damage caused by radical prostatectomy. In 1996, 27 men who had been left incontinent by surgery were given weekly sessions to retrain the pelvic floor muscles. Additional reinforcement sessions were given at one, three, six and 12 months. Outcomes were based on the men's reports of improvement as well as a doctor's evaluation of the pelvic floor muscle constriction. At the end of the evaluation period, 48 per cent of the men had completely recovered continence and 26 per cent experienced significant improvements. The following year another study at the University of Florida also concluded that biofeedback is an important aid to recovery after prostate surgery.

Constipation
This is another area of health where biofeedback has claimed substantial success. For instance, in 1999 a small study involving 36 people found that biofeedback may assist those suffering from chronic constipation.

Each individual was randomly assigned to one of four different types of biofeedback: (1) intra-anal electromyographic biofeedback training; (2) electromyographic biofeedback training plus intra-rectal balloon training (expelling a small balloon which is inflated in the rectum is a way of retraining the person's muscles to effectively expel faecal material); (3) electromyographic biofeedback training plus home training; or (4) electromyographic biofeedback training, balloon training and home training. Success was measured by increased unassisted bowel movements and reduction in the use of laxatives. Participants maintained a daily log with details of each bowel evacuation and laxative use. Groups 1, 2 and 4 showed a significant increase in the number of unassisted bowel movements and groups 1, 2 and 3 experienced a reduction in the use of laxatives. There was little difference between the outcomes of the four treatments and the authors concluded that electromyographic biofeedback alone was as effective as that used with balloon training, home training, or both.

In another study published in the *Lancet* in 1996, 192 children with constipation were already being treated by conventional means. The children were divided into two groups, one that continued to receive conventional medical treatment (laxatives, dietary advice, toilet training and keeping a diary of bowel habits) and one that involved conventional treatment plus five biofeedback training sessions. After six weeks those in the conventionally treated group experienced an increase in normal bowel movements from 41 to 52 per cent. In the biofeedback group the rate increased from 38 to 86 per cent. This is significant but there were problems. In reviewing the groups after one year, normal bowel movements were present in 59 per cent of the conventional group but in only 50 per cent of the biofeedback group. Such results caution us not to make sweeping assumptions for the long-term benefits of behavioural (and other) therapies based on the conclusions of short-term studies.

Hypertension

If you have moderate to severe hypertension, it is unlikely that biofeedback will make a significant difference. However, there is some evidence that for those with mild hypertension, using biofeedback techniques can help to lower blood pressure.

One study of 40 people with advanced heart failure randomly assigned participants to either a biofeedback or a control group. The people in the biofeedback group had one session of skin-temperature biofeedback, augmented by instructions on how to visualise hand warmth and on modified progressive muscle relaxation. Several bodily functions including skin temperature, heart rate, levels of stress hormone and respiratory rate were measured before and after the biofeedback session.

Those undergoing biofeedback relaxation experienced an increased finger temperature (a sign of relaxation), better heart rate and a decreased respiratory rate (again a sign of relaxation). None of the people in the control group experienced these beneficial changes.

Learning disabilities

Sophisticated brain imaging equipment has unlocked some of the secrets of the way our brains work. For instance, it is now known that the tasks of reading and maths computation require certain regions in the brain to become engaged and work with each other in unison. Some proponents of biofeedback believe that the combination of functional imaging and EEG biofeedback may one day provide a breakthrough in the remediation of various learning disabilities that have been relatively intractable. To date, studies in this area have not been vigorously pursued.

The first significant study of both attention and learning problems using EEG biofeedback was performed by Joel and Judith Lubar in 1984. The results were highly promising, but because several of the children were receiving other special academic support during the study, they could not be regarded as conclusive. In 1985 a small study of four children in which the focus was learning disorders was published and this was the first of many studies in which improvements in IQ score through EEG training were documented. In a follow-up study using 24 subjects with learning disorders, an average improvement of 19 points in IQ was documented after biofeedback training. While these are encouraging results, experts estimate that about 20 per cent of subjects with attention deficit disorder cannot be treated successfully by EEG neurofeedback.

Other problems

A whole rag-bag of small studies have hinted at possible other uses for biofeedback. Irritable bowel syndrome, for instance, can often respond to relaxation techniques learned through biofeedback. A study at the Royal Free Hospital, London, involved 40 people with irritable bowel syndrome who had failed to respond to conventional treatment. A computer biofeedback game based on animated gut imagery was used in a series of four 30-minute sessions to help patients learn to achieve progressively deeper levels of relaxation. By practising relaxation when bowel symptoms were troublesome, 50 per cent of individuals found relief in both general symptoms and those specific to the bowel. At long-term follow-up 64 per cent of those who had been helped by relaxation continued to use the technique, even though they had no further contact with the hospital.

Some small studies have shown that asthmatics trained in biofeed-back techniques have less severe attacks, fewer admissions to hospital and decreased need for medication. One in 1997 found that respiratory sinus arrhythmia (RSA) biofeedback was more effective than EMG biofeedback because it appeared to relax asthma sufferers more and thus help their breathing.

A stroke can often leave a person with a weakness on one side of his or her body. In one analysis of eight controlled studies, biofeedback helped to improve gait as well as grip and grasping abilities in the hands of stroke patients. Several studies have also shown biofeed-back to be especially helpful in treating kyphosis (a front to back curvature of the spine).

In Raynaud's disease (where poor circulation in the hands can lead to painfully cold fingers), psychological intervention, including biofeedback, may also have a useful role to play. Biofeedback involving relaxation techniques, guided imagery, in parallel with computer-assisted monitoring of sympathetic arousal (the sympathetic nervous system controls among other things constriction/relaxation of the arteries and circulation), may lead to the reduction in symptoms either as a stand-alone treatment or in conjunction with other treatment.

Biofeedback has also been used successfully to improve the circulation in the feet of diabetics. In one study published in the journal *Diabetes Care* in 1992, biofeedback, combined with a relaxation tape, helped the participants to elevate the temperature of their toes by 31 per cent – very significant since poor circulation in diabetics can lead to slow wound healing and, in extreme cases, the need for amputation.

Children suffering from anxiety could also benefit from biofeedback. In one study 150 children were randomly assigned to receive either biofeedback or no treatment. Those in the biofeedback group had six sessions of thermal training followed by six sessions of electromyograph training. Assessment at the end of the study period found that biofeedback brought about a 'significant reduction' in their anxiety levels.

Cautions
In biofeedback individual motivation is everything. Without a person's ability and willingness to understand what is being fed back to him or her, and a serious commitment to practising internal awareness and focused self-control, the therapy will not succeed.

There are no real contraindications for biofeedback therapy. It is not useful for chronic conditions where there has been structural damage or where there is an infectious disease. In addition, if you are using medication to maintain some form of homeostatic balance (e.g. insulin or antihypertensive drugs), you should consult both your physician and biofeedback therapist for advice as successful therapy may alter the amount of medication you need to take.

It is also thought that individuals with certain psychiatric disorders should not undergo biofeedback. This includes severe psychosis, depression or obsessive tendencies as well as those with multiple personalities. The sometimes intense inward focus of biofeedback may leave such individuals feeling as if they have 'lost touch' with themselves and their place in the world.

In the end what prospective users need to be most cautious about is interpreting the usually positive conclusions of biofeedback research.

Most studies into biofeedback are small, which in itself it not always a problem. But smaller study size also means that therapists can take more time counselling individuals. Also, in studies of behavioural therapies under trial conditions where there is a well-defined time limit, participants are often highly motivated to change. They may practise more and learn faster than they might do otherwise under real-world conditions, where support from a therapist may not be so consistent or intense.

What to expect
During a biofeedback session electrodes are placed on the skin at relevant sites and the patient is then given instruction on how to interpret the machine's cues and ways to begin to alter certain behaviours and bodily functions. This may include meditation, relaxation and visualisation. As the patient becomes more proficient the machine will feed back changes in the measured activity.

While some studies show results after just one session, the reality is that, at the very least, a series of 3–6 sessions is usually required to achieve lasting results for even simple problems. Chronic, severe or long-standing problems may require more, perhaps dozens of sessions to achieve change. Each session lasts between 30 and 60 minutes. In some cases biofeedback is available on the NHS. If you are interested in this therapy talk to your GP first, as private sessions can be expensive.

Chapter 8

Fasting & Detoxification

Commonly used for

Rheumatoid Arthritis • Allergies • Skin Disorders
• Digestive Disorders • Boosting Immunity
• Weight Loss • Depression • Detoxification

• *Professional supervision is recommended*

Traditionally, people fasted to attain discipline and spiritual enlightenment. Today we tend to fast for less admirable reasons, such as maintaining a youthful appearance or as a form of crash dieting. Fasting has long been a component of traditional ethnic healthcare systems such as **Ayurveda** and it is also used in **naturopathy** to detoxify the body and treat allergies, digestive problems, auto-immune diseases and even mental illnesses.

The success of a fast depends on many factors including the type and length of fast and a person's overall level of health. Contrary to popular belief, fasting is not a good way to lose weight or a permanent way to detoxify the body. Instead, it is a short-term intervention which must be followed up by good health practices in order to maintain any benefits.

There are several different types of fasting. The water fast is perhaps the most severe and should not be used over more than three to five days without supervision. Juice fasting, which allows freshly pressed fruit and vegetable juices throughout the day, is a popular alternative.

But because it provides nutrients and some calories it is really less of a fast and more of an elimination diet since it avoids common allergens such as wheat, dairy, nuts, eggs, chocolate, tomatoes and various food additives. In addition, during a juice fast the natural sugars in juice will be converted into energy by the body and you are much less likely to be burning fat and muscle.

Aligned with the juice fast is the mono diet, where only one food type is eaten. The most famous example of the mono diet is the grape fast. Anecdotes abound about the benefits of living on grapes. For instance, a man who lived on grapes for 50 days described his experience in this way: 'After the twenty-third day an abscess came away from my one and only kidney and I was completely cured after all medical treatment had failed and made my condition worse.' However, anecdote is not the same as evidence, and no scientific studies have ever proven that mono diets or juice fasts or any other type of fast can permanently cure anything.

How does it work?
Fasting works in several ways. One of the first benefits of fasting is that it allows the digestive tract to rest. The process of digestion – breaking down food into its component parts – requires an enormous amount of energy. During a fast, while the process of digestion is suspended, energy can be diverted to other functions of the body such as elimination.

Of course, this elimination process, which removes wastes and toxins from the body, is ongoing whether we fast or not. In a healthy person it is the job of the liver and kidneys to detoxify the body. Supported by a healthy lifestyle, these organs are supremely capable of doing their job. During a fast the body continues this natural process of excreting waste material and stored toxins (such as pollutants and allergens). However, because no energy is being used to digest food, and the person is not taking in any new toxins, the liver and kidneys may work more efficiently.

For someone who has a very poor diet, who may be regularly ingesting allergens and pollutants, a short fast may lighten the load on the digestive and immune systems. As the body is cleared of toxins and allergens, symptoms associated with toxic overload should also be reduced.

While recognising the short-term benefits of fasting, many naturopaths would recommend that a wholefood high-fibre diet, preferably comprised of foods that have been organically grown and are free from chemical additives, is the best way to provide prolonged benefit for the body.

What the research says

Although therapeutic fasting is probably one of the oldest known interventions, it has been the subject of only limited study by the scientific community. Research into fasting has been reported on and off since 1880. Since that time medical journals have carried articles on the use of fasting in the treatment of a variety of ailments such as skin conditions, obesity, arthritis, chemical poisoning, diabetes and mental disorders. However, no information exists on how fasting might help otherwise healthy individuals.

Rheumatoid arthritis

In one study of rheumatoid arthritis (RA) sufferers in 1984, their grip strength and functional ability in the hand were all improved and swelling and pain reduced after a week-long fast. Other evidence suggests that fasting followed by a vegetarian diet can be useful in relieving the symptoms of RA – reinforcing the idea that a fast, while useful, is only of short-term benefit and must be followed up by other healthful practices.

In one review article published in 1991, RA sufferers volunteered for a study conducted at the University of Lund, Sweden, and were fasted for 7–10 days and then examined for changes in arthritis-related symptoms. Symptoms of joint tenderness and severity of pain and stiffness, as well as blood analysis for chemicals specific to rheumatoid arthritis, were assessed after the fast. Significant improvement was found in all areas, although not until the fourth or fifth day of the fast. But as if to emphasise the short-term nature of the 'cure', the authors noted that these improvements were lost within approximately one week after return to the habitual diet, regardless of its composition.

Other inflammatory conditions may also benefit from fasting. In one study, 20 people with arthritis as well as those with a range of skin disorders, including atopic eczema, rosacea and psoriasis, were kept on a two-week fast. Afterwards, there were significant improvements in the skin complaints and a substantial reduction in arthritic pain.

Reducing cholesterol
People with heart conditions can also benefit by abstaining from food. Fasting has been shown to be helpful in relieving a range of cardiovascular diseases, including raised cholesterol, high blood pressure and clogged arteries.

Blood analysis of Muslims fasting during Ramadan showed that alternating periods of fasting with daily gorging, in place of the traditional three meals per day, may have a temporary but beneficial effect on HDL-cholesterol levels, but no effect on other types of cholesterol. Once again evidence of any long-term benefit is lacking.

Reducing toxins
In cases of extreme poisoning fasting may aid the process of detoxification. In a study published in the *American Journal of Industrial Medicine* in 1984, scientists studied Taiwanese people who had ingested rice oil contaminated with PCBs. After undergoing 7 to 10-day fasts, all reported improvement in symptoms and some reported dramatic relief of symptoms. This research supported past research of people poisoned with PCB and indicates the therapeutic effects of fasting. However, caution must be used with those known to be significantly contaminated with fat-soluble toxins, for example, DDT. Released into the bloodstream during a fast, these chemicals may reach levels known to cause damage to the nervous system.

Other conditions
While fasting enthusiasts claim that it can be used to treat anything, little research exists to back up such statements. Small studies have shown some benefits in specific cases, for instance, short-term weight loss and psychiatric disorders such as depression and schizophrenia.

In one trial published in *Digestion* in 1984 and involving 88 people suffering from pancreatitis (inflammation of the pancreas), fasting was shown to be just as effective as treatment with the drug cimetidine and other forms of medical intervention such as nasogastric suction (a surgical technique) for treating this condition.

Cautions

At its best, fasting can provide your body with a physiological break that enables it to divert more energy to the process of removing metabolic waste and restoring balance. Under proper supervision fasting can be constructive and uplifting. Gone into without forethought and for prolonged periods of time, it can weaken and even kill.

Most authorities say that fasting for a day or two is unlikely to harm the body and can even be healthful. However, some people should never fast, for example, pregnant and nursing women, people with diabetes, ulcers, liver, kidney, heart or lung disease, advanced cancer or a compromised immune system. Those taking medications should also not fast as this can alter the potency of some drugs. In people who take large doses of the painkiller acetaminophen, fasting has been shown to sometimes cause severe liver damage.

There are other aspects of fasting to be aware of. While the body tries to spare protein, and so does not automatically use it for fuel, even in short fasts some muscle will be lost. Also, while the myth is that fasting is good because it encourages the body to burn fat, there are problems to be aware of. During the first 24 hours of a fast, your body uses primarily stored carbohydrate, or glycogen, for fuel. When that is gone, fat becomes the preferred energy source. Unable to make use of its blood sugar in the normal way, the body metabolises fat and produces ketones – the toxic by-products of fat metabolism. If this goes on for a prolonged period, ketosis – the presence of excess ketones – develops. Ketosis is a particular risk in long water fasts and is a sign of profound malnutrition and exhaustion.

As a rule the body avoids ketosis by further processing ketones in other tissues. If, however, ketone production exceeds a certain level, the body tissues become overwhelmed and ketosis results. Apart from those who fast, ketosis is common in diabetics and in labouring women who have been denied food in hospital.

What to expect

There is no one specific 'right' way for everyone to detoxify his or her body, whether by fasting, drinking lots of vegetable juices, sweating or taking herbs or nutritional supplements. The method for detoxification may depend entirely on some particular factor that is quite peculiar to the individual. It will depend on the proper assessment of food sensitivities, whether or not the body is carrying an excess burden of particular toxins from exogenous (outside) sources or from exposure to harmful microbes or parasites, or whether or not the digestive tract is functioning properly.

During days 1 and 2 of a fast, most people feel symptoms of hypoglycaemia (light-headed, dizzy, headache, flu-like and fatigued). As the body starts to use fat as a fuel source, these feelings can intensify and many people continue to feel awful, if not outright sick. One reason for this is that the majority of toxic materials in our society are fat-soluble and are therefore stored in body fat. The best examples of this are the insecticides and pesticides on vegetables and fruit which need to be fat-soluble and not water-soluble, otherwise they would be washed off when crops are watered or when it rains. Once the body starts burning fat, these chemicals are released into the system.

As the body mobilises toxic materials either stored in the liver or in fat cells into the bloodstream, the eliminatory organs typically cannot handle the workload to which they are being subjected. The person feels ill until this backlog of toxic material is metabolised and/or eliminated. This temporary worsening of symptoms is commonly referred to as a 'healing crisis'. After the healing crisis has subsided, the person fasting notices a strong increase in energy, clear-headedness and a stronger sense of well-being. In some a feeling of euphoria can be experienced; indeed this feeling was the ultimate goal of religious fasts.

How to fast safely

Most people can safely fast for a short period without undue harm to their bodies. If you are considering a short fast of three to five days, there are some guidelines that will help make it more beneficial.

- Prepare for your fast the day before by making your last meal one of fruits and vegetables – some authorities recommend that your diet the day before a fast should be vegan.

- Only water should be consumed while fasting and the quantity of water should be dictated by thirst. You should not consume coffee, tea, juice, soft drinks, cigarettes or anything else by mouth. Herbal teas can be supportive of a fast, but they should not be sweetened.

- Fasting should not be combined with vigorous exercise. Conserve your energy to maximise healing. Short walks in the fresh air, however, may be useful. Try to have a nap or two during the day.

- Avoid exposures to chemicals such as those contained in toiletries as these add to your body's toxic burden. Instead, consider washing simply with lukewarm water.

- Try to avoid extremes of temperature. Your body temperature may drop during a fast so ensure you stay warm.

- If the sun is out try go get 10 to 20 minutes a day of exposure.

When you are ready to break your fast, do so slowly choosing small quantities of food (fruits and vegetables are ideal) at room temperature. Eat slowly and chew thoroughly.

Assisting detox

Two simple remedies have been shown anecdotally to help with short-term detoxification.

Activated charcoal is a medicinal form of charcoal that has the capacity to absorb whatever molecules it encounters. Supplying charcoal to the digestive tract not only absorbs gas and toxins, but also appears to aid detoxification anywhere in the body. ⊃

The reduction of toxins accomplished by the short-term use of activated charcoal takes some pressure off the whole detoxification system by diminishing the burden on the gut. However, charcoal is not a panacea and there are downsides to its use. Charcoal can cause constipation. It is also indiscriminate in what it absorbs. Therefore it should not be taken with food or medicines as it would absorb them, too, and it should not be taken for long periods of time.

Baking soda, or sodium bicarbonate, is another simple remedy (and commonly found in over-the-counter antacids) that appears to help by changing the acid/alkali balance of the body. When just about anything goes wrong with the body, there is a tendency for the system to become temporarily over-acidic. Sending a small amount of alkali through the system in the form of bicarbonate of soda may help to rebalance the system.

Healthy people can take a half-teaspoon of baking soda in a glass of water for occasional irritability, pre-menstrual syndrome or a hangover, or when coming down with a cold, and will usually find some relief. However, like charcoal, it is not risk free. Avoid using too much and too often. Do not use this remedy if you have a very full stomach or if you have kidney or lung problems. Since it is a source of sodium (salt), this remedy should also be avoided by those with high blood pressure or congestive heart failure.

Alternatives to fasting

Other forms of detox may work just as well as fasting. For instance:

• Consuming a nutrient-rich, wholefood diet high in fibre is also helpful. Fibre helps to remove toxic wastes from the gut. If you can, switch to an organic diet.

• Eating foods rich in antioxidants such as beans, whole grains, citrus fruits, berries, cruciferous vegetables (cabbage, Brussels sprouts, cauliflower and broccoli), nuts and seeds will help to improve your natural detoxification systems.

• Engaging in sweat-producing activities several times a week can aid the effective release of toxins through the skin.

- Not voluntarily poisoning your body will reduce the burden on your system. Cut down on alcohol and caffeine consumption, quit smoking, save over-the-counter medicine such as painkillers, antacids and cold remedies for when they are really needed (or better yet get to the root of what is ailing you, rather than suppressing symptoms with drugs).

- Removing mercury-containing fillings will significantly reduce your exposure to this toxic metal.

- Fitting a reverse osmosis water filter under the sink will reduce your exposure to toxins in the water supply, including pesticides, heavy metals, parasites and bacteria.

Steam detox

A regular sauna is a pleasant and effective alternative to starvation. Increased sweating increases elimination of salt and water through the skin. It also increases elimination of metals (such as nickel, copper, zinc and lead), toxic volatile hydrocarbons (including benzene, styrenes, toluene, trichloroethylene and PCBs), prescription and recreational drugs (such as cocaine, methadone, barbiturates and benzodiazepine) and other toxins.

Exposure to hot, moist air has been used to alleviate symptoms of many of the same disorders as fasting, for instance, asthma, arthritis and other rheumatic conditions.

Avoid using a sauna if you are a heavy drinker or alcoholic – there is an increased risk of death due to alcohol's effects on the body's thermoregulatory system. It is also not advisable if you are diabetic, suffer from kidney problems or high blood pressure. If you are pregnant, take care. Research varies on whether or not a long hot sauna can cause neurological damage to a foetus (how hot and how long appear to be the influential factors).

Chapter 9

Flower Essences

Commonly used for

Depression • Anxiety • Psychological Symptoms
• Stress • Menstrual and Menopausal Problems
• Assisting Life Transitions

• *Suitable for self-treatment*

It is said that there are no diseases, only sick people. This could best describe the philosophy of those who practise any type of energy medicine, and in particular those who use flower essences.

Ancient philosophers maintained that life, or matter, was composed of energy and that all body processes were simply patterns of energy. According to this belief, subtle movements and changes in those energy patterns ultimately directed the course of health and illness. Whereas modern medicine aims for stasis – a suppression of 'undesirable' symptoms, and indeed a body that is free of any symptoms at all – to ancient practitioners the ebb and flow of certain symptoms and body states was natural, even desirable, because where there is movement there is life.

The various forms of energy medicine – **homeopathy**, **acupuncture**, **spiritual healing** and **meditation** – see the life force as something that sustains and organises the physical body. Their aim is to transform energy patterns directly using various techniques to stimulate the body in the direction of greater balance and encourage the body's natural healing process. In contrast, most conventional doctors dispute the existence of a life force because it is difficult to measure scientifically. If it can't be measured, doctors argue, how do you know it's there and how can you be sure that whatever you are doing to it actually works?

Dr Edward Bach (pronounced batch), an English bacteriologist and homeopath, is generally credited with the discovery of the healing properties of potentised plant essences. In the 1930s he moved to the countryside in the hope of regaining his failing health. He walked daily in the woods and collected flowers and other botanicals near his home. Using his grounding in both conventional science and intuitive diagnosis, he began to develop his own individual theories on the way that personality types – first 12, then 19 and finally 38 different types, corresponding to the 38 remedies in today's Bach repertory – influenced disease and how this effect could be mediated by the use of certain plant essences.

Bach hypothesised that flower essences helped to rid the body of negative emotional states, much in the same way that homeopathy helps trigger the body's own physiological defence system.

Bach believed that chronic stress resulting from emotional states such as anger, fear, grief, worry and resentment had a role to play in lowering a person's resistance to disease. In his own practice he noted that his patients were prone to all sorts of infections when these emotional states prevailed. This affirmed his belief that a person's emotional outlook determined the length and severity of their illness. He also discovered that people with similar personality traits often suffered from the same types of diseases (something which modern psychology has begun to confirm) and responded to the same remedy, but those with different personality traits required different remedies to cure the same disease. At heart Bach's philosophy works along the same lines as other constitutional therapies – the homeopathy that he was so familiar with, but also older systems of healthcare such as **Ayurveda** and **traditional Chinese medicine**.

Today, there are literally hundreds of different types of plant essences. In addition to the 38 classical remedies of Dr Bach, there are 20 Master's Flower Essences made from fruit and vegetable blossoms, the 38 Healing Herbs (organic, hand-made versions of Dr Bach's remedies), the 72 Australian Bush Essences, 102 Californian Essences, the Alaskan Flower Essences, the Findhorn Flower Essences from Scotland, the Bailey Flower Essences from Yorkshire, the Himalayan Essences and more general combination essences from any number of media-friendly healers.

Too much choice?

In addition to plant essences, there are those made from almost every natural substance there is. On the fringe of flower essence therapy there are people all over the world making and using environmental, colour and light essences, gem and crystal essences, chakra essences, ocean essences and even animal essences.

It is hard to imagine that any of these could be very different from each other, and the sheer number of flower essences being developed and promoted is simply overwhelming. Nevertheless, their manufacturers claim subtle and not-so-subtle differences in their approach. Bach and the Australian Essences, for example, are both very much grounded in the day-to-day physical world, although the Australian Essences address more specific concerns, such as sexuality, communication, spirituality and learning, rather than personality type. The Californian Essences work on a more esoteric level, and the Himalayan and Alaskan Essences, rather like their places of origin, can only be described as targeting the more remote parts of the human psyche.

The various manufacturers also claim considerable differences in the therapeutic potential of essences made from the same species of plant. This begs a perfectly fair question: why, for instance, should the properties of a poppy from Europe be so fundamentally different from one grown in California?

The answer, according to devotees, would be that different parts of the world radiate different energy patterns. In addition, the varying climates and mineral content of different soils, a plant's ability to thrive, the time it is harvested and even the people involved in the harvesting, manufacture and prescribing of the remedy may all have a profound effect on its effectiveness. Considering how potentially complex the argument can get, it is easy to see why Dr Bach advised patients and practitioners alike to close off their minds completely to such explanations! It is also easy to see why many practitioners stick to the tried and tested, well-catalogued (and relatively few) remedies of Dr Bach.

How do they work?

Flower essences are thought to work through the emotions and the psyche to heal the physical body. In truth no one knows exactly how flower and other essences work. They have never been formally tested or proven scientifically to treat or cure anything. Nor is there any data on whether they produce measurable biochemical changes in the body. Unfortunately, Bach kept none of his research papers, lectured infrequently and preferred to diagnose intuitively, so his method of observing plants and ascribing various energies to them remains shrouded in mystery.

Nevertheless, it is a mystery that suits the esoteric healers who rely heavily on Bach and other flower remedies, since it has left the field wide open for a large diversity of practitioners to use and develop flower essences in their own ways – an intuitive and creative practice which sometimes creates more confusion than health.

Practitioners who use flower essences often use the symbolism of nature to explain the way they work. For a plant to produce flowers, an enormous amount of energy needs to be focused on the blossom. Believers in energy medicine would say that the blossom has an energy that resonates with the very essence of the plant. By making a remedy from the blossoms, a process which usually involves steeping the blossom in spring water and letting it sit in the sunlight for a few hours (see opposite), this essence can be preserved. A blossom is also symbolic of a plant in transition from one state of being to another and thus proponents of flower essences say that by using them we may also help ourselves in times of transition.

In clinical practice flower essences are sometimes used on their own and also in a complementary way with orthodox medicine. They are intended to work gently with the emotions and the psyche, enabling a person to deal with any conflicts or problems at a pace that suits them.

Many practitioners, nevertheless, report that chronic illnesses – everything from hay fever and asthma to ME and lupus – which do not respond to conventional treatment, do respond in varying degrees to flower remedies. Very little scientific literature exists, however, to back up these claims and that which does exist is general and anecdotal. In short, it appears that flower essences are best applied when emotional symptoms dominate or where they seem to be blocking the healing of physical symptoms. Certainly there are no known interactions with conventional medicine, making flower essences a good choice to complement conventional regimes.

Given the lack of evidence, it is surprising how many people find flower remedies genuinely useful. Lack of research into their effectiveness does not alter this fact. For practitioners wishing to integrate them into their work, the Bach Centre runs certificate courses. For others intuitive diagnosis remains the method of choice.

Making your own essences

While walking through the woods near his Oxfordshire home, Dr Bach gathered dewdrops from flowers, plants and trees. He used these to make remedies that he tested on himself. He began to notice that dewdrops exposed to sunlight were more potent than those that were not. This knowledge evolved into what is known as the 'sunlight method'. You can use this method to make your own simple flower essences. Here's what to do:

- Pick your flowers by hand, preferably in the early morning hours at the peak of their bloom.
- Place the flowers in a glass container of spring water or purified water. The flowers should cover the surface of the water.
- Leave the container in direct sunlight for around three hours or until the flowers begin to wilt.

- Remove the flowers with a clean utensil, or if you prefer the rustic approach, a twig.
- Pour the remaining liquid into an amber dropper bottle half filled with brandy or glycerine (which is used as a preservative).
- Shake vigorously and label.

The resulting liquid, called a 'mother tincture', will keep for many years if properly stored (in a dark bottle in cool conditions). To make a stock remedy from your mother tincture, place two drops of mother tincture into a 1 fl oz (30 ml) dropper bottle containing a teaspoon of brandy and then fill with spring water. This remedy can then be taken in water or on the tongue.

Cautions

Flower remedies can be taken by anyone including babies and even animals. They are also fairly inexpensive costing around £3 for a small bottle. Perhaps the biggest drawback in giving remedies this way (and this applies to other types of alternatives such as **homeopathy**) is that it reinforces the idea that you are taking or are being given a medication to directly cure an illness.

Some people do tend to think of flower remedies in the same terms as tablets that you take twice a day. But with flower essences, say practitioners, often small doses are needed frequently throughout the day. Flower essences are also very limited in what they can achieve. If the body is damaged, they will not cure or repair it. However, they may support the healing process by providing support for the emotions which either cause or are caused by illness.

If you make your own remedies, use your common sense. A great deal of literature exists to assist you in choosing only those flowers that are known to be non-poisonous and non-addictive. Avoid those which grow by busy roadsides and which have been treated with pesticides. To make sure you get the best and most appropriate flowers, consider turning a patch of your own garden into a medicinal, organic flower garden.

Taking flower remedies

So many people swear by flower remedies, no matter how they work (and even if the effect is that of a *placebo*), that they must be considered a valid choice in any natural medicine chest.

Flower essences are generally taken two to four drops at a time, four times a day – though they can be taken more often if needed. The drops are best placed under the tongue or if the brandy solution causes too much of a burning sensation, you can put the drops into a small amount of water. Some practitioners even believe they can be effective when applied topically, to the skin (usually on the wrist or temple). They are best taken 10 minutes before a meal or one hour afterwards.

Because they come in small bottles and can be placed directly on the tongue or sipped in a glass of water, flower remedies are among the most portable medicines you can use. There is a copious amount of literature to guide you in accurate self-selection of a remedy. Many chemists and healthfood shops keep guides under the counter or near the products themselves to help consumers in this regard. Nevertheless, since they work very gently and have no known side effects, it's worth experimenting to find a remedy that is right for you.

Most alternative practitioners will recommend that you choose your remedy intuitively according to your needs. Some will recommend flower remedies either on their own or in conjunction with any other remedy they may prescribe.

To learn more about flower essences contact Bach Flower Remedies or the Flower Essence Fellowship.

Use the following brief guide to help you select a useful remedy.

The Bach remedies

Flower remedy	Emotional state
Rescue remedy (a combination of cherry plum, clematis, impatiens, rock rose, star of Bethlehem)	Fear, panic, apprehension, inconsolable crying, anxiety, tension, night terrors, unexplained screaming
Agrimony	Outwardly smiling and brave, inwardly anguished and suffering
Aspen	Fearfulness of an unknown origin, apprehension
Beech	Impatience, intolerance, judgmental
Centaury	Shyness, easily intimidated
Cerato	Need for constant affirmation, doubts own ability
Cherry plum	Fear of losing control, doing something desperate
Chestnut bud	Fails to learn by experience, repeats past mistakes
Chickory	Need for constant attention, selfishness, possessiveness, easily hurt feelings
Clematis	Indifference, apathy, short attention span
Crab apple	Excessive neatness, compulsive behaviour
Elm	Feelings of incompetence, strives for perfection
Gentian	Easily discouraged, self-doubt
Gorse	Deep despair, usually after serious family trauma
Heather	Self-centredness
Holly	Anger, fits of temper
Honeysuckle	Obsession with happy times from the past, homesickness
Hornbeam	Weary in body and mind, too tired to cope
Impatiens	Impatience, nervousness, hyperactive behaviour
Larch	Lacks confidence, anticipates failure
Mimulus	Fear or anxiety of a known origin
Mustard	Black depression, gloom
Oak	Constant business and bustling, even when depressed
Olive	Complete exhaustion resulting from illness, mental fatigue
Pine	Feelings of guilt
Red chestnut	Inappropriate worrying
Rock rose	Absolute terror, panic
Rock water	Self-repression, self-denial, a martyr
Scleranthus	Feelings of uncertainty, indecision
Star of Bethlehem	Emotional shock following a life-changing experience
Sweet chestnut	Mental anguish and torment
Vervain	Over-effort leading to stress and tension
Vine	Dominating, inflexible, ambitious
Walnut	Tendency to be very easily influenced, a link breaker
Water violet	Aloof, proud
White chestnut	Persistent unwanted thoughts, mental arguments

Chapter 10

Herbal Medicine

Commonly used for

Skin Complaints • Digestive Disturbances
• Constipation • Urogenital Complaints
• Infections • Headache • Respiratory Infections
• Inflammation • Anxiety/Depression • Haemorrhoids
• Insomnia • High Blood Pressure

• Requires a professional therapist • Suitable for self-treatment

Before there were 'experts' and self-help books there were medicinal plants. Herbal remedies are part of a tradition that stretches back long before our first human ancestors. Animals instinctively turn to certain plants when they are ill and perhaps watching these animals is how humans first learned to differentiate between toxic and curative plants.

Palaeontologists often discover bunches of herbs, seeds and flower fossils at ancient dwelling sites, confirming the belief that plant life has long been considered necessary to support human life. Some sceptics dismiss herbal remedies as nothing more than witches' brew and therefore not worth serious exploration; but others believe there is real benefit in looking to the past and understanding how central herbal medicine has been to so many ancient cultures. In so doing we can begin to appreciate how herbs exert such a powerful influence over us and why herbal medicine is to this day the most widely used medicine in the world.

Many plant, animal and mineral remedies were part of the pharmacopoeias of ancient Egyptian, Chinese and Indian civilisations. Four hundred years before Christ, Hippocrates, the father of modern medicine, utilised the medicinal properties of local plant life to support the healing process in his patients. A new interest in preventative medicine grew and herbal remedies continued to be used throughout Roman times. The Persians and Arabs added new remedies of their own and the knowledge of herbal medicine eventually extended to the New World.

But the New World wasn't so new after all and early settlers in places like America and Australia often received valuable education regarding the medicinal use of local vegetation from the natives. Such has been our faith in healing plants that in the mid-19th century traditional healers were still giving stiff competition to orthodox physicians.

It was not until the early 1900s that the active ingredients in natural substances began to be isolated in the hope that they could eventually be synthesised in the laboratory. Even today chemists turn to nature for inspiration. Many familiar medicines have been copied from natural blueprints. Ergometrine was copied from ergot of rye, morphine and codeine from opium poppies, atrophine from deadly nightshade, digoxin from foxglove, aspirin from white willow bark and quinine from cinchona bark. We have copied anti-ulcer drugs from liquorice and anti-cancer drugs from periwinkle and yew, and herbal medicine continues to evolve in our culture. Today there is a great interest in plants as the basis of energy medicine. The ongoing development of a vast array of **flower essences** that purport to cure the body by addressing the mind and emotions is testimony to this. **Homeopathy** too makes use of highly diluted plant materials.

Of all the trends in healthcare the increase in the use of herbal medicines in recent years has been one of the most remarkable. Whereas herbalism was once viewed as a fringe interest or a poor man's form of healthcare, these days you will find learned medical journals such as the *Journal of the American Medical Association* and the *British Medical Journal* discussing the latest research on the antidepressant effect of St John's wort or the anti-cancer properties of garlic.

This blossoming interest in herbal medicine, however, has not had much support either from conventional medics or the government. Indeed, the problem of knowing how to choose an effective herbal remedy has been made more difficult since the implementation of the 1968 *Medicines Act*. Since that time manufacturers of herbal remedies in the UK have not been able to make medicinal claims for their products. This means that you may get a nice picture of a flower on the box and some vague guidelines about how much to take, but otherwise you are on your own.

Following a 1990 review, many herbal products which could not prove their efficacy were taken off the shelves. Those that survived were granted a licence by the Medicines Control Agency and were given a code number (usually beginning PL . . .). These products can make carefully worded general statements about their use, such as 'A herbal remedy traditionally used for the symptomatic treatment of . . .' But because most licences are normally only granted on a limited basis – usually that a particular remedy can be used to treat a minor self-limiting condition – what is printed on the label may impart only a partial description of the herb's uses.

These laws are supposed to be protective of the consumer, but what has resulted is that people are taking herbs without really knowing what they can and cannot do, often relying on media misinformation rather than good evidence to guide them. A good example would be taking ginseng as a general tonic – unaware that it is a powerful stimulant which can cause a wide range of adverse effects such as headaches, tremors and nervousness and, for women, hormonal imbalance.

Another example would be using ginkgo biloba, a potent vascular stimulant, as a kind of herbal Viagra – a use for which there is no convincing evidence. Yet another disturbing trend is one that could be described as the 'echinacea syndrome', where otherwise healthy individuals take large doses of herbal preparations prophylactically – as a preventative – when there is no convincing evidence that the herb works in this way (and also little information about what happens when a healthy person takes a particular herb in quantity over long periods of time).

Another problem that bedevils the consumer is the fact that, in spite of all the laws and restrictions placed on herbal supplements, they are not well regulated. Many manufacturers frankly get away with murder producing sub-standard products which contain little or none of the active ingredient stated on the label. Or they manufacture products which genuinely do contain the advertised herb, but in such small quantities that they could not possibly have a therapeutic effect.

Taking herbal remedies
Herbs can be used as medicines in their own right or to complement other types of healthcare. Most work in the same multitude of ways that conventional medicines do, albeit more slowly. In other words, they can ease pain and inflammation, relax or stimulate organs, act as antidepressants, fight bacteria and boost the immune system.

Many different alternative disciplines use herbs in a variety of ways. These include **naturopathy**, **traditional Chinese medicine** and **Ayurveda**, and **fasting and detox** therapies. In addition, when you are using **flower remedies** or **aromatherapy** you are also harnessing the therapeutic properties of herbs.

Herbal remedies can be prepared in a variety of ways and taken internally or applied externally. For internal use, the most common preparation is the *infusion* in which fresh or dried leaves, flowers and stems are steeped briefly in boiling water to make a 'tea'. Harder parts of the plant, such as the bark, roots, nuts and seeds, need to be boiled in a saucepan to release their therapeutic properties. This process is known as *decoction*.

Many herbal preparations also come in tablets and capsules made from the dried herb. Opinion is divided about which type is best, but generally speaking the herbs in a capsule have not been subjected to the same amount of processing as those in tablet form and so may be more potent.

Herbal preparations are also available as *tinctures*, made by steeping the raw herb in water, vinegar, glycerine or alcohol. Tinctures are concentrated remedies, so you will only need to use very little each day. The usual way to take a tincture is to put a few drops in a glass of water and drink it. How much and how often will vary according to the instructions on the bottle or the advice of your practitioner. Some herbalists even prefer tinctures to infusions and decoctions since the dose can be more easily controlled. A tincture can also be easily absorbed, even in a body system that is very run down.

Herbs can also be used externally. You can make a herbal bath by tying some fresh herbs in a muslin bag and steeping them in your bath water or by making a strong infusion or decoction and adding this to your bath. They can also be applied locally in creams and ointments or by soaking a wash cloth in a herbal brew and using it as either a hot or cold compress. Similarly, herbal poultices – pastes made from herbal mixtures – can be applied to specific areas of the body.

Whichever way they are used, herbs can be very powerful medicine and should be taken with the same caution and respect you would take with any conventional medication. Whether you are self-prescribing or going to a qualified herbalist, you should be prepared to ask questions. What is the herb? Is it from an organic source? What effect is it expected to have? What are the potential side effects?

Everyday medicine

Many herbs can be eaten as part of your daily diet. The restorative properties of oats, barley, horseradish, mustard, garlic, onions, alfalfa spouts, seaweeds, celery, asparagus, chicory, endive, potato, carrot, artichoke, walnuts, pumpkin seeds, almonds, sesame seeds, watercress, fresh dandelion leaves, young nettles, parsley, dill, chickweed and coriander can be used – even by the most reluctant individual – as daily herbal tonics. If you are new to the idea of herbal medicine, you might want to begin your exploration of herbs by combining some of these familiar ingredients into a health-promoting and delicious daily herb salad.

What the research says – 11 of the best

Herbal remedies are an effective and valid way of self-treating many day-to-day health complaints. But right now there are probably more than 1,000 over-the-counter herbal remedies to be found in healthfood shops and more recently in mainstream chemists around the country. Knowing which herb to choose and how much to take (and when not to take them) can be difficult for the uninitiated.

Herbs are among the most widely researched of alternative remedies and it would be impossible to comprehensively review the evidence for all available herbs in a single book, let alone a single chapter. The following list – an 'A' list of useful herbs – is comprised of the best researched and commonly used herbs. If you are new to the use of herbs, it will provide a good basis for understanding the actions of some of the most popular and easily obtainable herbal products. Even those who regularly consume herbal products may find some surprising information about their favourites.

Echinacea (immune stimulant)

This immune stimulating herb is among the most widely used of natural remedies. Numerous studies in Germany in the last 20 years have shown echinacea to be extremely valuable in boosting immune system function. Root extracts of echinacea have also been shown to possess interferon-like activity as well as antiviral activity against difficult-to-treat conditions like herpes. The most recent potential use for echinacea is in the prevention of sun damage to the skin by blocking the transmission of pain from burn receptors. But in the main echinacea is used to prevent and treat colds, flu and catarrh.

Several studies have shown that echinacea can work to relieve the symptoms and reduce both the severity and duration of colds. One trial in Sweden looked at 246 otherwise healthy adult volunteers who caught a cold and took one of several *Echinacea purpurea* preparations or a placebo. The volunteers took two tablets three times daily for seven days – or until they felt better. The echinacea preparations were found to be significantly more effective than a placebo in treating the common cold. Other trials have also found that echinacea can shorten the duration and reduce the severity of colds.

But while there is good evidence that its use can relieve cold symptoms, opinions are divided about whether echinacea is really an effective form of prevention. German researchers studying echinacea as a prophylaxis gave the liquid root extract of either *Echinacea purpurea* or *Echinacea angustifolia* – two of the most popular types of echinacea – or a placebo to 302 healthy volunteers in a controlled, double-blind, randomised trial. Results showed that both types of echinacea were only slightly more effective than the placebo in preventing colds over the 12-week period, although compared to the placebo group, participants taking the herb reported feeling better. The authors concluded that at best echinacea might slightly reduce the risk of getting a cold by about 10 to 20 per cent. This finding was confirmed by Swedish researchers a year later who found that the herb shortens the duration of a cold but did not prevent it from occurring.

The key with echinacea, as with other remedies, may be to treat at the first signs of cold or flu. In a recent review of 13 trials for echinacea in the treatment and prevention of colds, it was concluded that, while it may not prevent colds, early treatment appears to be beneficial for relieving symptoms.

Dose Echinacea contains many active constituents and can be equally useful taken in many different forms. Doses are best spread out over the day, so three times daily try taking either: 2–4 ml tincture, 325–650 mg freeze-dried plant or 100–250 mg solid dry powdered plant. Experts are divided over which type is more effective. Most recently opinion has swung in favour of *Echinacea angustifolia* over the more common *Echinacea purpurea*. But reviews into the effectiveness of echinacea draw no conclusions about this. The simplest advice is, if one type does not work for you, try the other.

Shortly after drinking an echinacea preparation, particularly a tincture, your tongue may feel a little numb or tingly. This temporary effect disappears within a few minutes and is not only harmless but is valuable as a form of in-your-mouth quality control. If you don't get the 'tongue effect', you may not have used enough echinacea, or you may have used an inferior product.

Take care Echinacea has a very low toxicity, though some people may experience raised temperature, nausea and headache after using it (these should subside within a couple of hours). One Australian study estimated that as many as 20 per cent of atopic individuals may experience an allergic reaction to echinacea. Since it is an immuno-stimulant it should not be given at the same time as immuno-suppressants (e.g. corticosteroids and cyclosporin). Some therapists believe that it should not be used by individuals with auto-immune diseases such as lupus, rheumatoid arthritis and AIDS. Because of the herb's ability to stimulate the production of white blood cells, it may also be contraindicated in leukaemia and related diseases.

Like all immune-stimulating herbs, it should only be used when it is needed, for instance, when you are run down or find you are catching one cold after the next, after a hard business trip or during prolonged periods of stress. Don't take it as a general tonic as its long-term use can result in a form of rebound immuno-suppression. In addition, heavy use in men is reputed to result in temporary infertility, though evidence of this effect is slender.

Herbs for kids

Everywhere a parent turns today there is some new herbal elixir for kids – to relieve coughs, cure colds, reduce fevers, reduce anxiety, beat insomnia and clear parasites. Children can, of course, benefit from herbal remedies, but adults should be aware of certain issues. Children are not just small adults: their bodies are very different, their immune systems function differently and they respond differently to medicines. In common with most conventional medicines, there are few studies of the effectiveness of herbs in children and certainly no long-term studies exist.

It is vitally important that parents don't simply use alternative remedies as a substitute for unnecessary conventional ones. More than 90 per cent of childhood illnesses are self-regulating. They will heal whether you use medicine or not. Parents have a responsibility to discourage their children from the habit of taking a pill for every ill – even a herbal one – as it creates poor habits in adulthood. What is more, many commercial childhood herbals contain so little of the active ingredient that parents can end up paying for empty promises rather than effective medicine. ⊃

The opposite can also be true, however. Children can sometimes get too much and this can profoundly upset their systems. As a general rule of thumb, the child's dose should be one-quarter to one-third that of an adult dose. But it's not just the dose that can cause problems. Herbal medicine, particularly **Ayurvedic** and **traditional Chinese medicine**, can contain toxic heavy metals which can permanently damage internal organs such as the liver and kidneys. All medicines should be used with caution where children are concerned and parents, wherever possible, should stick to the tried and tested. Keep herbals out of the children's reach and never give more or more often than is recommended.

Garlic (healing infections)

This tiny bulb is potentially nature's most perfect medicinal food. Garlic, which is rich in alliin and other sulphur compounds, has been used throughout the world and throughout history to treat a huge number of conditions.

Garlic has been shown to thin the blood and raise levels of 'good' HDL cholesterol while lowering 'bad' LDL cholesterol and triglycerides (blood fats), thus making it useful in the treatment of heart disease and stroke. This fact was confirmed by an analysis of several research articles into garlic. In 1993 in the US medical journal *Annals of Internal Medicine* researchers reported that taking the equivalent of a half a clove of garlic daily could lower cholesterol levels by nearly 10 per cent. In a 1999 study from New Zealand an aged garlic extract supplement was found to be more effective than raw garlic in the diet at preventing atherosclerosis.

However, not all garlic studies have shown this positive effect. One famous and controversial study which looked at the effects of steam-distilled garlic preparations found no benefit at all. This study was a good example of how important it is to use the right preparation: steam-distilled garlic preparations have virtually no beneficial alliin in them, so a negative result was a foregone conclusion.

Research into garlic's potential anti-tumour activities are mixed and it is probably fair to say that garlic is not a cancer cure but may be a potential preventative for certain types of cancer. Though clinical trials are lacking, population studies in China and Italy have found that people who regularly eat a lot of garlic have less risk of developing stomach cancer than those who eat little or none.

A study in Iowa in the US also looked at the diets of over 40,000 women and found that those who consumed the most garlic had the lowest risk of colon cancer. However, a Dutch study of over 120,000 men and women found no relationship between the consumption of garlic supplements and the incidence of breast, colon, rectal or lung cancers, which seems to reinforce the view that it is fresh garlic that provides the most effective protection.

Where garlic really shines is in dealing with infections such as those caused by *Staphylococcus* (staph infection), *Streptococcus* (strep infection), *Vibriocholerae* (cholera), *Corynebacterium diphtheriae* (diphtheria), *Rickettsia rickettsii* (typhus) and *Shigella enteritides* (bacillary dysentery). In a review in the journal *Medical Hypothesis* as far back as 1983, it was found to be effective against a broad spectrum of bugs including bacteria, viruses, worms and fungi. What is more, garlic appears to be effective against harmful organisms at very low doses – in one study garlic juice diluted to one part in 125,000 still had an inhibitory effect.

Garlic has proven particularly effective against fungal infections such as candida and athlete's foot. In a review in 1993 in the journal *Phytotherapy Research* it was shown to be more effective than the antibiotic cream nystatin, gentian violet and six other reputed antifungal agents in treating candida.

Dose The best way to take garlic is fresh, in your diet. Oil-based products are generally inferior to those made from the dried herb and contain little or no alliin and alliinase (which are converted into therapeutic allicin in the body). Commercial preparations with an alliin content of 8 mg appear to be the most effective. Follow the manufacturer's instructions about daily dosage.

Take care A standard dose of around 200 mg daily – the equivalent of around 70 cloves – has no known toxic side effects. To produce toxic effects on the stomach and liver you would have to eat around 300 to 500 mashed cloves in one sitting. Because of garlic's low toxicity, many people 'overdose' on fresh garlic in the belief that it is good for them – but eating four or more cloves of garlic in one sitting is only likely to make you vomit. Because of their blood-thinning properties, garlic supplements should not be taken with blood-thinning drugs such as heparin, warfarin and coumarin derivatives, and should not be taken before surgery where over-use can lead to uncontrollable bleeding.

Ginkgo biloba (prevents dementia)

The therapeutic actions of this ancient herb are supported by more than 280 scientific studies. Ginkgo biloba has been shown to contain a range of bioflavonoids that act to clear the body of free radicals and limit the damage caused throughout the body by these toxic by-products of metabolism.

Clinical and laboratory tests have shown that standardised ginkgo biloba extract (GBE) can be of significant benefit in the treatment of increased intestinal permeability, ulcer, Raynaud's disease, chronic cerebral and peripheral vascular insufficiency, senile dementia, depression, tinnitis, diabetic retinopathies, macular degeneration, glaucoma, cataracts and bronchitis. The vital link between many of these disorders is circulation and ginkgo has been shown to thin the blood (thus preventing clots) and improve circulation in all parts of the body.

So far, the most promising use has been in the treatment of dementia and symptoms of cerebral dysfunction such as memory impairment and poor concentration. A review in the *British Journal of Clinical Pharmacology* in 1992 looked at more than 40 clinical studies of ginkgo in the treatment of many forms of dementia such as Alzheimer's and concluded that the research standard was high and that ginkgo was an effective way to treat dementia.

In another review, 11 good-quality trials were evaluated in order to investigate the effectiveness of a GBE, standardised to contain 24 per cent ginkgo flavonglycosides, in the treatment of cerebral vascular insufficiency (poor blood flow to the brain). Most of the trials used

150 mg of the extract and compared it to a placebo. The overall results clearly demonstrated the therapeutic effectiveness of GBE for this condition which can cause, among other things, impairment in short-term memory and mental performance.

An Italian study also found encouraging results. The authors state that the most promising indication for the ginkgo extracts, apart from symptoms of poor cerebral circulation, is in the treatment of intermittent but severe pain that causes limping or lameness (known as claudication). Controlled trials have shown that after six months' treatment with ginkgo extract, walking distance increases and pain at rest decreases significantly.

Dose The usual dose of ginkgo biloba extract, standardised to contain 24 per cent ginkgo flavonglycosides (the herb's active components), is 50 mg three times daily.

Take care Ginkgo is probably best taken when there is a genuine indication and not as a general tonic, and not as a herbal detox. It can alter bleeding time and should not be used with blood-thinning drugs such as heparin, warfarin and coumarin derivatives. Anecdotal evidence also suggests it should not be used with over-the-counter blood thinners such as aspirin. Like garlic, it should not be taken before surgery.

St John's wort (lifts depression)
If you believe everything you read in the press, this herb is the Prozac of the new millennium. There is no doubt that good research exists to back up its use in cases of mild to moderate depression and anxiety. In one German study in 1993, two-thirds of depressed individuals experienced positive effects from taking St John's wort (also known as *Hypericum perforatum*) as opposed to just over a quarter of those who took a placebo. In another randomised, placebo-controlled study a regime of 300 mg hypericum three times daily resulted in 70 per cent of the treatment group being symptom free within four weeks. Hypericum is also of benefit to those suffering from seasonal affective disorder (SAD).

Unusually for an alternative remedy, St John's wort has been involved in several trials comparing it to conventional antidepressants. For instance in 1994, two German studies compared hypericum to conventional drugs. In one, comparing it to maprotiline, researchers found that the herb was more effective over the longer term. Though improvement showed earlier in those taking maprotiline, long-term side effects such as tiredness, dry mouth and heart complaints were common with the conventional drug. In the other, a study of hypericum and imipramine for severely depressed individuals, the herbal remedy performed as well as the conventional drug. This finding was particularly surprising since St John's wort is not always effective in severely depressed individuals.

Similarly, a 1995 review analysed the data from 12 controlled clinical trials and concluded that St John's wort was more effective than a placebo and comparable to standard antidepressant medications. It has also been found to be as effective as amitriptyline in cases of mild to moderate depression, and another more recent study compared the herb with Prozac in elderly individuals and found it was just as effective.

Another review in the *BMJ* looked at 23 randomised controlled trials in which hypericum was compared to a placebo and conventional drugs and found to be superior to the placebo and at least as effective as conventional drugs. Generally speaking, taking St John's wort results in fewer adverse effects such as tiredness, mouth dryness and heart complaints. However, side effects of St John's wort in this study were high. They occurred with 19.8 per cent of those taking the herb and 5.8 per cent for those on antidepressant drugs.

Dose The most effective St John's wort preparations usually contain 250 to 300 mg standardised hypericum extract, delivering between 0.1 to 0.3 per cent hypericin. A daily oral dose of 500 to 900 mg St John's wort extract, corresponding to 1.0 to 2.7 mg total hypericin, is typically recommended. The usual length of treatment is one to six months.

As with many other herbs, St John's wort preparations can vary enormously in how much of the active ingredient they actually contain (despite what the label may say). Stick to well-known

WHAT WORKS, WHAT DOESN'T

manufacturers and brand names and avoid 'bargain' products in order to ensure you get a credible product.

Take care Side effects are mild and uncommon, but in one major study included gastrointestinal irritation, allergic reactions, fatigue, restlessness and irritability. To cure depression you need to discover its cause, and depression has many causes. Deficiency in virtually any nutrient can result in depression. Other common causes include the use of certain drugs including caffeine, nicotine and oral contraceptives, as well as corticosteroids, beta-blockers and other blood pressure medications. Abnormal thyroid function, hypoglycaemia and dysfunction of the adrenal gland, as well as allergies, exposure to toxic substances in your environment and systemic candida infection, can all cause depression. St John's wort, which works in part by reducing levels of the brain chemical serotonin, is unlikely to improve depression in these cases.

St John's wort should probably not be used with conventional antidepressants such as monoamine oxidase (MAO) inhibitors and selective serotonin reuptake inhibitors (SSRIs) whose actions it mimics. In rare instances, individuals taking St John's wort may experience increased photosensitivity. Like all herbs (and conventional medicines) it is best avoided during pregnancy.

Because it is so widely used and so well researched, we know more about St John's wort and its potential interactions with other medications than about most other herbal preparations. In April 2000 the American FDA issued a warning to St John's wort users detailing the herb's many adverse interactions with conventional medications. Taken with any of the following drugs, St John's wort may reduce the effectiveness of these medications:

- ***Heart drugs*** – digoxin (Lanoxin), diltiazem (Cardizem), nifedipine (Procardia) and beta-blockers (Inderal, Lopressor, Levatol)

- ***Antidepressants*** – imipramine (Tofranil), amoxapine (Asendin) and amitriptyline (Etavil)

- **Anti-seizure drugs** – carbamazepine (Tegretol), phenytoin (Dilantin) and phenobarbitol (Luminal)

- **Anti-cancer drugs** – cyclophosphamide (Cytoxan), tamoxifen (Nolvadex), paclitaxel (Taxol) and etoposide (Toposar, Etopophos, VePesid)

- **Anti-transplant rejection drugs** – cyclosporin (Neoral, Sand-immune, SangCya), rapamycin (Rapamune) and tacrolimus (Prograf)

- **Birth control drugs** – ethinyloestradiol (Demulen).

Aloe vera (wound healer)

Aloe vera's use as an aid to skin health is certainly not new and we have benefited from its use for at least 4,000 years. Over the centuries there have been many references to aloe vera in the literature of many traditional cultures, including the ancient Egyptian, Greek, Roman, Indian, Chinese and Arab peoples. The name 'aloe vera' or true aloe probably stems from the Arabic word *alloeh*, meaning 'shining, bitter substance'.

Although there are more than 300 species of this plant, there are only four types with known medicinal properties:

1. *Aloe barbadensis Miller* – also known as *Aloe vulgaris*, or the Curaçao aloe

2. *Aloe perryi Baker* –Socotrine aloe or Zanzibar aloe

3. *Aloe ferox* – sometimes called Cape aloe

4. *Aloe arborescens* – a species favoured largely by the Japanese.

Of these *Aloe barbadensis Miller* is considered the most potent and is usually the aloe referred to in scientific literature.

There are more than 75 different chemical compounds that occur naturally in this desert plant, including vitamins, enzymes and minerals, amino acids and sugars. Aloe gel is thought to have a complex action that includes the ability to act as an anti-inflammatory, moisturiser, emollient and antimicrobial.

Applied topically, aloe vera has been shown to be an effective treatment for psoriasis. It has also been shown in studies and reviews throughout the last decade to heal burns of all kinds, from simple sunburn to radiation burns to frostbite. It can also help heal minor wounds and grazes. Its ability to heal wounds may be also because of its ability to kill germs including *Pseudomonas aeruginosa, E. coli, Staphylococcus aureus, Candida albicans* and other fungi such as those involved in ringworm, athlete's foot and the herpes virus (both simplex and zoster), as well as its ability to moisturise and provide the skin with nutrients.

Dose There is no standard dose of aloe. However, consumers should be advised that many products which state that they contain aloe often contain only minute non-therapeutic quantities. A product may contain only a fraction of a percent of aloe and still be called an aloe cream or gel. To get the best out of topical aloe preparations, look for products made from 100 per cent pure *Aloe barbadensis Miller* and follow the instructions.

Take care Side effects from topical aloe vera are uncommon, but be aware that aloe can cause allergic reactions and has been shown to delay wound-healing in cases of surgical wounds such as those produced during laparotomy and Caesarean section. It should therefore not be used in the treatment of deep wounds. Aloe should not be taken internally except under the guidance of a qualified practitioner since it is a severe purgative which, if taken for more than a week, can lead to laxative dependence and considerable damage to the bowel. Taken internally during pregnancy, it may produce miscarriage or premature delivery.

Panax ginseng (energy tonic for men)
Health-conscious individuals have long regarded Panax, or Korean ginseng, as a kind of miracle cure-all. Certainly millions of people around the world consume ginseng regularly, usually to relieve fatigue, anxiety, nervousness and poor concentration, or as a general tonic and restorative.

Ginseng is popular but also problematical in that, like caffeine-containing products, it is commonly used to prop up people who really need to take a vacation. In addition, Panax is indiscriminately recommended to tired women, often without any mention that it can disturb menstrual function and/or make menopausal symptoms worse. The upshot is that women should probably avoid Panax, whilst for men it is best used as an energy aid alongside a time-management plan that allows for reasonable rest.

There are different types of ginseng available, each with a slightly different action. If the one you want is Panax ginseng, that scientific name should be printed on the label. If this does not appear on the packaging, it is usually because the product does not contain Panax.

Panax ginseng root is available in two varieties, 'red' or 'white'. Both come from the same plant, *Panax ginseng C.A. Meyer*, but each is preserved differently. White ginseng is bleached with sulphur dioxide after harvesting and subsequently dried either in the sun or artificially at 100 to 200°C. Red ginseng is treated with hot steam before drying (the reddening occurs as a result of chemical reactions to the heat). In spite of the different preservation methods, as yet no essential difference has been established by chemical analysis or pharma-cological tests between the two types of commercial ginseng. American ginseng, taken from the roots of *Panax quinquefolius*, is similarly marketed as white or red ginseng.

Unfortunately, results of the few human studies that exist on Panax are conflicting. While some have reported specific health benefits, there are an equal number of studies that provide contradictory evidence. Moreover, it is difficult to assess something as subjective as an energy level. Many, however, have tried. Several well-designed US and Canadian studies have failed to find any connection between ginseng and energy.

There's so little human evidence that ginseng counters stress that a small three-day study completed 20 years ago remains the most frequently cited by proponents. In it 12 British nurses who were switching from day shift to night shift work were given ginseng or a placebo to see if the herb would help them handle the stress of disrupted sleep patterns. After taking the ginseng the nurses reported feeling more energy and better able to adjust to their new routines.

In another double-blind, placebo-controlled trial of Panax ginseng, involving people between the ages of 25 and 60 who were suffering from occasionally disabling fatigue, significant improvement was noted in symptoms such as tiredness, anxiety, nervousness and poor concentration, while side effects were minimal.

More recently, a randomised, double-blind, placebo-controlled study recruited 19 healthy women who, for eight weeks, added either a concentrated ginseng extract or a placebo to their otherwise supplement-free diet. The women's level of physical activity was similar before, during and after the study. At the end of the study there were no significant subjective or biochemical differences between the women taking the supplement and those who did not in terms of their work performance, resting and exercise (and recovery from exercise).

There is also little evidence that ginseng can substantially improve your mood or well-being. A recent study of people taking 60 mg of ginseng daily found it had no appreciable effect on their mood whatsoever.

In study after study people had no better memories after taking ginseng than after taking a placebo. A recent British study of 32 middle-aged people found that a ginseng-ginkgo biloba combination improved the memory in the morning but worsened it in the afternoon. A more recent study by the same team found that the same combination had only a small beneficial effect on memory.

In experiments with animals, ginseng generates the release of nitric oxide. So does the anti-impotency drug Viagra. On this basis some have theorised that ginseng may help improve sexual performance. In the only published human study, 30 Korean men with erectile dysfunction who took 300 mg a day of Korean red ginseng for three months reported significant improvements in their sexual performance. Thirty similar placebo-takers reported less improvement. Men should, however, refrain from reading too much into such limited evidence.

Studies purporting to show that ginseng prevents cancer are usually large observational studies (or reviews based on medical records) of oriental people who have been taking the fresh herb or supplement over the long term. In one five-year study involving 4,634 people over 40 years of age, ginseng users had a slightly smaller risk of developing cancer than non-users. Among ginseng users, those using the fresh extract had a significantly decreased risk of developing gastric cancer.

These results should be interpreted with caution because they are simply based on participants completing a questionnaire and are not the result of careful study. The oriental diet as a whole – rather than a single component of it such as ginseng – may hold the key to the lower rates of certain types of cancer in that population.

Dose Most experts recommend looking for a product labelled as Panax ginseng, standardised to contain 4 and 7 per cent ginsenosides. A typical dose is 100 to 200 mg a day. Occasional use is generally recommended, or alternating two to three weeks on and one to two off. While Panax ginseng possesses immuno-stimulating activity, it should not be used in large doses during an acute infection, as an opposite effect may occur.

When it comes to quality, ginseng has one of the worst track records of any popular supplement. Different preparations can vary wildly according to how much ginseng or ginsenosides they have, and the amount in each product can be very different from what is stated on the label. According to industry insiders, as many as 15 per cent of ginseng products tested contain no ginseng at all. There is almost no way for a consumer to be 100 per cent sure that the product they are taking contains enough Panax to be effective. As a general rule, if a product looks too cheap to be true, it probably is.

Take care Each individual's response to ginseng is unique and ginseng toxicity is a risk with long-term use or large doses. Signs of toxicity include headaches, tremors, anxiety, irritability, nervousness, hypertension, breast pain, menstrual changes, insomnia and, rarely, diarrhoea and skin problems. Ginseng should not be used with estrogens and corticosteroids because it may potentiate their effect; nor should it be taken by those with heart conditions. It may also affect blood glucose levels and should not be used, or should only be used under professional supervision, by those with diabetes. Those taking antipsychotic medications should also seek medical advice before starting ginseng. Women who take Panax ginseng may experience variations in their menstrual cycle and increased breast tenderness.

Siberian ginseng (energy herb for men and women)

Siberian ginseng (*Eleutherococcus*) is a somewhat milder stimulant than Panax ginseng, with a more limited range of uses. Also, comparison of the chemical compositions of eleutherococcus with the more familiar Panax or 'true' ginseng has underscored the fact that they are two completely different herbs from two completely different plant species and so cannot be justifiably considered as mutually interchangeable.

Siberian ginseng has been used primarily for fatigue and to stimulate the immune system and has been the subject of intense study in its native Russian Federation. It is what is known as an adaptogenic herb, which means it can help the body maintain balance under adverse physical conditions such as heat, noise, motion, stress and exertion. It is also thought to increase mental alertness.

Although ancient records indicate that the Chinese may have used Siberian ginseng for thousands of years, it was the Soviets who brought it to worldwide attention. As many as 1,200 Soviet scientists researched the properties and requirements of the herb over a 40-year period. As a result, in 1962 the Soviet government approved eleutherococcus for clinical use.

In the West little published study exists on Siberian ginseng. In fact there is next to nothing to back up claims for its efficacy. Such research that does exist is all from the Soviet Union in the early 1970s, and nearly all of this is positive – something which suggests a possible bias and therefore a need for cautious interpretation.

Several of these experiments appear to demonstrate that eleutherococcus extract, given prophylactically, can reduce the overall disease incidence by up to 35 per cent. For example, between 1973 and 1975, 1,200 drivers at a Russian automobile plant were given 8–12 mg eleutherococcus extract with tea daily for two months annually, in spring and autumn. These individuals were then compared to others at the plant who did not take the herb. After one year the percentage of workers who fell ill in the control group was unchanged, whereas in the group given eleutherococcus the number decreased by 30 per cent.

In this study rates of hypertension and ischaemic heart disease among the workers was also monitored. The proportion of the individuals suffering from these conditions was approximately the same at the beginning of the study. But by the end the number of drivers with hypertension had been reduced by 3.5 times in those taking eleutherococcus. A later analysis showed that blood pressure continued to drop even after the study had ended.

At the same auto plant during November/December 1975 a mass experiment in disease prevention was carried out: 13,096 individuals were involved in experiments in which 2 ml eleutherococcus extract was given as a daily supplement. At the end of the experiment the total incidence of disease had decreased by 30–50 per cent in those who had been taking the extract, compared to those who had not.

In a seven-year experiment in the (then) USSR it was shown that eleutherococcus extract reduced the incidence of flu in truck drivers by more than 90 per cent over the total period of the experiment. In a further study approximately 1,000 workers in a Soviet mining/ smelting works received 22 ml eleutherococcus extract daily for two winter months. The incidence of acute respiratory diseases and flu decreased by 2.4 times, compared to those working in the same conditions who did not receive the supplement.

Dose The standard dose of fluid extract of Siberian ginseng is 2–4 ml up to three times daily. As with the more powerful Panax, it is important to take periodic breaks when taking this herb. Most experts recommend a two to three-week interval between each 60-day course.

Take care Siberian ginseng is virtually non-toxic but in rare instances can produce adverse effects including insomnia, irritability, melancholy and anxiety. If you experience any of these symptoms while taking this herb, discontinue its use.

From a 'master herbalist'?

When buying commercially made herbal products, try to avoid those which are mega-blends of dozens of herbs. Often such products are advertised as being created by 'master' herbalists, but the claim rarely stands up to scrutiny.

A really good herbalist will choose no more than a handful of appropriate herbs in any blend. The 'everything but the kitchen sink' approach is more likely to be the approach of a master salesman or marketing executive than a master herbalist. What is more, should you have a bad reaction to a product containing multiple herbs in it, it will be almost impossible to say which herb or herbs caused the reaction. As far as possible keep your choices simple and you can't go wrong.

Feverfew (migraine relief)

The main uses of this ancient herb are in the treatment of fever, migraines and arthritis. Among these its effectiveness in the treatment of migraines is the most remarkable.

The action of feverfew on migraines is still not widely understood, though recent research suggests that individuals who have low levels of circulating melatonin may be more prone to migraine attacks. Feverfew, according to some scientists, contains melatonin and may work to boost circulating levels of this hormone. It is also thought to work by inhibiting the release of blood vessel-dilating substances and the production of inflammatory substances and by re-establishing good blood vessel tone.

Studies have shown that, in those with intractable migraine, as many as 70 per cent improved while taking the herb and as many as one in three had no further attacks. In all, more than 50 scientific papers have been published in the last 15 years which confirm its usefulness.

Several carefully conducted trials have conclusively demonstrated that those who take feverfew experience fewer episodes of migraine headache and undergo a marked reduction in nausea and vomiting during attacks. The most famous of these was conducted at the University of Nottingham in 1988, comparing feverfew with a placebo over a period of four months. Those taking the feverfew experienced a 24 per cent drop in the number of attacks they experienced, while the placebo group experienced no change.

Another study in Israel involved 57 people selected at random and treated for two months with daily doses of 100 mg feverfew leaf as a means of preventing migraine attacks. These individuals were compared to another group who were given dried parsley leaf in capsule form as a placebo. Those taking the feverfew experienced a significant reduction in pain intensity and the severity of other typical symptoms of migraine such as nausea, vomiting and sensitivity to noise and light. No mention was made, however, of any beneficial effect on the frequency of attacks.

While feverfew is a worthwhile option for many migraine sufferers, the elimination of food allergies and intolerances plus the correction of any nutritional imbalances may be the best way to make long-term gains in the reduction of the number of migraine attacks and their severity. Putting some effort into these kinds of lifestyle changes also helps avoid long-term analgesic drug dependence.

Dose Feverfew is best taken in tablet or capsule form since the dried leaves can be bitter and with tea there is no way of guaranteeing consistent strength. Studies showing efficacy for migraine have all been done with leaves, not liquid extracts. One study which used liquid feverfew extract rather than the dried leaves showed disappointing results and seemed to highlight the importance of taking the herb in the correct form.

How well any feverfew supplement works depends on adequate levels of its active ingredient, parthenolide. Unfortunately, when researchers in Nottingham tested dried preparations in 1992, they found that parthenolide levels varied enormously between products and was not detected in some at all. In clinical trials the effective standard parthenolide content was 0.4 per cent and the effective dose has been between 25 and 82 mg of the dried herb twice daily. While these low dosages of feverfew may be effective in preventing an attack, a higher dose (2–4 mg parthenolide) is necessary during an acute attack.

Take care Feverfew is generally well tolerated but there is little information about adverse effects associated with taking this herb over the long term. Taking it alongside NSAIDs (such as paracetamol and ibuprofen) may negate the effectiveness of the herb. Feverfew can also alter bleeding time and should not be used at the same time as blood-thinning drugs such as warfarin or before surgery.

Goldenseal (digestive tract infections)

Goldenseal was used widely by the practical Native Americans as both a herbal medicine and a clothing dye.

Its medicinal value is thought to be because of its berberine content (an alkaloid that is also found in Oregon grape root and barberry). It is this active component which has been most widely studied and laboratory tests have shown that berberine has broad antibiotic effects and can be useful in the treatment of acute diarrhoea caused by a range of nasty bugs including *E. coli, Giardia, Salmonella* and *Vibrio cholera* (cholera).

Tincture of goldenseal is typically recommended for all types of infections, but such broad usage may be unwarranted and experts believe that an amazing 90 per cent of goldenseal use is clinically inappropriate. This is because berberine is poorly absorbed into the bloodstream from the small intestine. The amount typically absorbed is only about 1/200 of that necessary to kill most bacteria. As a result, goldenseal taken orally can only treat infections of the digestive tract; externally or as a douche it may be useful for skin and vaginal infections. However, it does not work as a systemic (whole body) antibiotic.

This fact is important not only for human health, but because goldenseal is a seriously endangered plant. Threatening its existence further by using it to treat conditions against which it is ineffective seems very foolish indeed.

Assuming that it is being used appropriately, goldenseal can be a highly effective remedy. It is reported to have a beneficial effect on the digestive tract and laboratory studies suggest that berberine is effective in the treatment of bacterial, fungal and protozoan infections, confirming its long history as an antibiotic gastrointestinal remedy. Berberine kills many bacteria that cause infectious diarrhoea (*Salmonella, Shigella* and *Klebsiella*) and other infections. It may also be effective against the protozoa that cause amoebic dysentery (*Entamoeba histolytica*) and giardiasis (*Giardia lamblia*), and several reports show berberine to be effective against cholera (*Vibrio cholerae*).

In a controlled study of diarrhoea due to gastroenteritis, 100 children were treated with antibiotics or 25 mg berberine orally four times daily. Both groups had equivalent success and recovery rates. In another randomised controlled trial of 165 adults, using 400 mg berberine in a single oral dose, measurement of stool volumes showed that berberine was safe and effective for acute diarrhoea caused by toxins secreted by *E. coli*. In one study in the 1960s researchers found berberine effective against micro-organisms resistant to the antibiotics penicillin and chloromycetin.

Other reviews suggest that it can be used to treat haemorrhoids, nasal congestion, mouth and gum sores, wounds, sores, acne, ringworm and other ailments. It is reputed to stimulate the secretion of bile in humans, as well as lower blood pressure in laboratory animals.

Dose For best results use goldenseal extracts with a standardised berberine content of between 8–12 per cent and take between 250 and 500 mg three times daily. Goldenseal is best taken in small doses throughout the day – 10–15 drops of a tincture or fluid extract in a glass of water. It should begin to take effect in a few days to a week. Larger doses or longer duration can cause adverse effects.

Take care Do not use more than the recommended amounts, and like any potent medicine, use goldenseal cautiously for brief periods. Goldenseal (and other berberine-containing plants) should be avoided by those with high blood pressure. It should not be given to children under 2 years of age and is also not recommended for use during pregnancy as it can stimulate strong uterine contractions. Higher doses may interfere with B-vitamin metabolism, may irritate the skin, mouth and throat, and cause nausea and vomiting. In addition to the risk of pelvic inflammatory disease (PID), goldenseal douches may cause vaginal irritation. Hydrastine (another alkaloid in goldenseal) stimulates the central nervous system, and while extremely rare in humans, in animals large doses have caused death from respiratory paralysis and cardiac arrest.

Liquorice (anti-inflammatory)

This sweet root is one of the most extensively investigated botanical remedies. It has been shown in well-conducted studies to heal peptic ulcers and aid menstrual irregularities. There is also some evidence that it can be used to fight influenza and common cold viruses and as an expectorant and decongestant. Taken in small amounts, it can be used to decrease sugar cravings. Liquorice may also exert a protective effect on the liver, in part because once in the body it enters what is known as an 'enteric loop', and is reabsorbed by the system and represented to the liver before being excreted from the body.

Liquorice has also been found to have other benefits. Animal and laboratory studies have shown that a component of liquorice, glycyrrhizin, has immune-stimulating properties as well as anti-microbial action.

However, its main action on the body is as an anti-inflammatory shown to reduce symptoms of a number of conditions such as inflammation of the digestive tract including peptic ulcers, esophagitis, heartburn and gastritis. Inflammatory conditions of the skin, especially eczema, may also respond to topically applied liquorice extract. A synthetic derivative of glycyrrhizinic acid (GA, one of liquorice's main components), carbenoxelone, has been shown to be useful in the treatment of oral herpes lesions.

Early research into the benefits of liquorice for the treatment of ulcers showed that while it was an effective treatment it also created problems. In the body GA acts like the adrenal hormone aldosterone, which is involved in salt and water metabolism. Large amounts can cause a potentially serious condition, pseudoaldosteronism, symptoms of which include headache, lethargy, water retention, elevated blood pressure and possible heart failure.

However, scientists keen to capitalise on the encouraging results, particularly in the treatment of ulcers, discovered they could retain the herb's healing benefits but eliminate its hormonal side effects by removing 97 per cent of its GA, creating a new herbal medicine, deglycyrrhizinated liquorice (DGL). The usefulness of DGL in treating ulcers has since been widely proven. What is more, it is effective for both duodenal and gastric ulcers. In comparisons it has been proven to be just as effective as conventional medications such as Tagamet, Zantac or antacids for both short-term treatment and maintenance and peptic ulcers.

Recently liquorice extract, with both the glycyrrhizinic acid and the glabridin (another active compound found in liquorice) removed, was also shown to significantly inhibit LDL cholesterol oxidation as well as remove toxic free radicals in both humans and mice.

DGL research in Europe has continued to show benefits for those with ulcers. Nevertheless, some herbalists remain unconvinced, believing that DGL is just weird science masquerading as herbalism.

Dose Liquorice is probably best taken three times a day either as 1–4 mg of the powdered root, 1–6 ml (1½ teaspoons) of the fluid extract or 250–500 mg of the solid extract. Discontinue use after four to six weeks to prevent side effects. Taking the deglycyrrhizinated form (DGL) appears to be safer over the longer term than taking the whole herb.

Take care Herbalists contend that adverse reactions to liquorice have been limited to over-indulgence in liquorice candy and gum rather than from herbal preparations. Several reports from medical literature verify this. Still, as with most medicinal herbs, liquorice root is not advised for long-term use. Liquorice can cause potassium loss, sodium retention and suppression of the renin-angiotensin-aldosterone system (which regulates blood pressure and water balance). Taken together, these effects are known as apparent mineralocorticoid excess (AME) syndrome.

Pregnant and nursing women and anyone with a history of diabetes, glaucoma, high blood pressure, stroke or heart disease should steer clear of liquorice because it might raise their blood pressure and cause potentially serious problems. And anyone with an adrenal disorder or anyone taking cortisone or other adrenal hormones should not use liquorice because of its potential hormonal effects.

Much of the evidence for the adverse effects of liquorice is based on case histories. Nevertheless, taken together they show the range of potential problems. Hypertension is one of the main adverse effects, but water retention, abdominal pain, amenorrhoea, muscle weakness, headache and even fatal cardiac arrest have also been noted.

Several recent studies have also shown just how powerful a hormonal effect liquorice can have. In men it has been shown to reduce serum testosterone levels. When Finnish scientists studied the liquorice habits of more than 1,000 women, they found that pregnant women who eat large amounts of black liquorice may be raising their risk of a preterm delivery. The researchers noted that consuming at least two and a half 100 g packages of black liquorice on a weekly basis more than doubled the risk of giving birth before 38 weeks. Liquorice contains natural plant steroids which researchers believe may boost the production of prostaglandin (a naturally occurring hormone that stimulates labour). Liquorice use has also been found to cause reversible growth retardation (Addison's disease, another hormone-related effect) in children.

Choosing herbs wisely

The debate rages on as to whether whole plant extracts or those standardised to contain a certain amount of the plant's known active component are best. There is probably merit in both, depending on what you want to treat. Researchers and scientists love standardised extracts because they are easy

⊃

to research. But many herbalists believe that there is too much we do not know about all the chemicals in plant remedies and how they interact to say that a single component is responsible for its healing action. If you are confused about what kind of product to take, it may be worth consulting a professional.

When considering self-treatment always be suspicious of:

- Any herbal mixture which contains more than three or four herbs. In general, it is only possible to get 1–3 herbs into a standardised capsule in doses which have any therapeutic effect. Also, if you have an adverse reaction to the mixture, it will be very difficult to tell which herb is causing it.

- Any product where the labelling seems incomplete. Does the label say how much of the herb you will be getting? If you are taking a standardised herb, does it include standardisation information. If not, don't buy it.

- If any herbal supplement seems too cheap to be true – it probably is.

- Herbal tablets or tincture which don't have a taste. Whether dried or liquid, a herbal mixture should taste like a herbal mixture. Each herb has a distinct taste and smell. If not, it is likely to be of inferior quality.

- Exotic sounding herbs you've never heard of. Unless you are an expert, stick to names you know. Leave prescriptions for the weird and wonderful to professionals and even then always ask what the plant is and what it does.

Saw palmetto (for prostate problems)

Saw palmetto was once considered a nuisance by early European settlers in America because it grew everywhere, was resistant to burning and therefore had to be removed by hand, making land-clearing difficult. The saw palmetto is a dwarf palm tree native to the West Indies and the south-eastern United States (Florida, Georgia, Louisiana, Mississippi and South Carolina.) The fruit, a reddish-brown berry, is the part that is harvested for its extract. It is widely used in the treatment of benign prostatic hyperplasia (BPH) – a non-malignant enlargement of the prostate gland.

BPH is a condition that can result in the gradual compression of the urethra by the prostate, hindering urine flow and causing a frequent urgent desire to urinate. Saw palmetto works by the same mechanism as conventional BPH drugs – by blocking the production of an enzyme called 5-alpha-reductase in human tissue. This enzyme is required to change testosterone into dihydrotestosterone (DHT), the altered hormone that causes prostate cells to grow.

In 1998 researchers at the VA Medical Center in Minneapolis conducted a meta-analysis – a technique that allows the results of many small studies to be mathematically combined as though they were all part of one big study – of 18 studies of saw palmetto for BPH involving 2,939 men. Their analysis showed that saw palmetto significantly improved BPH symptoms. Men who used it for an average of nine weeks showed improved urine flow and less need to get up at night to urinate. The benefits were comparable to those produced by one of the major pharmaceuticals used to treat BPH, finasteride (Proscar).

A three-year study in Germany examined the effect of 160 mg saw palmetto extract twice daily in 315 men with mild or moderate symptoms of BPH. The urgent need to urinate in the middle of the night (known as nocturia) decreased in 73 per cent of the men and daytime urination decreased in 54 per cent. The amount of urine left in the bladder after voiding also decreased significantly from an average of 64 ml to 32 ml. These benefits were maintained at the six-month evaluation, and only 14.7 per cent of the men had a deterioration of symptoms over the three-year study. Once again these results compare favourably to those of conventional drugs such as finasteride and terazosin.

Then in a 1999 American trial, saw palmetto proved beneficial in reducing swelling of prostate tissues in men with BPH. While numerous studies have confirmed the ability of saw palmetto extract (SPE) to reduce BPH symptoms, this small trial was the first evidence that it might actually work to shrink enlarged prostate tissues. What is more, there were no effects on hormone levels or other blood parameters with the use of saw palmetto.

Saw palmetto is often combined with nettle root and the combination appears to be effective. In one six-month, placebo-controlled study the effect of a saw palmetto and nettle root combination in 40 men over the age of 50 with mild to moderate BPH was examined.

The men randomly received either the herbal mixture (containing 160 mg saw palmetto and 120 mg nettle root) or a placebo for six months, followed by a six-month observational period in which all the men received the herbal product. During the first part of the trial, those taking the saw palmetto/nettle root combination showed a significant improvement in the amount of urine they voided, compared to those taking the placebo. Those taking the herbs also had significant improvement in a range of BPH symptoms. During the second part of the trial, men switching from placebo to the herb showed similar improvements.

Two studies have compared finasteride with either saw palmetto alone or in combination with nettle root. The first in 1996 involved 951 men with mild to moderate BPH and compared 320 mg saw palmetto extract with 5 mg finasteride daily. At six months there was a 38 per cent decrease in the symptoms in both groups, with no other significant difference between the groups, indicating that saw palmetto was as effective as the drug.

Another study comparing finasteride (5 mg/day) to a saw palmetto (320 mg/day) and nettle root (240 mg/day) combination over 48 weeks in 543 men with mild to moderate BPH symptoms found similar results. The researchers noted also that the herbal combination produced far fewer side effects with no reports of impotence or headache. The saw palmetto/nettle root product did not affect prostate-specific antigen (PSA), high levels of which are associated with an increased risk of prostate cancer.

Dose Saw palmetto extract is commonly taken in doses of 320 mg, split into at least two daily doses to treat mild to moderate BPH.

Cautions Side effects appear to be few and far between. Saw palmetto can occasionally produce headache, but there have been no reports of sexual dysfunction, a common adverse effect with conventional medicines. In one large German study involving more than 1,300 men, mild gastrointestinal disturbances reported in 29 (2.2 per cent), of which only 10 were viewed as possibly being related to the saw palmetto extract.

Take care Herbs are the closest things in the natural world to the conventional medicines we use today. But herbs also have a complex nature; often they are made up of hundreds of active compounds. Adverse side effects from herbal remedies are still rare – much more rare than with conventional drugs – but they are not unheard of. The more we begin to research herbs, the more the list of potential adverse effects grows.

It is hardly surprising then that the use and misuse of herbal medicine has become associated with a wide range of adverse effects such as nausea, fatigue, skin eruptions, allergic reactions, headache and damage to the liver and other internal organs. In some individuals the herb may cause a deterioration of their condition rather than remediation. There are also a number of interactions with other drugs (see Appendix 2). Because of this, they should be taken with respect and not in a naive 'natural equals best' way.

There are a surprising number of herbs which should be avoided during the first trimester of pregnancy and if possible throughout the whole pregnancy. Some of the herbs which follow such as squaw vine and blue and black cohosh may be prescribed by a qualified herbalist towards the end of pregnancy (and for a short time) to initiate an overdue labour. If you are pregnant, exercise caution with: angelica, arbor vitae, autumn crocus, barberry, beth root, black cohosh,* blue cohosh,* broom, celery seed,** cotton root bark, fennel,** feverfew, goldenseal,* greater celandine, juniper, lovage, meadow saffron, mistletoe, motherwort, mugwort, nutmeg,** oregano,** pennyroyal,* Peruvian bark, poke root, rosemary,** rue, sage,** sassafrass, squaw vine,* tansy, thyme,** vervain and wormwood.

These herbs can be used in labour and may be effective in cases of threatened miscarriage. Consult your practitioner.

** These common culinary herbs are generally safe, especially when used in culinary quantities. However, if you are prone to miscarriage, you may wish to avoid them.

What to expect

Your herbalist will want to know as much about you as possible. Your initial consultation will consist of a lengthy history-taking and talking about those health concerns which you feel are most important. Subsequent consultations will probably not last more than half an hour unless your herbalist also combines other disciplines such as **massage, fasting & detox** or **acupuncture** into his or her practice. How long it takes to find relief with herbs depends on several factors, including the type of condition you are treating and your overall level of health. In general, herbalists believe that most people will get results within a few months.

Because they are so powerful, many practitioners would exercise particular caution in prescribing herbs during pregnancy (see opposite). Before making a recommendation, any practitioner should take into account the woman's general state of health, her lifestyle, her character, the quality of support she has around her and her domestic and working environments. As pregnancy is a time of growth and nourishment, only herbs that support this process should be used.

At the moment anyone can set up shop as a herbalist, whether they have had any training or not. To find a reputable herbalist in your area, contact the National Institute of Medical Herbalists. Members of this organisation must have completed a four-year B.Sc. course in herbal medicine and adhere to a code of ethics. Another useful organisation that can help is the International Register of Consultant Herbalists and Homeopaths.

Chapter 11

Homeopathy

Commonly used for

Respiratory Problems • Insomnia • Pain Relief
• Skin Complaints • Colds and Flu • Stress-Related Conditions
• Depression/ Anxiety • Injury • Pregnancy and Birth •
Digestive Disorders • Constipation • Headache • Heartburn

• *Requires a professional therapist* • *Suitable for self-treatment*

In the West, bigger is always considered better, so the concept of a therapy that employs infinitesimal doses of substances derived from a variety of plant, mineral, chemical and even animal sources seems very foreign to many. Yet homeopathy is increasingly proving itself to be a gentle, non-toxic way of treating a whole range of health problems in both children and adults.

Homeopathy is based on the idea that like can cure like, or the 'law of similars'. This idea was well known to the ancient Greeks but only became resurrected in Western society in the 18th century when a German physician, Samuel Hahnemann, began looking for a more humane way to treat his patients.

During his years as a physician, Hahnemann became increasingly distressed by the often barbaric cures of his day, which included bleeding, purging and the use of leeches. Eventually he chose to leave the medical profession altogether, supporting his family by translating medical, scientific and botanical texts. While engaged in this work he rediscovered the ancient law of similars. His first application of this principle was to test the effect of chinchona bark which was, at the time, a common treatment for malaria. During his research he noted that in healthy individuals the bark could produce malaria-like symptoms; but when minute doses of chinchona were administered to malaria patients, their symptoms abated.

Hahnemann's approach was, and still is, in complete contrast to conventional medicine, which treats a person's symptoms with medicines which have the opposite effect. So, for example, someone suffering from insomnia would be given something to induce an artificial sleep. In homeopathy, this same person would be given a minute dose of something such as *Coffea* (derived from unroasted coffee) which would normally act as a stimulant and in a healthy adult could produce sleeplessness.

Having rediscovered the law of similars, Hahnemann spent the rest of his life developing and cataloguing the relationship between diseases and symptoms and the toxic effects of natural medically active substances.

Today, more than 2,000 substances, which can imitate the symptom patterns of common conditions, including infectious diseases such as flu and colds, chronic conditions such as allergies, asthma, migraines and PMS, as well as more acute disorders such as arthritis and cancer, have been catalogued. Professional homeopaths use relatively few of these in their day-to-day practice and you certainly do not need to be an expert in all 2,000 to learn to diagnose and prescribe safely and effectively for yourself.

How does it work?

Doctors and scientists have developed many different theories in order to explain how such infinitesimal doses of a pharmacologically active substance can produce such profound results. One of the more intriguing is the 'memory of water' theory. Chemists believe that when the active ingredient is mixed in the water/alcohol base and shaken vigorously it makes an imprint on the water. Even though none of the active ingredient remains after this process, the water retains information about the active ingredient in this imprint even after millions of dilutions. What is more, repeated dilutions, known as potentisations, make the imprint stronger, not weaker, which is why in homeopathy higher dilutions are considered stronger medicine.

While such a view challenges everything we have been brought up to believe and everything modern science is built on, increasingly modern scientific testing is being used to show that it is true. For example, in 1968 a study using nuclear magnetic resonance (NMR) imaging demonstrated distinctive readings of subatomic activity in 23 different homeopathic remedies. But no such activity was found in the placebos tested. It is only a small leap from such findings to understanding homeopathy as a form of quantum or energy medicine. If this is the case, then it may be that homeopathy works by matching the frequencies of the plant extract with the frequency of the person's illness.

The memory of water theory was first put forward by a French biologist, Dr Jacques Benveniste. In the 1980s Benveniste began experimenting with human white blood cells, called basophils, which produce among other things histamine, which is released in an allergic response. In 1988 a study published in the respected journal *Nature* by an international team of researchers, which included Benveniste, found that even when exposed to homeopathic dilutions of immunoglobulin E (a substance known to stimulate the release of histamine), the basophils reacted by releasing histamine.

The results caused a major panic in the scientific community and *Nature* took the precautions of not only distancing itself from the findings but setting up a team of experts (which famously included a professional magician, a journalist and a scientific fraud expert) to reinvestigate the original findings. Not surprisingly, this inexperienced and motley crew could not reproduce the findings of the more experienced scientists. Nevertheless, this study was greeted with open arms, and with not a little relief by the wider scientific community.

A British attempt in 1993 to reproduce Benveniste's results (funded by London's University College and also published in *Nature*) also failed. Benveniste's theory continued to be so derided by other scientists that going public lost him his laboratories, his funding and some would say his international credibility.

But more recently a large pan-European team – originally with the aim of proving the French scientist wrong (again) – has found that water does indeed retain a memory of things dissolved in it. Their findings were published in the journal *Inflammation Research* in the spring of 2001.

In a refinement of Benveniste's study, the team used histamine to test the theory. Histamine solutions in both pharmacological concentrations and diluted to the point where no active ingredient remained in the solution (known as ghost solutions) were tested in the laboratory for their ability to inhibit a process known as basophil degranulation – a biochemical reaction to large amounts of immunoglobulin E which causes the cell to first release histamine and then restrict its release.

Three of the four labs involved in the trial reported a statistically significant inhibition of basophil degranulation by the ghost solutions, when compared with controls. The fourth lab found results that almost reached significance. The initial results which relied on human assessment were then checked by a totally automated process in order to rule out any human error. The results were the same.

Scientists are still clamouring for more research to confirm this data. But if confirmed, it would be much more than a simple validation of homeopathy; it would quite literally require a complete re-evaluation of how we understand the workings of chemistry, biochemistry and pharmacology. Given that it represents a threat to all they know, it is not surprising that so many scientists are resisting further investigation into the field of homeopathy or give only the most grudging acknowledgments to studies which show positive results.

What's in a name?

Most homeopathic medicines are referred to by their Latin names. This makes them sound rather more exotic than they really are. Use the table below to decipher the origins of some of the most commonly used homeopathic remedies.

Latin name	Common name	Latin name	Common name
Aconitum napellus	Monkshood	Ferrum phos	Iron phosphate
Allium cepa	Onion	Gelsemium	Yellow jasmine
Apis mellifica	Crushed bee	Hepar sulphuris	Hahnemann's calcium sulphide
Arnica	Leopard's bane or mountain daisy	Kali carbonicum	Potassium carbonate
Arsenicum album	Arsenic trioxide	Lachesis	Venom of the bushmaster snake
Belladonna	Deadly nightshade	Ledum	Marsh tea
Bellis perennis	Daisy	Lycopodium	Club moss
Berberis vulgaris	Barberry	Magnesia phosphorica	Magnesium phosphate
Bryonia	Wild hops	Mercurius	Mercury
Calcarea carbonica	Calcium carbonate	Natrum muriaticum	Salt
Calendula officinalis	Marigold	Nux vomica	Poison nut
Cantharis	Spanish fly	Opium	Dried laytex of poppy
Carbo vegetabilis	Vegetable charcoal	Oscillococcinum	Duck heart and liver
Caulophyllum	Blue cohosh	Pulsatilla	Windflower
Chamomilla	Camomile	Rhus toxicodendron	Poison ivy
Cimicifuga racemosa	Black snakeroot	Sarsaparilla	Wild liquorice
Cina	Worm seed	Sepia	Cuttlefish
Colocynthis	Bitter cucumber	Silicea	Silica, pure flint
Cuprum metallicum	Copper	Sulphur	Sulphur
Dioscorea villosa	Wild yam	Thuja occidentalis	Arbor vitae
Drosera	Sun dew	Urtica urens	Stinging nettle
Euphrasia	Eyebright	Zincum metallicum	Zinc

What the research says

Given the general level of scepticism about homeopathy among conventional practitioners, there has been what appears to be an almost disproportionately concerted effort to research homeopathic remedies. A quick look at much of the research reveals why. Most studies into homeopathy are designed to show that it does not work, that it could not possibly work and that it is simply a fancy type of *placebo*.

Many of these studies employ the double-blind, placebo-controlled design – pitting an active remedy against a placebo without the participants knowing which they are taking – that 'real' scientists hold in such high regard. And yet the majority of these studies do show that homeopathy works and, more importantly, that it works better than a placebo.

While most studies into homeopathy are small, taken together they show an impressive trend towards efficacy. For instance in 1991, the *British Medical Journal* published an analysis of 107 clinical studies into homeopathy published between 1966 and 1990. The authors found that in 81 (75 per cent) of the experiments, the homeopathic treatments were successful. Even when they re-analysed the data, using only the 23 studies they considered to be of the highest quality, the majority of these, 65 per cent, showed positive results.

Results showed that in 13 out of the 19 trials of respiratory infection treatment homeopathy proved effective; 6 out of 7 were positive for other infections, 5 out of 7 were positive for digestive system treatment, 5 out of 5 were successful for hay fever, 5 out of 7 showed quicker recovery after surgery, 4 out of 6 helped in rheumatological disease, 18 out of 20 were beneficial for pain or traumatic injury, and 8 out of 10 worked for mental or psychological problems.

In 1992, in the *Canadian Medical Association Journal*, Dutch researchers reported that a review of 105 published papers over a three-year period showed that 85 of the 105 studies favoured a homeopathic treatment for a variety of illnesses, with most showing 'statistically significant advantages over a placebo'. Similarly in 1997 the UK medical journal, the *Lancet*, published a much larger and more thorough review of all the properly conducted clinical trials into homeopathy published between 1943 and 1995. It concluded that 77 per cent of these studies yielded a positive result. In addition, while some conventional practitioners poo-pooed the effectiveness of homeopathy as a mere 'placebo effect', in this review homeopathy was 10 times more effective than a placebo.

In spite of research that shows that homeopathy works, and the continued popularity and success of the five NHS homeopathic hospitals in the UK that treat a wide range of conditions using homeopathy, the medical profession continues to be reluctant in its acceptance of the therapy.

Respiratory conditions

Of all the conditions which homeopathy treats, respiratory conditions such as asthma and hay fever are the most commonly researched. For instance, one of the most significant analyses on the homeopathic treatment of asthma was published in the *Lancet*. The researchers performed a meta-analysis (a pooling together of the results from different trials) on a series of three studies and found that, taken together, the evidence showed that homeopathy had made a substantially significant difference in the treatment group. The researchers boldly concluded that either homeopathic medicines work or controlled studies do not.

A later analysis of trials into asthma and homeopathy, published in the *Lancet* in 1997, concluded that there was only mixed evidence for its effectiveness. But it also noted that the use of standard remedies, rather than individually chosen ones, may have influenced those trials where outcomes were poor. This seems to be reinforced by recent trials showing positive results when remedies are chosen according to classical homeopathy on the basis of constitutional type for the treatment of a variety of conditions.

In a recent analysis of conventional medical practitioners in four countries using homeopathy to treat upper and lower respiratory tract infections and glue ear, homeopathy was at least as effective as conventional treatments for these conditions. Among the 456 patients studied, those taking homeopathy recovered somewhat faster than those in the conventional group and the rate of adverse events related to treatment were much lower in the homeopathy group (7.8 per cent compared to 22.3 per cent).

In another study published in 1986, a team of researchers compared the effects of an isopathic hay fever remedy with a placebo. Isopathy is a branch of homeopathy that uses dilutions of the substance that causes the disease (in this case pollen), rather than a substance that produces similar symptoms. In this double-blind, controlled study, those who received the homeopathic remedy had six times fewer symptoms and were able to cut their use of antihistamines by half.

Individual commercially available remedies, however, can also be effective. An analysis of seven randomised, double-blind, placebo-controlled trials and four non-placebo controlled trials involving 1,038 people with hay fever found that the use of the homeopathic preparation, Galphimia glauca, was an effective way to relieve itchy eye symptoms associated with hay fever in 79 per cent of cases. This success rate was comparable with that of conventional antihistamines, with the added bonus that the Galphimia glauca produced no adverse side effects.

Hay fever sufferers also appear to benefit from using the homeopathic nasal spray Luffa Comp-Heel. In 1999, when German researchers tested it against a standard cromolyn sodium spray in 146 people, they found that Luffa (which is made from a homeopathic combination of Luffa operculata, Galphimia glauca, histamine and sulphur) brought quick and lasting relief comparable to that given by conventional treatment. The researchers noted that many in the Luffa group experienced an almost complete remission. Only three people in the Luffa group experienced mild nasal irritation from the use of the remedy.

In yet another trial published in the British Medical Journal in 2000, researchers from the Homeopathic Hospital, Glasgow, studied 50 people with perennial allergic rhinitis. The subjects were randomly given either a 30C dose of an ISO remedy made from inhaled allergens or a placebo. After three and four weeks the researchers compared changes in symptoms and ability to breathe freely among the participants.

The homeopathic group showed a significant improvement in free breathing compared with the placebo groups. And when the researchers then combined their results with those of three previous trials (bringing the number of individuals studied up to 253), the reduction in uncomfortable symptoms was 28 per cent for the homeopathic groups, compared to just 3 per cent in the placebo groups. This success was roughly equivalent to those a patient could expect with a steroidal nasal spray, only without the side effects.

Not all studies are positive, however. A randomised, placebo-controlled study of 175 Dutch children with recurrent upper respiratory infections found that those receiving individually chosen homeopathic remedies did not fare any better than those who received the placebo.

Tissue salts

The remedies known as tissue salts exist on the border between homeopathic and nutritional medicine. Although they are diluted in the same way, they are not diluted to the same degree. Instead, they come in a decimal potency (usually 6X), as opposed to the centesimal, or C, potencies common to other homeopathic remedies. This means they have been diluted six times, one part remedy to nine parts water and alcohol (see *Taking homeopathic remedies*, p. 158). At this level of dilution there is a theoretical possibility that some of the original material remains.

Your body tissues are made up, in part, of various inorganic minerals known as biochemical cell salts. There are 12 tissue salts in all, each of them playing a role in maintaining the health of our bodies. During times of stress, if your diet is poor, if you have been ill, and during pregnancy, the balance of tissue salts in the body may change. Occasionally this can result in a 'deficiency' (a descriptive term rather than a diagnosis as true deficiency of these minerals can be difficult to assess) which can show itself as uncomfortable physical symptoms such as cramp or constipation. ⊃

Tissue salts have never been proven to cure anything, though many people swear by them. The individual salts are:

- **Calc fluor (fluoride of lime)**
Found in all your body's connective tissues. Imbalance can result in varicosities, muscle tendon strain, cracked, dry skin and deficient tooth enamel. This remedy is often recommended to prevent stretch marks.

- **Calc phos (calcium phosphate)**
Constituent of bones, teeth, gastric juices. Imbalance can cause impaired digestion, teething troubles, itching, chilblains, simple anaemia.

- **Calc sulph (calcium sulphate)**
A constituent of blood. Helps to relieve skin symptoms such as pimples during adolescence, sores that are slow to heal, sore lips.

- **Ferum phos (phosphate of iron)**
A constituent of the blood and other body tissues. Imbalance may cause diarrhoea, constipation and even spontaneous nose bleeds. Useful for chills, fevers, inflammation congestion and rheumatic symptoms. Occasionally helpful in cases of anaemia.

- **Kali. mur (potassium chloride)**
Blood constituent and conditioner. Used sometimes in combination with ferum phos in cases of coughs, colds, respiratory ailments and children's feverish ailments.

- **Kali. phos (potassium phosphate)**
Necessary for the proper function of the nervous system. Thus this remedy is indicated in cases of nervous exhaustion, nervous indigestion, nervous headaches and insomnia. Eases stress due to worry or excitement.

- **Kali. sulph (potassium sulphate)**
Necessary component of healthy skin. Eases rough, dry, scaly skin, hastens wound healing. Also useful for hair loss and nail disorders.

- **Mag. phos (phosphate of magnesia)**
A component of the teeth, bones, brain, blood, nerves and muscle cells. Deficiency can cause cramp, flatulence, neuralgia and shooting pains.

- **Natrum mur (chloride of soda)**

Regulates the body's water balance and carries moisture to the cells. Imbalance may result in salt cravings, hay fever and watery discharges from the eyes and nose. This remedy may also prevent heartburn, swollen ankles and dry skin.

- **Natrum phos (sodium phosphate)**

Neutralises acid, thus good for over-acidity of the blood, gastric disorders, heartburn, rheumatic symptoms.

- **Natrum sulph (sodium sulphate)**

Known as the 'liver' salt. Helps eliminate excess water, relieves liverish symptoms, bilious attacks, watery infiltrations and symptoms of flu.

- **Silica (silicic acid)**

Exists in all connective tissue as well as in hair, skin and nails. Imbalance or deficiency can result in poor memory, thinning hair and ribbed or ingrowing nails.

Tissue salts can be purchased as single remedies or in combination in most chemists and healthfood shops. The tablets dissolve quickly when placed under the tongue. There is not one simple correct dosage for mineral tissue salts, as the amount you take will reflect the type and severity of your symptoms. Tissue salts are finely balanced in the body and you may not need to take more than one tablet daily on alternate weeks to effect change. However, the usual dose is four tablets three times a day before meals. When symptoms are very severe, you may take them more frequently. Alternatively, for longer-term illnesses a low daily dose such as two tablets twice daily may be more beneficial. If unsure, consult your practitioner.

Colds and flu

Each year as the weather changes and the cold and flu season comes around, sales of over-the-counter remedies increase several-fold. In homeopathy individually chosen remedies may help to strengthen the constitution against invading viruses, but there is little study to show this. However, one remedy *Oscillococcinum* (derived from duck heart and liver) has been the subject of scientific interest.

A controlled study, published in 1989 in the *British Journal of Clinical Pharmacology*, found that two-thirds more of those with flu who took Oscillococcinum recovered within forty-eight hours, as compared to the placebo group.

A recent analysis of the use of Oscillococcinum in the treatment of colds and flu notes that, while there have been too few studies to draw definite conclusions, the remedy does appear to reduce the duration of illness in individuals with influenza. It is not, however, effective in preventing flu.

Headaches
While often recommended for chronic headaches, studies into the use of homeopathy in this area show mixed results. For example, one study of eight different remedies (singly or in a combination of two) or placebo used on 60 volunteers determined that homeopathy significantly reduced the number of headaches. In the homeopathy group this represented a reduction from 10 attacks per month to 1.8 at the end of four months. In the placebo group the reduction was less marked, from 9.9 per month to 7.9.

However, in Sweden 68 people with migraine participated in a placebo-controlled study designed to test the efficacy of home-opathy in preventing attacks and relieving symptoms. Both groups experienced a reduction in the frequency and intensity of attacks, but the final evaluation performed by a neurologist, who did not know which results belonged to which remedy, concluded that while more individuals in the homeopathy group experienced a reduction in frequency and severity of attacks, the difference was too small to be significant.

Similarly, when researchers at the Princess Margaret Migraine Clinic in London undertook a four-month, double-blind, randomised, placebo-controlled trial of homeopathy for migraines in 1997, both groups improved (homeopathy 19 per cent, placebo 16 per cent). Eleven different homeopathic remedies were used in all. Interestingly, the placebo showed its most marked effect on mild migraine attacks, while homeopathy seemed more effective on moderate to severe attacks. However, improvement in the placebo group began to reverse itself after the fourth month, while slow improvement continued in the homeopathy group. The authors concluded rather reluctantly that homeopathy was not without effect, but could not be recommended because (a) it was slow to work and (b) traditional prescribing methods, matching the remedy to the individual, were too unreliable – and then, as if to hedge their bets, they also acknowledged that this is also a problem in conventional medicine!

And yet reviews of the long-term effectiveness of homeopathy in treating headaches show that, even if it is slow to work, the effects can be long-lasting with approximately 30 per cent of patients maintaining improvements in severity and frequency of headache pain a year after being treated. Why isn't the figure higher? Probably because headaches and migraine are of multi-factorial origin, in other words, they have multiple causes including allergies, stress and hormonal factors. No single remedy, even a homeopathic one, can address all of these.

Childhood ailments

Parents who do not wish to give conventional medicine to their children often opt for homeopathic remedies instead. There is no evidence to show that homeopathic remedies cause adverse side effects in children, and many studies show that for some childhood illnesses homeopathy can be very effective.

One significant study published in 1994 was conducted in Nicaragua and included 81 children with acute diarrhoea. All the children received standard anti-dehydration treatment for diarrhoea, consisting of water containing salt and sugar. In addition, half the children received homeopathic treatment, while the other half received a placebo. The recovery time for children receiving homeopathic treatment was 20 per cent faster than those receiving the placebo, reducing the bout of diarrhoea on the first day of use.

Several studies have shown that homeopathy can be more effective than conventional medicines for treating middle ear infections (otitis media). In 1997 a study of 131 children with recurrent otitis media received individually chosen homeopathic remedies and were compared with another group receiving conventional treatments such as nasal drops and antibiotics. In the homeopathic group 70.7 per cent were free of recurrence within a year, compared to only 29 per cent in the conventional treatment group.

Another small study in 1999 also found that homeopathy can be an effective way of treating glue ear. The researchers studied 33 children in two locations in southern England. The children were aged 18 months to 8 years. They all had otitis media with significant hearing loss. They found that a higher proportion of children receiving homeopathic care had regained their hearing over the 12 months follow-up, compared with those who received standard GP care (64 versus 56 per cent). Referrals to specialists and antibiotic consumption was also lower in the homeopathic group.

Pain relief

Study in this area is small, but in what was considered a well-conducted study published in the *British Medical Journal* in 1989, fibromyalgia was found to respond to homeopathic treatment with *Rhus toxicodendron 6X*. The double-blind, controlled trial was also 'crossed over', meaning the treatment lots were switched after one month so the subjects could be compared not only with each other, but also with themselves. The results were evaluated by a rheumatology professional who was not a homeopath and the conclusion was that the homeopathic remedy provided highly significant improvement in both subjective and objective symptoms.

Research into homeopathy for osteoarthritis has shown few positive effects. But in 1980 a small double-blind controlled study conducted in Britain found that 82 per cent of those receiving an individually prescribed homeopathic remedy experienced improvements in painful symptoms of rheumatoid arthritis versus 21 per cent of the control group on a placebo.

The same author had earlier compared aspirin to a variety of homeopathic medicines for rheumatoid arthritis and found homeopathy to be much more effective. By the end of the year-long trial, 43 per cent of the homeopathic treatment group had stopped other treatments. Another 24 per cent of the homeopathy group improved but carried on with other treatments. In contrast, only 15 per cent of the aspirin group either maintained or improved on their treatment. All those on placebo dropped out of the trial within six weeks of starting because their condition deteriorated.

While some practitioners maintain that bruising can be healed more quickly with the homeopathic remedy arnica, studies show mixed results. In one conducted in 1978 volunteers received identical bruises on both arms, one of which was treated with arnica and the other with a placebo. The arm treated with arnica was judged to heal more rapidly than the one treated with the placebo. But a more recent study of 93 women recovering from abdominal hysterectomy found no difference in terms of post-operative recovery between arnica and a placebo. What might be more useful in this area would be the comparison between a standard remedy like arnica with an individually chosen remedy to see if one was more effective in treating a major trauma such as abdominal surgery, but this has not yet been done.

Taking homeopathic remedies
Unlike conventional drugs, homeopathic remedies do not generally cause adverse effects and you cannot become addicted to them. Although some people report swift and profound relief from their symptoms with homeopathy, most studies show that homeopathy tends to work slowly but produces long-lasting results.

Homeopathic remedies are available in a wide range of doses from specialist suppliers. However, the remedies which you can buy in most healthfood shops are commonly sold in two strengths, 6C and 30C (though occasionally the C is omitted on the label). The 'C' stands for centesimal – meaning that one part of the active ingredient has been diluted in 99 parts water and alcohol, then shaken vigorously to release its energy. To make a higher potency remedy one part of this newly diluted solution will then be mixed with 99 parts water and alcohol and shaken vigorously. This process can be repeated any number of times to achieve the desired potency (in a 6C remedy, for example, this process will have taken place six times). Less is more in homeopathy and although the 30C remedy has been diluted more times, it is considered more potent.

It is important, if you are self-diagnosing and buying homeopathic remedies over the counter, not to use them as you would a conventional remedy. Often a single dose is all that is required. This is very difficult to take on board if you have spent years taking medicine on a three or four times daily schedule. If you are uncertain about how to take a remedy and the remedy's label is unclear, it is best to consult a qualified therapist for advice.

If you or your homeopath select the wrong remedy, it simply won't work and you are unlikely to suffer any unpleasant side effects. If the right remedy has been chosen, some change may begin to take place within a relatively short space of time. It is important to remember that once a change does occur, you should stop taking the remedy (don't be tempted to take another dose 'just in case'); your body will take over the process from then on.

Both 6C and 30C potencies are appropriate for most of the conditions. As a general guideline, the higher 30C potency acts more quickly and deeply than the lower 6C potency, but requires a more precise selection of an appropriate remedy. If after selecting a remedy you are unsure about which potency to use, start with the lower one. For many conditions the right choice of remedy may be more important than its potency. Nevertheless, a useful guideline when self-prescribing is to try to match the potency to the nature of the symptoms; select a 6C potency for chronic conditions which have been slow to develop and which seem neither to improve nor get worse, and 30C for those which come on quickly and are more intense.

How frequently you take the remedy depends on the urgency of the situation. Thus for mild conditions you may only need to take one tablet day and night and for other chronic conditions no more than three 6C tablets daily. Higher potencies should be taken less frequently. For example, in cases of a severe backache or a headache that comes on suddenly, a single 30C potency would be appropriate.

In urgent, changeable situations such as sudden anxiety, you could conceivably take one 30C tablet every five or ten minutes for up to four to six doses or your homeopath might prescribe a single very high potency (200C or more) tablet.

Selection of the right remedy, in the right potency, is only one part of the process. Taking your remedies under the right conditions and storing them properly will also ensure that your homeopathic remedies work optimally for you. Homeopathic remedies are very delicate and certain things will act as an antidote to them. Try following these guidelines to get the best out of your remedies:

- You should not touch homeopathic remedies with your bare hands. Always tip them straight into the bottle top and from there into your mouth. To make this process easier, some commercially available remedies now come in special dispensers. Remedies should always be stored in a cool, dark place. Do not store them near any essential oils and/or electronic devices.

- You should leave 20 minutes before or after food before taking a remedy. Also avoid strong, highly flavoured foods and other items such as mints (toothpaste, gum, mouthwash), cloves, garlic or onions immediately before or after taking a remedy. Products containing eucalyptus and camphor will also antidote your remedies, as will cigarette smoke and caffeine. While you are taking a homeopathic remedy it may be wise to switch to a non-mint toothpaste. It is also advisable not to wear strong perfumes while taking remedies, since these can sometimes act as an antidote.

- Electromagnetic fields generated by telephones, cell phones, headphones, computers and by machines with large motors such as automobiles can also antidote homeopathic remedies. It's probably best to avoid these things for five minutes before taking a remedy and for 25 minutes afterwards. Take care also not to store remedies close to sources of electromagnetic radiation.

Cautions

There are very few cautions with homeopathy. Most homeopaths do not recommend taking daily doses of any remedy for extended periods of time. Generally speaking, if there has not been some form of improvement within a week or so, you may want to consider another remedy. Homeopathy is also safe for people who might otherwise need to be cautious about what medications they take, including those on conventional medicines and pregnant women. While there is absolutely no evidence that homeopathic remedies can cause any adverse effects to a mother or her unborn child, women with a history of miscarriage are advised to avoid taking the remedies *Apis*, *Silicea* or *Thuja*, as these can theoretically increase their risk of another miscarriage.

What to expect
Your homeopath will want to take a full medical history from you and this will take up most of your first session together. Once the history-taking is completed, your practitioner will study your pattern of symptoms and choose a remedy that is best for you.

Classical homeopaths maintain that certain individuals have an affinity to particular remedies. These remedies are 'constitutional remedies' – single remedies given in a single very high dose or in a lower potency taken over a period of days. The theory is that if you get the constitutional remedy right, it will strengthen the whole system and help to heal a variety of ailments. Such remedies are prescribed according to the person's 'constitutional type', which is determined by the lengthy process of history-taking and the practitioner's own observations.

The 'Ignatia type', for example, is nervous, apprehensive, tearful, and usually a woman. The 'Nux vomica type' is fiery, hyperactive, ambitious, thin and regularly over-indulges in stimulants such as coffee and alcohol. The limitations of this type of prescription are obvious, since the homeopath is treating a person, not a 'type'. Strict adherence to this kind of diagnosis can easily lead to stereotyping (the very thing that many people find so frustrating about conventional care) and the inability to see the patient as an individual.

Other homeopaths, believing that there are no 'true' types, prefer to address symptom patterns and may prescribe combination remedies.

There is disagreement among practitioners about which method is officially best and which one reflects true homeopathic practice. In self-prescribing you can treat constitutionally or in a symptom-oriented way, since over-the-counter remedies are available both singly and in combination form. A great deal of literature exists to help self-prescribers identify major symptom patterns and personality types and assist you in your choices.

Professional homeopaths generally distinguish between acute symptoms – which they see as representing self-protective efforts by the body and/or psyche to deal with some kind of recent stress or infection – and chronic symptoms – recurrent, unsuccessful efforts by the body to re-establish health and balance. Chronic symptoms may persist if you are weakened by stress, lifestyle or environmental factors, or because of some inherited weakness. Sometimes what appears to be an acute condition is really the manifestation of an underlying chronic condition. This is one example where a 'constitutional remedy', which matches the *totality* of the symptoms, may be particularly appropriate.

In most cases, once a remedy is selected, you will not need to see your practitioner again too soon. It will be apparent if the right remedy has been selected, since you will begin to note an improvement in your condition and your practitioner may only need to see you again in two weeks or a month's time to check your progress.

Because the profession is not regulated, anyone can claim to be a homeopath. Some practitioners in other disciplines (both alternative and conventional) 'prescribe' homeopathic remedies with no (or minimal) training in the field.

To contact a qualified homeopath in your local area, get in touch with the *British Homeopathic Association*, who can supply you with a list of medically qualified doctors who are also homeopaths, or the *Society of Homeopaths*, whose members have trained at approved colleges.

Chapter 12

Hypnotherapy

Commonly used for

Fear/Anxiety • High Blood Pressure • Respiratory Problems
• Labour Pains • Relaxation • Depression • Headaches
• Digestive Problems • Irritable Bowel Syndrome
• Quitting Smoking • Resolving Childhood Traumas
• Relationship Difficulties

• Requires a professional therapist • Suitable for self-treatment

The power of suggestion can be powerful medicine. It is also one of the oldest forms of therapy. Ancient writings confirm that the Sumerian priest-doctors used hypnotic suggestion as a therapeutic tool, as did the later Hindu fakirs, the Persian magi and the Indian yogi.

The Ebers papyrus tells us that ancient Egyptian priest-doctors would often approach the task of healing by asking those who consulted them to fix their gaze upon a glossy piece of metal to help induce a trance-like state – a technique which is commonly used by modern practitioners. The modern practice of hypnotherapy also has links with other mind-body therapies such as ***meditation, spiritual healing, biofeedback*** and even ***yoga***. Today, hypnotherapy is considered so powerful that it has been used by dentists and doctors in lieu of an anaesthetic. There is even a case of a 15-year-old girl undergoing a heart operation while under hypnosis.

Although hypnosis can induce powerful feelings of relaxation, objective research suggests that being hypnotised is not the same as being asleep. When the brainwaves of hypnotised subjects are being monitored, an increase in alpha wave activity – the electrical impulses which are produced when humans are in a relaxed but mentally alert state – is revealed. When a subject is asleep, slower delta waves are the predominant type of brainwave activity.

Hypnotherapy is also not the same as the stage hypnotism you see on TV. The common confusion between the two means that many people feel unable to take hypnotherapy seriously. Yet research continues to show that, under the right circumstances, hypnotherapy can be a very powerful catalyst for change.

Unlike stage hypnotism, your therapist is not controlling your thoughts or making you act in a certain way. On the contrary, in hypnotherapy you direct the course of the therapy. The therapist's role is to help you gain insight into your everyday actions, to achieve your goals and feel confident in the decisions you make. When an individual feels comfortable with their therapist, the benefits of increased relaxation and the control and management of problems such as chronic pain can be very significant.

Mesmerised

In Victorian England, the idea that an electromagnetic influence could pass between people and influence their behaviour was widely taken for granted. This invisible force called 'animal magnetism' was introduced into Europe in the 18th century by the physician Franz Anton Mesmer. The technique of manipulating animal magnetism came to be called mesmerism, the forerunner of modern hypnosis.

Mesmer used animal magnetism to treat a variety of psychological and psychophysiological disorders such as hysterical blindness, paralysis, headaches and joint pains.

Because he was also something of a showman, his experiments also contributed to a widespread scepticism about the use of hypnosis. He was, however, the source of a new word in the English language – the trance-like state of his patients came to be known as being 'mesmerised'.

How does it work?

The mind is divided into two parts, the conscious and unconscious. Some practitioners liken it to an iceberg, with the conscious mind being the tip and the unconscious being the large mass that lies beneath the surface. We cannot live in the unconscious; it is too vast and complex. To function on a day-to-day basis we need to remain in the realm of consciousness. Nevertheless, what goes on below the surface is relevant and important since the conscious and unconscious mind are constantly interacting in subtle ways of which we are largely unaware. Because of the strong connection between body and mind, what lurks in the unconscious can often be at the root of our health problems and anxieties.

Hypnotherapy uses the power of suggestion to induce a trance-like state that enables an individual to explore the hidden levels of their mind and emotions. Positive suggestion can then be made, and heard by the patient at a very deep level, to help bring about change.

While some view hypnotherapy as an opportunity to shine a light on the dark corners of the mind, others find it a frightening prospect, almost like having to walk down a dark, unfamiliar street in the dead of night. But the unconscious does not only hold our scariest, darkest secrets and memories; it also holds all our potential for good, for instance, our under-used creative talents and unexpressed emotions. Hypnotherapy, then, can be seen as a way to tap into the good as well as the unfamiliar and uncomfortable in a safe, supportive space.

Under hypnosis you enter a state of consciousness somewhere between sleeping and waking. Many of us have already experienced this powerful state, for instance, at night when we are drifting off but have not yet fallen asleep. Some people recognise this as a time when insight seems to come out of nowhere or when they suddenly identify a solution to a problem which has been plaguing them for some time.

If you are deeply absorbed in a book, task or hobby you are in some form of a light trance state; aware of what you are doing, but also able to shut out a significant amount of external stimuli. Many of us fall into this kind of trance without knowing it. Others use trance states in a more conscious way. People with cancer, for instance, often use techniques such as visualisation and hypnosis as ways of managing pain and keeping a meaningful connection between body, mind and emotions.

For hypnosis to work you must have the desire to be hypnotised. Your willingness is what opens the door to a dialogue with your own subconscious. For instance, people who have lived with physical or emotional pain for years often forget what it is like to live without that pain. The pain becomes deeply ingrained as part of their personality. They may even believe, on some level, that they need their pain to make them feel alive. Hypnotherapists believe that hypnosis can take you back to a time when you were generally pain free and help you to re-experience that feeling. It can provide positive supportive suggestions that can help you create new patterns in your life. It can also help to free you from uncomfortable physical symptoms. For instance, if you are experiencing headaches as a response to stress, you can begin to build new, pain-free responses to help you deal with stress. Given this, it's perhaps not surprising that the overwhelming experience of hypnotherapy is one of relaxation and relief.

What the research says
In medical settings, hypnosis has been used to provide pain relief, lower patient anxiety and nausea during medical procedures and to reduce blood flow to a surgical site. The use of hypnosis has also been documented in cases of allergy, asthma, heart disorders, insomnia, gastrointestinal problems, headaches and skin conditions.

Studies into all these areas are limited, but among those who use hypnotherapy, more than 90 per cent appear to derive some benefit, particularly if their condition is related in some way to stress and/or anxiety.

Relaxation
Most people view hypnotherapy as a way to manage stress and aid relaxation. For instance, it may benefit those who are about to have surgery by helping them to relax and feel in control. In one study 32

adults due to have coronary bypass surgery were either taught self-hypnosis or given no therapy. Those who were taught self-hypnosis relaxation techniques were significantly more relaxed following the operation, compared with the control group. They also required significantly less pain medication. There was no difference in the surgical outcomes between the groups.

While relaxation is a good end in itself, it also has deeper benefits for the body, including better immune response. Evidence suggests that there is a continual interaction between the central nervous system, the immune system and the endocrine system, so much so that a new field of medicine, psychoneuroimmunology, has been developed to study this relationship. There are thought to be two main communication pathways: the first is via the hypothalamus-pituitary-adrenal axis; the second is via the network of nerves found in the lymph tissue.

Through these pathways what happens in the mind is continually influencing the function of the immune and hormonal systems and vice versa, and this relationship can be measured scientifically. For example, a German review of many different types of studies conducted between 1958 and 1993 suggested there was strong evidence for a two-way interaction between the central nervous and the immune systems. Not all studies in the analysis found evidence for a direct link between psychological stress, mood states and immune function. Nevertheless, the reviewers concluded that, overall, the evidence did suggest that the immune system can be influenced by hypnosis and relaxation.

More specific studies on the use of hypnotherapy to influence immunity have shown interesting results. In one 57 children were randomised to one of three groups to: (1) learn self-hypnosis to suggest to themselves, in their own words, that they increase an immune substance in their saliva called immunoglobulin-A, or IgA; (2) learn self-hypnosis with specific suggestions for the control of salivary immunoglobulins; or (3) spend equivalent time with an instructor without learning any hypnotic procedure.

The children were all given general instruction in the function and production of saliva and the immunoglobulin role in saliva. Two samples of saliva were collected before practice to provide a comparative measurement. Samples were then collected after each 30-minute self-hypnosis session. Compared to their first measurements, subjects in group 2 were found to have a significant increase in salivary IgA from 7.75 to 12.6 units after three 30-minute practice sessions. Groups 1 and 3 increased from 7.85 to 8.5 and 7.8 to 9.25 units, respectively.

In a trance

Hypnotherapists generally recognise three levels of hypnosis:

Light trance – where the eyes are closed and the person is deeply relaxed.

Medium trance – where the person is fully hypnotised, physiological processes slow down, allergic reactions subside and the person is less aware of pain.

Deep trance – where the person is in a sleep-like state and age regression can be attempted or simple operations such as the removal of warts can be carried out without anaesthetic.

Headaches

Hypnotherapy can be performed with a practitioner or the method can be taught to individuals suffering from specific conditions such as headaches. The person can then practise self-hypnosis as either a form of prevention or to provide pain relief in the event of getting a headache. Both hypnosis and self-hypnosis appear to work equally well at reducing the frequency and sometimes the intensity of headaches. In addition, a small German study in 1999 noted that hypnotherapy also improves people's confidence in their own ability to keep their headaches and well-being under control. This too may have a therapeutic effect.

There have been several studies into the use of hypnosis for headaches. In one, published in 1985 in the *American Journal of Clinical Hypnosis*, 23 individuals who received hypnotherapy all reported significant improvement in their headache pain. In 1991, when researchers from Brigham and Women's Hospital in Boston, Massachusetts, used hypnotherapy to ease chronic tension headaches among adult sufferers, they discovered that the duration of the headache and its intensity was significantly reduced by the therapy.

When hypnotherapy was compared to the dopamine antagonist/ nausea drug prochlorperazine (Stemetil) in a group of 47 migraine sufferers randomly assigned to either treatment, 10 out of 23 in the hypnosis group reported complete remission, compared with only 3 out of 24 in the drug group.

In another comparison with drug treatment, children aged 6 to 12 years with classic migraine were given either the beta-blocker propranolol or a placebo and then after six months taught self-hypnosis. During the first six months of the trial the average number of headaches per child did not differ significantly between the drug (14.9 headaches on average) and the placebo (13.3 headaches). But after being taught self-hypnosis the average number of headaches dropped to 5.8 over the three-month period in both groups. However, while hypnosis was useful at lowering the number of migraines, it was not found to alter their severity.

One study by researchers at the Catholic University in Nymegen, the Netherlands, compared autogenic training (a method of mental, meditative-type exercises that promote relaxation) to self-hypnosis and found no differences between the two techniques in terms of their overall effectiveness in treating headaches. They did, however, find what may be an important difference between subjects who improve and those who do not. Those who attributed the reduction in pain experienced during therapy to their own efforts (in other words, those who felt some measure of control over their own health) experienced longer-term headache pain reduction.

Pain relief
Hypnosis has been found to significantly reduce pain and anxiety – both before and after a surgical procedure – and many other kinds of pain, including back and dental pain, respond well to the use of hypnosis.

In a Belgian study in 1997, 60 people were randomly allocated to use either stress-reducing strategies or hypnosis during elective plastic surgery under local anaesthesia. They were also given intravenous sedation on request. A psychologist observed each patient during the procedure. In addition, each person was asked to judge their pain, anxiety and perceived control before, during and after the operation. Post-operative nausea and vomiting, patient satisfaction and surgical conditions were also recorded. Results showed that the hypnosis group required less sedation and felt they had greater control over the proceedings. The psychologist observed fewer signs of discomfort in those who were hypnotised, and noted that their vital signs were significantly more stable during the operation. Post-operative side effects were noted in 6.5 per cent of those using hypnotherapy, compared with 30.8 per cent in the stress-reduction group.

Pain management through hypnosis may also be an effective way of dealing with back pain for which no physical cause can be found. In a small 1998 study hypnosis significantly lowered perceived pain and sensory distress in a group of 15 adults with chronic lower back pain. The patients were also taught self-hypnosis and were then able to successfully use what they learned to reduce their own pain. After just three sessions the participants reported less pain, improved sleep and greater psychological well-being.

A review of the evidence for the use of hypnosis in the treatment of burn pain found that case reports provided strong anecdotal support for treating pain from severe burn injuries in this way. Evidence from controlled studies, while also positive, was less emphatic. The researchers noted that the way hypnosis works in treating burn pain is poorly understood, as it is with pain in general. It could be, for instance, that some people with burn injuries and in need of urgent pain relief are more motivated and receptive to hypnosis than the general population, and this could account for some of the reported success stories.

Can anyone be hypnotised?

Practitioners believe that 90 per cent of people can be helped into a hypnotic state. But research shows that around 4 per cent of the population are especially susceptible to entering a trance-like state, often without any outside help or suggestion. A person's susceptibility to a hypnotic suggestion may also be related to heightened states of confusion or emotion.

Under the right conditions, whole crowds of people can be hypnotised and, for instance, mass hypnosis of people by the Indian fakirs has been well documented. During one such occurrence, a crowd believed they were watching the Indian rope trick. Later, still photographs revealed that the rope had fallen and the fakir was just standing there doing nothing.

Pregnancy and birth

Women who use simple self-hypnosis during labour experience less pain and may even have a lower risk of medical complications.

In one study US researchers assigned 42 pregnant teenagers to receive either counselling or instruction in self-hypnosis for birth. The hypnosis group learned deep relaxation and imagery techniques as well as receiving suggestions to help them respond to potential complications and improve their confidence under stress. The results were surprising – only one of the 22 women in the hypnosis group remained in hospital longer than two days after birth, compared to eight in the counselling group. More intriguing, none of the women practising self-hypnosis required surgical intervention during labour, compared with 60 per cent of those in the counselling group.

In another study 100 pregnant women with babies in breech position at 37–40 weeks of gestation received one or more sessions of hypnotherapy with suggestions for general relaxation and the release of anxiety and fear. During the therapy they were also encouraged to talk about why they thought their baby was in breech presentation. Hypnosis was repeated as regularly as possible until birth or until the baby changed to a head-down position either on its own or through external cephalic version, or ECV (where the physician applies gentle pressure on the abdomen to turn the baby). ECVs have a patchy success rate, yet among those who received hypnotherapy and/or ECV, 81 per cent of the babies spontaneously turned head down. The women receiving hypnosis were then compared with 100 carefully matched women whose success rate with ECV and standard care was only 48 per cent.

Respiratory problems

Breathing difficulties may respond somewhat to hypnotic suggestion. In a small US study of 16 children suffering from dyspnea – a medical term that describes difficulty breathing as it relates to asthma, allergies, cystic fibrosis and other lung problems – hypnosis resulted in subjective improvements in breathing in 13 out of the 16 studied. Obviously such a small study is not conclusive, but it points the way towards future areas where study might turn up useful information.

In another study published in the *Journal of the Royal Society of Medicine* in 1988, involving 16 asthmatic children whose condition could not be controlled by drugs, hypnotherapy produced amazing results. In just a year there was a drop in the number of hospital admissions in the group from 44 to 13. Six of the youngsters were able to come off the steroid asthma drug prednisolone and eight were able to reduce their dosage. In an earlier study in 1986 after 39 adults suffering from asthma were treated with hypnotherapy, 12 showed almost 74 per cent improvement in respiratory function as measured by an objective breathing test. These individuals had a 41 per cent reduction in symptoms as well as a 26 per cent drop in their use of bronchiodilators.

Other conditions

Hypnosis may be an effective way to help as many as 70 per cent of those who suffer from post-operative nausea and vomiting after general anaesthesia, even if they have already been given an anti-vomiting/nausea drug. In one study of a group of 50 women undergoing breast surgery, a combination of an audiotape (which provided hypnotic suggestion) and hypnotic induction prior to surgery had dramatic results. The women in the hypnosis group experienced significantly less vomiting – 39 per cent compared with 68 per cent in the control group – as well as less nausea and less need for post-operative painkillers. Hypnosis has also been used success-fully to relieve the pain and nausea cancer patients feel when undergoing chemotherapy.

Stomach and bowel disorders often respond to hypnosis too. For instance, when 30 individuals suffering from irritable bowel syn-drome (IBS) were given either hypnotherapy or psychotherapy, the hypnotherapy group showed dramatically better results. Another study of 33 people with IBS, published in the *Lancet* in 1989, found that four 40-minute sessions over a seven-week period improved symptoms considerably. In all 20 individuals improved and 11 of these lost their symptoms entirely. This improvement continued for at least three months without further treatment. Duodenal ulcers too may show some improvement with hypnotherapy treatment.

Impotence, which can have a physical cause but is often psycho-logical in origin, may also respond to hypnosis. In one study 60 men with impotence related to psychological causes were put into one of four groups. The first group was treated with electro-acupuncture twice weekly for six weeks. The second was treated with sham electro-acupuncture (meaning the needles were inserted into non-functioning acupoints) with the same frequency. The third group underwent hypnosis (initially three sessions a week, then once monthly; some also learned self-hypnosis). The fourth group took vitamins as a placebo. After six weeks, 60 per cent of those receiving electro-acupuncture were cured, compared to 43 per cent of those receiving sham electro-acupuncture. But in the hypnosis group 75 per cent were considered cured. Among those receiving vitamins 47 per cent reported complete resolution of difficulties. No adverse effects were reported for any of the groups.

While it is well known that hypnosis can be used to address psychological conditions, there is emerging evidence that it may also be useful in physical healing as well. In the journal *Archives of Dermatology* in 2000 researchers at the Department of Internal Medicine, College of Medicine, University of South Florida, reported the findings of their review of studies in which hypnosis was used to treat skin conditions.

To their surprise the results showed that hypnosis has been used successfully to aid the treatment of a wide array of skin problems, among them acne excorie, alopecia areata, atopic dermatitis, herpes simplex, lichen planus, pruritis, psoriasis rosacea, trichotillomania urticaria and vitiligo. While it is unlikely that hypnosis alone will cure many of these disorders, this review suggests that it may be a useful adjunct to other therapies for some individuals.

Even more unusual, a US study published in *Alternative Therapies in Health and Medicine* in 1999 found that hypnosis aided bone healing. The study involved 12 healthy adult subjects with fractures, all of whom received standard orthopaedic treatment including serial radiography and clinical assessments throughout the 12 weeks following injury. However, half were also given a hypnotic intervention in the form of individual sessions and audiotapes designed to augment healing.

To provide an objective assessment radiographic pictures were used. These revealed a notable difference in fracture healing at six weeks and a trend towards faster healing in the hypnosis group that continued through the ninth week. In addition to faster healing, the hypnosis group also had a lower use of painkillers and improved mobility. Although only a provisional study, its implications are large and, like so many studies into healing alternatives, may warrant further investigation in the future.

Cautions
Hypnotherapy is not really a cure. It is simply a way of helping patients deal with whatever situation they find themselves in. This increased sense of control, however, may have the knock-on effect of accelerating healing in some individuals. Adverse effects of hypnosis are rare but not unheard of, and the best way to avoid these is to recognise that they can occur.

As with all types of medicine, the skill of your practitioner is paramount. A 1998 review of the literature about the safety of hypnotherapy revealed what the researchers suggested was a long-standing inattention by therapists to the potential harmfulness of hypnotic interventions. These can include clients' unexpected reactions which have resulted in clinical complications such as amnesia, sudden uncontrolled expressions of emotion, paralysis, disorientation, responding too literally to hypnotic suggestions, becoming emotionally dependent on the therapist and the altering of a patient's memory. Complications, noted the reviewers, may also arise from a practitioner's unchecked need for power over others and from an inappropriately narrow focus upon the hypnotic process itself, which can distract from the more fundamental problems a patient may have.

As with any psychological therapy, it is important that your therapist is supervised (that is, has a peer or group of peers to regularly discuss his or her caseloads with). Supervision, which is still more common among psychotherapists and counsellors, provides a safety net for both client and therapist, and for your own peace of mind you may wish to enquire whether your therapist is regularly supervised.

Although hypnotherapy employs several mechanical methods to help the client reach a state of altered consciousness, your therapist should not approach the business of hypnotherapy like a mechanic. Preferably, your therapist should have some training and skill in counselling or psychotherapy. You should be given an opportunity at the end of each session to talk about what you have experienced and integrate it into your everyday consciousness. You should feel fully supported emotionally and safe in the process of entering and emerging from this other consciousness, and in exploring this 'other' side of yourself. Leaving the session with unresolved issues can make you feel worse, not better.

What to expect
Hypnotherapy usually takes place in a quiet room. Some therapists prefer to use dim lighting. At the first session your therapist will ask you about your life, the reason why you have sought this particular therapy and what you hope to achieve through the practice of hypnotherapy. He or she will take a detailed case history. During this initial session you will probably not have a therapeutic session but your therapist may try to induce a trance-like state to see how well you respond to hypnotic suggestion.

At the next session you will be asked to sit or lie down – sometimes you are given a choice – and the therapist will help you into a hypnotic state. Sometimes he or she will do this by simply speaking quietly to you. At other times you will be asked to fix your gaze on something in the room and focus on this until a change in your consciousness becomes evident.

You will probably have discussed beforehand what issues you would like to explore. While in this trance-like state, your therapist will ask you questions specific to these areas. For instance, if you wish to quit smoking, your therapist may ask you to talk about smoking, asking why you smoke and when you smoke. If smoking is a coping strategy, your therapist may help you explore more positive ways to cope with stress and reinforce the positive message that your willpower is strong enough to make such a change.

Owls and larks

According to one 1992 study different personality types are susceptible to hypnotic suggestions at different times of the day. The researchers divided people up into what they termed larks and owls. Larks are bright and fresh in the morning, whereas owls are at their best in the evening. By scheduling hypnotherapy at a time whey you are at your least best and your normal psychological defences are more fragile – larks in the evening and owls in the morning – you may derive more benefit.

If you are seeking to use hypnotherapy for pain relief, your therapy may consist of an exploration of what 'pain' means to you and may include positive reinforcing statements such as 'My body will never give me more pain than I can cope with.' Your therapist will also spend some time teaching you simple self-hypnosis techniques that you can use. Your therapist should, however, be honest with you about what can and cannot be achieved in this area. The success of such therapy depends, to some extent, on your own personality type. Some people are more susceptible to suggestion than others and some, for instance those suffering long-standing emotional pain, can require many sessions over months or years to shift.

There is no regulatory body for hypnotherapy and training tends to be short – anything from a weekend to six months. You can be referred to a hypnotherapist on the NHS or you may wish to seek private help. The British Hypnotherapy Association, the British Society of Experimental and Clinical Hypnosis and the British Society of Medical and Dental Hypnosis can all help you find a qualified practitioner in your area.

Self-hypnosis

If you are seeing a hypnotherapist, the chances are that he or she will give you some self-hypnosis suggestions that you can practise at home. These usually involve taking a few moments each day to relax and reinforce the positive suggestions you have received during your formal session.

Anyone can practise simple self-hypnosis at any time. You will need to be somewhere quiet where you can be assured of few distractions. You should be sitting comfortably in a chair. You should also be clear about what you would like to achieve, for instance, whether it is the complete relaxation of tense muscles, letting go of obsessive thoughts or steadying your nerves.

Begin by focusing on a point in front of you. It can be anything – a picture, a pattern on the wallpaper, a place where the light is reflected on the wall. Let everything except that object drop away from your mind. Stare at the object until you begin to see it change. That's the signal to close your eyes. Now focus your attention on your body. Identify somewhere in your body that you are particularly aware of at that moment. It could be your heavy eyelids or the way your lungs expand and contract as you breathe; it could even be an itch or an ache somewhere. Let everything else drop away and focus on this place until you feel a change – for instance, your breathing may slow down, or a tense muscle may begin to relax.

Once you reach this stage, you can help yourself go into a deeper trance by counting slowly backwards from 10 to zero. Some people like to imagine that they are descending a staircase and that with each step they are becoming more relaxed and receptive. Using the opposite method, counting up and ascending the staircase, is a good, gentle way of coming out of hypnosis.

When you are in this trance-like state, find as many different ways of saying the same constructive things to yourself as you can. It may help to write out a few statements you can use during self-hypnosis beforehand. Try to keep these positive; instead of saying 'I will not be tense', say 'I am relaxed and calm.' Or instead of saying 'I won't let the pressure get on top of me', say 'I am coping well with all the things I have to do.'

Try also to make good use of your imagination. For instance, if you are tense about something you have to do at work, imagine yourself coping well and with confidence at each stage of the day: getting up, travelling to work, arriving at work, seeing your colleagues, taking meetings and so on. Let yourself explore all the possibilities of the day and your reactions to them, reminding yourself at each stage that you are coping in a relaxed and positive way.

Remember that negative patterns take a long time to build up and they can take an equally long time to knock down. Doing this type of exercise just once or twice is unlikely to produce significant results. You will need to practise each day for a month or more to even begin to feel a change occurring in yourself and the way you respond to outside forces. Like many alternative therapies, hypnotherapy requires a commitment to yourself and your own well-being. It also requires a commitment of time in order to restructure the less constructive aspects of your personality and to bring out your best qualities.

Chapter 13

Massage

Commonly used for

Improving Circulation • Boosting Immunity • Lowering Stress
• High Blood Pressure • Depression and Anxiety
• Headaches • Constipation • Establishing Intimate Contact
• Skin Conditions • Detoxification

• *Requires a professional therapist* • *Suitable for self-help*

Although it has been practised for thousands of years and is the ancient origin of many modern types of bodywork including **shiatsu**, **aromatherapy** massage and **reflexology**, massage is a therapy almost by default since it requires no tools, no specific methods and no philosophy. What is more, quite apart from any physical benefit of the laying-on of hands, comforting and sensitive touch, stroking and soothing provides a profound form of spiritual nourishment for the body.

In days gone by massage was an integral part of medical care. Hippocrates, the father of modern medicine, believed all doctors should be trained in the art of 'rubbing'. Since then scientific studies have shown that a good massage really can be good medicine, providing emotional consolation, reducing pain and physical discomfort and enhancing feelings of well-being.

Today it is a widely accepted therapy; so much so that at the 1996 Summer Olympic Games the United States officially included massage therapists in its medical services team. Therapists from all 50 states converged on Atlanta to provide therapy for the athletes there.

Massage has, of course, been used for years at the Olympic Games. However, this was the first year that massage therapy was put on a par with other medical services which included MDs, physical therapists, osteopaths, nurses, athletic trainers, emergency medical technicians and physicians' assistants.

Massage can be performed at home or by a professional therapist; each has its own unique advantages. Going to a professional therapist can become a part of your life, helping you establish a regular nurturing routine for yourself. Similarly, receiving a massage from, or giving a massage to, your partner can be a way of establishing and maintaining deeper intimacy.

Because massage has been an integral part of healthcare in almost all cultures throughout the ages, many different varieties of massage now exist. In the West the most common types include:

- Deep tissue massage
- Esalen and Swedish massage
- Manual lymph drainage
- Myofascial release
- Neuromuscular and trigger point massage
- Sports massage.

Popular types of massage imported from the East include:

- Acupressure
- Tui na
- An mo, or anma
- Jin shin do
- Jin shin jyutsu.

Bodywork, body movement

Within the wider context of massage there also exist a number of other types of 'bodywork' such as Reiki, which do not require actual skin contact, but instead are similar to the therapeutic touch used in *spiritual healing*.

Body movement can also produce a sense of physical and psychological well-being. It could also be described as a form of self-massage. Through body movement we 'massage' internal organs, increase circulation, lower stress, regulate breathing and maintain muscle elasticity. Popular types of bodywork include yoga, the Alexander technique, Rolfing, Hellerwork, Aston patterning, Feldenkrais method, Pilates and Tragerwork.

There are also several East-meets-West types of massage that mix techniques from both cultures. These include:

- Shiatsu

- Reflexology

- Therapeutic touch

- Reiki

- Polarity therapy.

Among these alternative types of massage, *shiatsu* and *reflexology* are the most popular and bring an extra dimension by working on specific meridians throughout the body and in the feet and hands.

Shiatsu is sometimes described as Japanese physiotherapy. This ancient form of massage evolved from an even earlier form of massage called anma, which was brought into Japan from China (where it was known as amma) as early as the 6th century. The Japanese adapted the principles of amma while still adhering to the basic tenets of oriental healing. Often anma was used in conjunction with acupuncture, healing herbs and lifestyle modifications in order to encourage health.

It wasn't until the 1960s that shiatsu was recognised in Japan as an entity in itself, separate from anma. The shiatsu which we know today is still evolving, but typically involves many different kinds of pressure applied with the practitioner's fingers, palms, elbows and knees. Shiatsu has much in common with **acupressure**, since it also stimulates acupoints with pressure. But it is also different since pressure is sometimes applied to other areas as well.

In common with other oriental therapies, shiatsu works on the flow of energy in the body, which in Japanese is called *ki*. In shiatsu, touch is used to assess the flow and distribution of ki in the body. Once assessed, your practitioner can then begin to aid the process of restoring balance.

Some doctors may dismiss this as mumbo-jumbo, but research in Japan has shown that the energy channels or meridians used in shiatsu lie in the connective tissues. The connective tissues form a continuum throughout the body, a kind of undercoat that connects all the important body systems – circulatory, nervous, musculoskeletal and digestive, as well as all the internal organs. Every movement of the body, no matter how small, creates bioelectric signals that run through the connective tissue. Some points on the body generate more electricity than others. In oriental medicine these are known as *tsubos*. Pressure on the tsubos generates small electric currents that are then conducted along specific pathways away from their point of origin.

But pressure is not the only technique used. Shiatsu also involves gentle stretching and manipulation techniques – perhaps the result of Western influence. A therapist may press, hook, roll, sweep, shake, rotate, pat, pluck, lift, pinch and brush. Even so, there are differences between shiatsu and, say, Swedish massage. For instance, while a Swedish massage therapist may use long sweeping movements, shiatsu practitioners apply light, rhythmic movements and gentle but increasing pressure to meridians and sensitive pressure points. Sometimes the practitioner will 'hold' a hand over an area until he or she can feel a change. Often a hand may be passed over an area without touching it, either to heal or assess that area.

Reflexology, sometimes called reflex zone therapy, is a particularly sophisticated form of foot massage which has its roots in an ancient

Chinese therapy which makes use of pressure points and energy pathways similar to those used in **acupuncture** and **acupressure**. Until fairly recently there was very little written about this type of therapy, but there is evidence that ancient civilisations believed in an interaction between the feet and the rest of the body. For instance, certain African tribes practised some form of foot therapy and ancient Egyptian tomb paintings depict scenes of what appear to be foot massage.

The practice of reflexology emerged in the West in the early 1920s when an American ear, nose and throat doctor, William Fitzgerald, found that by applying pressure to a certain area of the foot he was able to anaesthetise the ear, enabling him to perform minor operations without an anaesthetic. After discovering that certain native American tribes used a similar technique, he refined his views further, using pressure on certain other foot points to alter his patients' perceptions of pain.

His research led him to divide the body into ten longitudinal zones running from the head to the toes and fingers (he called his therapy zone therapy, a term still used by some practitioners today). At this time the feet had not yet been singled out as the optimum place for treatment, so hands and the tongue were also used. Eventually word of this new technique spread throughout the US and the UK and other practitioners began refining their own techniques.

Reflexologists believe that the soles of the feet, when viewed together, represent a map of the entire body. Reading the map of the body in reflexology is fairly simple. The right foot represents the right side of the body and the left foot the left side. The reflexes, or pressure points, which are stimulated are mostly on the soles of the feet, although there are a few on the top and sides of the feet as well. The reflexologist will draw an imaginary line across the middle of the feet representing the waistline. The big toes will represent the head, the little toes the sinuses and the heart point is found in the left foot just above the waistline.

Through stimulating the feet the reflexologist aims to stimulate the body's own healing powers and its ability to rebalance itself. Study using ultrasound imaging has shown that reflexology really does increase blood flow to the organs targeted on the feet. And although it is not a diagnostic tool, some reflexologists claim to be able to detect areas of disorder or disease that may be present in the body.

Similar reflex points to those found in the feet are also found in the hands. However, the feet are normally used because the reflex points are larger. Also, the fact that feet are protected day to day in socks and shoes means they are more receptive to massage. For self-treatment, however, the hands are more convenient.

While some therapists still hold to Fitzgerald's zone theory, others see reflexology as a Western way of interpreting and understanding the Chinese meridians and their energetic connections to the rest of the body.

Metamorphosis

A related therapy to reflexology is metamorphic therapy, which makes use of the oriental principle that certain parts of the feet correspond to life in the womb. Practitioners of metamorphic technique believe that massaging each foot with a vibratory motion along a line stretching from the big toe to the heel on the inner side of the foot can help heal any physical and emotional traumas which occurred in the womb. Although originally developed to help handicapped children, this gentle technique can be used by anyone and might be supportive to those considering rebirthing. Contact the Metamorphic Association for more information.

Massage basics

Whatever type of massage you have, there are some basic techniques that all therapists use. Different therapies give them different names but overall the basic techniques used are:

Stroking Using the flat of the hand, fingertips or thumbs to create flowing, relaxing movements. Stroking is sometimes likened to performing a ballet on the skin. It is most effective when a variety of strokes are used in combination, thus strokes can be light or firm, straight or circular, brisk or slow. Stroking is usually done in the direction of the heart, except on the legs where stroking down from the thigh to the feet will provide the sensation of removing tension. When working on the head and face, the stroke is upwards, taking tension out of the top of the head. Stroking aids circulation, calms the emotions and tones the muscles.

Kneading This involves, grasping the flesh between the thumbs and fingers in a flowing motion from one hand to another. It is particularly effective on the shoulders, hips and thighs, but can also be used on other fleshy parts of the body to relax muscles, aid circulation and encourage the release of toxic build-up. If the muscles are very tense a therapist may knead them briefly and move on to another area, returning intermittently to the tense area until it begins to loosen up.

Pressure Using fingers and thumbs to work directly on specific muscles. Using small circular movements may be beneficial and very pleasurable, especially on either side of the spine during a back massage. The knuckles can also be used effectively to apply a wider area of firm pressure.

Percussion This is the name used for a variety of techniques such as cupping, hacking and pummelling (as in Swedish massage). These techniques are appropriate on the fleshy, muscular areas of the body in order to stimulate and improve circulation. Because they are stimulating, these techniques should be avoided in those who are stressed out and require a relaxing massage.

The environment of the massage is also important. Those elements which make massage a more relaxing experience include:

- a room that is warm, peaceful and, perhaps, softly lit

- a firm, but padded surface – a futon is ideal but a floor padded with towels and blankets and covered with a sheet is also suitable

- towels to cover the receiver and pillows to support the body

- massage oils are nice, but not always necessary

- the giver should have short fingernails, clean hands and no watches, bracelets or rings.

How does it work?

Almost any form of massage can improve circulation, reduce stress, relieve pain, lower heart rate and blood pressure, boost immunity, reduce swelling, strengthen muscles, promote healing, restore range and motion to the joints and help the body get rid of waste.

How it does these things is still a subject debate, but studies have shown that massage may enhance immune function by reducing the level of stress hormones in the body while increasing the number of endorphins (the body's natural painkillers and mood lifters) in the bloodstream. Reducing stress can have a profound effect on health since high levels of stress hormones such as cortisol can lower immunity. It may also increase white blood cells and natural killer-cell activity – both necessary for the body to fight off harmful micro-organisms such as viruses and bacteria.

Massage may be of short-term benefit for pain relief because it can warm and relax muscles. Often pain is made worse by the tensing of muscles against the pain. The same may apply for the relief of anxiety, since anxiety also produces muscle tension throughout the body.

There are psychological benefits from massage as well. Many of us suffer from touch deprivation and a sense of isolation. Massage fills that space. It can also make us more body aware and thus encourage us to pay closer attention to our body's needs and the signals it sends out.

What the research says

In the last decade research into the benefits of massage as a therapy for specific physical ailments has increased significantly, though many studies into its benefits are still psychologically/emotionally oriented. Specific areas which have been investigated include massage for infants or children, sports massage, massage during childbirth, anxiety or stress in otherwise healthy subjects, massage for psychiatric patients and massage on a particular body part such as the hand, foot or arm. Invariably studies are small and often observational, which means that massage is not often compared against other types of therapy. So there is little to enlighten us as to whether massage is better than herbs or conventional drugs or even a placebo in treating headache or whether hypnotherapy might be a better way to treat anxiety. Nor is it common for different types of massage to be compared to each other, so there is little information to show whether, for instance, shiatsu is more beneficial than Swedish massage.

What researchers have also failed to do is investigate over the longer term whether there are cumulative physiological as well as emotional effects of regular massage – though those who regularly give and receive massage would argue that there are.

Pain

Several small studies have examined the effect of massage on pain. One small study in 1986 looked at the effect of back massage for cancer patients receiving radiation therapy and found that the subjects reported fewer symptoms of distress, a higher degree of tranquillity and vitality, and less tension and tiredness. Yet another found that two 30-minute sessions of massage on consecutive evenings significantly reduced levels of pain in cancer patients.

An Australian study of massage for post-operative pain in 1997 suggested that individuals receiving back massage had a decreased perception of pain over the 24-hour period following surgery. Hospice patients too have reported benefits from a form of slow-stroke back massage.

Individual trials sometimes show that massage can provide effective relief for low back pain. In one US study in 2001, published in the *Annals of Internal Medicine*, it was more effective than acupuncture. However, a review of several trials into massage for low back pain concluded that on its own massage is unlikely to be consistently useful, but that it could be helpful as part of a multifaceted approach to the problem.

Most studies into massage are small and short and the clear conclusion is that the pain-relieving benefits of a single massage are short term. Relief from pain can also vary from individual to individual. In one study of subjects with soft tissue injuries, massage provided pain relief for periods of 20 seconds to 48 hours. The average period of relief was 26 hours. Another in 1990 reported that male cancer patients reported a significant decrease in pain level immediately after one 10-minute massage but, unusually, female patients did not. Nobody has yet to adequately answer why some individuals respond while others don't.

Anxiety

Other studies have examined the impact of massage therapy on anxiety, stress, sleep, rest and vitality among hospitalised patients. There is some evidence that back massage decreases anxiety and pain in this group of people. Results, however, can vary and what appears to be clear is that any therapy that focuses attention on the patient helps to reduce anxiety. For instance, in a study of anxiety in elderly residents in a long-term care facility, massage lowered anxiety but not more than conversation. Another study in 1995 found no significant differences in physiological stress or ability to cope between subjects in an intensive care unit who received massage, aromatherapy or periods of rest. In this study those subjects receiving aromatherapy reported the greatest improvement in mood and perceived anxiety.

Another study focused on the effects of back massage on sleep, anxiety and improved energy levels for elderly males in a critical care environment. Sixty-nine men were randomly assigned to a relaxation, massage or a usual-care group. Both the relaxation and massage groups experienced less anxiety and there was a significant differ-ence in the quality of sleep experienced in the massage group, as compared to the relaxation and usual-care groups.

Another study on child and adolescent psychiatric patients found that a massage was more effective at relieving anxiety than watching a relaxing videotape.

Chronic fatigue

Chronic fatigue syndrome is characterised by severe, prolonged exhaustion, as well as symptoms such as mild fever, sore throat, muscle weakness, pain and/or tenderness, headache, irritability, inability to concentrate, depression and sleep disturbance.

One study found that twice-weekly massage for people with chronic fatigue syndrome had many benefits including decreases in depression, anxiety and pain, better sleep patterns, lower cortisol (stress hormone) levels and higher dopamine (a neurotransmitter that plays a role in movement as well as in feelings of pleasure) levels.

Other conditions
A few studies have shown that massage can improve chronic tension headaches, probably by reducing stress and enhancing a general feeling of well-being.

One small study published in the *Journal of Pediatric Psychology* in 1999 revealed that children with cystic fibrosis, who were massaged daily by their parents, experienced decreased levels of anxiety, better moods and improved breathing capacity. Interestingly, anxiety levels among parents who performed the massage also decreased.

Colic can affect as many as 20 per cent of infants, though it usually resolves itself, with or without treatment, by age 4 months. However, while the baby is suffering, it can have a shattering effect on the confidence of new parents. While baby massage is sometimes promoted as the optimal way to soothe fussy or colicky babies, this has not been entirely borne out by what little research there is on the subject.

For instance, a study in the journal *Pediatrics* in 2000 compared a group of 58 infants suffering from colic. Half were massaged by the parents, while the other half were soothed only with crib vibrators. The difference, measured by a decrease in colicky behaviour, was only slightly in favour of massage. After four weeks colicky crying had decreased in 64 per cent of the babies receiving massage and 52 per cent of those in the vibration group. Around 60 per cent of parents in both groups felt that their allocated treatment had helped cure their baby of colic. But the researchers believed that what was most helpful in both groups was probably the passage of time.

Another study conducted in India in 2000 found that infant massage with sesame oil improved growth rates and sleep of healthy full-term infants. Another study showed that women suffering from postnatal depression felt a greater connection with their babies and so had less depression when they practised baby massage. Evidence for the benefits of massage on premature infants is also inconsistent.

Massaging individuals with bronchitis, especially if it involves tapping their back and chest, has been shown to help remove mucous and improve breathing. This type of therapy is commonly used on hospitalised pneumonia patients. However, another small study of reflexology for people with bronchial asthma in 1992 did not find any benefit.

Finally, one study found that ear, hand and foot reflexology significantly reduced premenstrual symptoms when compared to a sham treatment and that the benefits lasted for two months after treatment had stopped.

Cautions

There are very few contraindications for massage. In general, it should not be practised on those who have:

- a high fever

- just eaten – leave two hours after meals

- varicose veins – pressure should not be applied directly

- a history of high blood pressure

- a history of stroke or brain haemorrhage

- blood-borne cancer.

If you are pregnant, you must seek out a therapist with a full knowledge of the physiology of the pregnant woman and what is appropriate in labour and birth. Some practitioners believe that massage is not appropriate during the first trimester. Certainly, your practitioner should avoid putting pressure on certain points, and work on the lower back and sacrum should always be gentle. Certain areas on the lower leg should also be avoided at this time. If you have a history of miscarriage inform your practitioner, and if there are signs of an imminent miscarriage you should avoid massage altogether.

Similarly, there are times when it is inadvisable to apply a home treatment. Use your common sense and don't work over broken skin or sites of infection, inflammation or swelling since you run the risk of spreading infection to other areas of the body. Massaging varicose veins can release blood clots into the circulation and should be avoided. You should also seek advice if you feel you may have torn a ligament or tendon, or if you feel that you have pulled a muscle or put your back out. In such cases massage, however loving its intent, may only make the condition worse. Always seek professional advice if you are in acute pain.

Not everyone will benefit from massage. Those who could be described as being 'out of touch' with their bodies or emotions often don't feel any immediate benefit. Such people may only be aware that something is wrong when there is a pain; more subtle body symptoms, which arose before the pain became chronic, tend to pass them by. For them the sometimes subtle beneficial effects of massage may also be missed. Sometimes, however, failure to feel any benefit from the therapy can be due to the practitioner's lack of skill or that the particular style of massage does not suit the receiver (for instance, not everyone would feel comfortable with a massage that requires them to remove all their clothes). When choosing a therapy, it is best to fit the therapy to the personality. When the match is good, health has a better chance of improving.

What to expect
A good holistic massage therapist will want to establish some understanding of who you are, what is important to you and what your immediate and long-term needs are. Your initial consultation may involve a process of answering questions about all these things.

Follow-up treatments, which usually last 45 minutes to an hour, will build on what comes out of this first session. Your therapist will 'listen' to your body and sense how it reacts, for instance, whether you tense up when touched in certain places, the noises you make as the massage progresses and any feedback you have after the session and at the beginning of the next.

During shiatsu or reflexology you will remain clothed, but be sure to wear light, loose, comfortable clothes to help your therapist work and you to relax. However, an effective full body massage is difficult to give even through light clothing, therefore other types of practitioners will generally ask you to strip off your clothes and lie down either on the floor, a special mattress or a massage table. Your therapist will cover with a towel those parts of your body which are not being worked on. The towel will be repositioned as he or she works along your body. Some therapists use aromatherapy or massage oil and some do not, often according to their client's wishes.

After massage treatment a sense of well-being is common. But some people experience other effects. Be aware that massage can bring up powerful feelings in the receiver. Our bodies often 'hold', or store, emotional pain within the muscle tissues. Before beginning treatment with a professional therapist, you might want to discuss their views on this and whether they are sufficiently trained in basic counselling skills to help you talk about any feelings which come up during treatment. You should never have to leave a massage session feeling strung out, upset and unsupported.

Because of the deep relaxation that massage encourages and the stimulus to the major body systems, you may experience some 'healing reactions'. These are generally transient and can include coughing, mild headache, chilliness, aches and pains, tiredness and/or unexpected emotions. These symptoms are often a sign that the body is responding to treatment and should disappear with each successive treatment. As a general rule, you should consider a course of six to eight treatments to begin to see real change. Long-standing health problems will, of course, take longer to treat.

'Beauty' massage is not the same as therapeutic massage. Neither is relaxation massage. For you to gain real therapeutic benefit, you need to seek out a therapist who is a qualified masseuse (or masseur). Unfortunately, there are no regulations which stipulate how long or how comprehensive a massage therapist's training should be. The British Federation of Massage Practitioners has a list of 20 organisations and training schools and can supply a list of local practitioners in most areas. The Massage Therapy Institute of Great Britain also holds a large list of qualified practitioners. The Shiatsu Society can help you find a practitioner in your area. The Institute of Complementary Medicine and the British Reflexology Association keep lists of qualified reflexologists.

Chapter 14

Meditation

Commonly used for

High Blood Pressure • Anxiety • Insomnia • Headache
• Migraine • Digestive Complaints
• Menstrual and Menopausal Symptoms

• Suitable for self-help after instruction

The ability to quiet the mind has long been perceived as an effective way to keep the body healthy. The practice of meditation provides an effective way to achieve a quiet mind as well as providing a deep form of relaxation that puts the practitioner in touch with usually untapped resources for creating health, energy and mental balance.

Many of the techniques used in modern meditation such as focused awareness and sitting in a particular position have their roots in spiritual practices. What is more, many alternative therapies, among them **acupressure**, **aromatherapy**, **biofeedback**, **massage**, **yoga**, **hypnotherapy** and **spiritual healing**, involve meditation of one type or another. Given the known interactions between body and mind it is reasonable to expect meditation to produce important physiological benefits – and many studies show that it does. There are literally hundreds of ways to meditate and yet in spite of its widespread use the practice of meditation still has a kind of fringe image.

No form of meditation has been so widely researched and documented as transcendental meditation (TM), thus most of what we know about the benefits of meditation comes from research into this specific form of meditative practice.

Transcendental meditation first came to prominence in 1959 when the Maharishi Mahesh Yogi made his first visit to America. By 1975 TM was a household term. This form of meditation is an easily learned mental technique practised for 15 to 20 minutes twice daily, usually sitting comfortably with the eyes closed. Unlike hypnosis there is no suggestion and, unlike other forms of relaxation, it requires no special postures or procedures. Although the practice of TM inevitably gets lumped in with the increasing jumble of Eastern spiritual disciplines, TM is not a religion, a philosophy or a lifestyle. It does not involve any codes of conduct, value systems, beliefs or worship.

While the original goal of meditation was to lead the practitioner to a more absolute, unconditional or sacred state of consciousness – known in some Eastern cultures as enlightenment – today there is nothing inherently spiritual about meditation (unless of course the practitioner wishes it). The same techniques used to connect with one's divine self can be used to promote restful sleep, relief from stress or anxiety and improvement in a variety of health conditions.

How does it work?
Most of the benefits of meditation are subjective – feeling 'better', more 'confident' and 'healthier'. This makes them extremely difficult to research using conventional scientific research. Indeed, most scientific research strives to eliminate subjective things like feelings in the belief that these can only obscure facts. Nevertheless, and almost in spite of themselves, scientists who have investigated meditation have produced some useful objective cross-validation of the 'felt' benefits of meditation. For example, the feeling that TM reduces stress and anxiety can be validated by studying physiological changes in the body as it relaxes, such as a drop in levels of the stress hormones, decreased muscle tension and normalisation of blood pressure.

Meditation – the basics

There are four elements basic to most traditional types of meditation. They are:

A quiet place – somewhere with a minimum of distractions, conducive to rest and relaxation. This is particularly important for those just beginning to meditate. With experience you may be able to meditate easily in places where more is going on – launderettes, trains and doctors' or dentists' waiting rooms.

A comfortable or poised posture – A sitting posture is better for meditation than lying down. In the traditional meditation postures of Hindus, Buddhists, Christians, Taoists, Egyptians and others, the back is normally kept erect, though not rigidly so, in what is called a poised posture. A poised posture promotes the right state of attention/awareness for successful meditation. A lying down posture is not generally recommended because it could easily lead to sleep. However, if you are not a person who drops off easily during the day, you may try meditating in a semi-reclining position on a sofa or large armchair with the back of your head supported.

Something to focus on – Central to the benefits of meditation is the ability to attain a state of focused awareness. As in *self-hypnosis*, practitioners use a variety of things to focus on, including a physical sensation such as breathing or a part of the body, a thought or word which can be silently repeated, the process of attention itself or an external object such as a candle's flame or a statue. By deliberately focusing on a single thing a practitioner can modify the way the mind functions and its relationship to the body, as well as rest the attention in the present moment. With practice, this state can be maintained for longer and longer periods of time.

A passive attitude – The ability to let go of tension in the muscles of your arms, legs, trunk and face and of thoughts that invade your mind is essential to meditation. In this passive state things that would normally be considered distractions have less power to intrude. Beginners often try to force distracting thoughts or noises from their minds. More experienced practitioners are able to let them come and go without fighting them or letting them take over. Eventually everyday distractions will not invade your meditation time.

Studies of TM practitioners also show that brain activity, metabolic and respiratory rates all slow down during meditation. In one representative study of experienced meditators, for instance, there was a 50 per cent decrease in respiratory rate and a 40 per cent decrease in oxygen consumption during meditation. Experienced meditators can also change their body temperatures – in one study published in 1990, by as much as 61 per cent.

What the research says

Because so many disorders can be caused or made worse by stress it is not surprising that meditation claims to heal such a wide variety of health problems. Conditions such as depression, insomnia, digestive disturbances, PMS and headaches have all been shown to respond to regular meditation.

Some of the most interesting data about the overall benefits of meditation has come out of research done by insurance companies in the US and Canada, whose main concern is their bottom line. Anxious not to pay out more in claims than they have to, these companies have funded several studies into what makes a person healthy.

In 1987 a five-year study identified approximately 2,000 TM partici-pants from a database of 600,000 kept by one health insurance carrier. Analysis showed that this group used medical care, both in-patient and out-patient, half as often as other non-meditating individuals of similar age, gender and occupation. The TM group had lower sickness rates in all categories of disease, including 87 per cent fewer hospitalisations for heart disease and 55 per cent less cancer. What is more, the difference between the TM and non-TM groups was greatest for individuals over 40 years of age – the ones statistically most likely to fall ill from these diseases.

Another study of 677 TM participants, both men and women, enrolled in a health insurance programme in Quebec, Canada, showed similar results. In the three years before starting the technique, the group's medical expenses had been typical for their age and sex. After taking up TM there was a 5 to 7 per cent reduction in medical expenses cumulatively every year. After seven years, health costs in the group had dropped by almost 50 per cent.

Stress
Most of those who take up meditation do so because they are looking for a way to cope with or manage stress in their day-to-day lives. Stress stemming from work, family, illness or environment can contribute to a wide range of conditions such as anxiety, hypertension and heart disease. During meditation respiratory and pulse rates slow down placing less strain on the lungs and heart and doing this regularly may have a cumulative beneficial effect on health.

Practitioners of TM believe that meditation takes them to what is sometimes referred to as the fourth state of consciousness – a type of 'restful alertness' which is very different from sleep. One meta-analysis that compared TM with other forms of relaxation and meditation found that TM was the most effective technique for reducing anxiety and improving psychological health. However, while some research has shown that meditation is different from eyes-closed resting, other research suggests there is little difference between the two.

High blood pressure and heart disease
TM can be an effective non-drug technique for reducing high blood pressure, though often reductions are small. Nevertheless, meditation is a key component of Ornish therapy, a multifaceted approach to heart disease devised by US doctor, Dean Ornish. Dr Ornish's studies have shown a significant reduction of coronary artery narrowing in those practising one hour of stress management, including meditation, daily.

Other studies have found that meditation has a beneficial effect on hypertension and other risk factors for heart disease. In one 1998 study of 127 African Americans aged between 55 and 85 researchers concluded that meditation was as effective in lowering blood pressure as most antihypertensive drugs. In this study regular meditation produced an average reduction in systolic blood pressure of 10.7 points – more than double the reduction experienced by another group practising progressive muscle relaxation.

A year later researchers at the Medical College of Georgia found that meditation lowers blood pressure by reducing blood vessel constriction. This small study compared a group of 14 healthy non-meditating adults with 18 people who practised regular TM. In one test the meditators' veins were 6.5 per cent less constricted, while in the other group, who were told simply to relax, constriction of the veins increased by 1.6 per cent.

Another 11-month study in 1979 showed that cholesterol levels decreased significantly in individuals practising TM, compared to those who did not meditate. Similarly, after conducting an 11-month study with a group of African Americans who were at risk of developing cardiovascular disease, researchers from the University of California, Los Angeles, and the College of Maharishi Vedic Medicine in Fairfield, Iowa, concluded that a state of restful alertness may trigger self-repair mechanisms in the body that can lead to the regression of atherosclerosis. In this study those practising TM showed a decrease of 0.098 mm in artery wall thickness, compared to an increase of 0.054 mm in those who did not meditate. This was the first controlled study to suggest that stress reduction alone could reduce atherosclerosis without changes in diet and exercise.

High levels of lipid peroxide, a sign that oxidative stress due to the presence of free radicals (toxic by-products of metabolism known to damage the vascular system), have been shown to be an important factor in the formation of atherosclerosis and are directly associated with the ageing process. Until recently researchers have not paid much attention to the fact that psychological stress may be linked to physiological stress. However, data from a 1998 study showed that by lowering stress with TM, levels of lipid peroxide could also be lowered by as much as 15 per cent.

Cancer

A question mark will always hang over meditation as a cancer treatment. This is because, among other things, it is considered unethical to conduct large-scale randomised trials – where one group of people with a potentially lethal disease receives treatment and another doesn't – into the subject. Therefore, proponents of cancer regimes which involve meditation rely solely on case histories.

Such reports, however inspiring, are few and far between. In one story, included in a collection of anecdotes about spontaneous remission, a 64-year-old man developed cancer of the rectum. He was a psychologist by profession and refused surgery, pursuing instead a course of intensive meditation at home for one or two hours a day. He noted subjective improvements in his condition within two weeks. By six weeks he no longer needed enemas to relieve the partial obstruction of his colon. One year after beginning treatment his meditation practice averaged three hours per day in 'divided doses' and he was totally free of symptoms.

For this patient, like so many others, dedication, a strictly positive attitude, support from care-givers and physicians who believe in the possibility of recovery, were the essential ingredients leading to cure. For the majority of cancer patients, however, it may be that meditation and other approaches to relaxation are most useful in helping them stay calm and focus on how best to handle the illness and proceed with life.

Ageing
No technique (or drug) can promise eternal life or ageless ageing. But there is some evidence that those who practise meditation may help their bodies maintain greater vitality for longer. For instance, a 1982 study compared a TM group (average age 50) to a similar non-meditating group using a measure called the Adult Growth Examination (a test measuring indicators of biological age such as systolic blood pressure, hearing and eyesight). It found that the biological age of long-term (five years or more) participants on the TM programme was, on average, 12 years less than their actual chronological age.

Another way of marking biological age is by measuring blood concentrations of the hormone dehydroepiandrosterone sulphate (DHEAS), levels of which decline with age. In one study levels of DHEAS were found to be significantly higher in a group of 326 adult

TM practitioners than in a similar group of 972 individuals who did not meditate. The differences were largest for the oldest age categories.

In another study 73 residents of homes for the elderly (average age 81 years) were randomly assigned to one of three apparently similar treatments: TM, another technique to increase self-awareness and a relaxation programme. A fourth group received usual care. The TM group improved significantly more than all the other groups on all measures tested, including blood pressure, mental health and cognitive function. Moreover, after three years the survival rate for the TM group was 100 per cent, compared to 88 per cent and 65 per cent for the other treatment groups, respectively, and 77 per cent for the untreated group.

Addictions

Meditation may be similarly useful in treating addiction to cigarettes, alcohol and drugs. The transcendental meditation technique may be useful on many levels, for instance, as a coping strategy in helping to deal with drug addiction, a useful tool through which individuals can control the immune system, and an effective manager of stress and pain.

A statistical meta-analysis of studies totalling 198 independent treatments for both heavy and casual users found that TM produced a significantly larger reduction in tobacco, alcohol and illicit drug use than either standard substance abuse treatments (including counselling, pharmacological treatments, relaxation training and the Twelve-Step programme) or prevention programmes (such as that to counteract peer pressure and promote personal development).

Another review of 24 studies on the benefit of TM in the treatment and prevention of the misuse of drugs confirmed the multi-level benefits of TM. When taken together TM did appear to address the problems of addiction on many levels providing some immediate relief from symptoms as well as long-range improvements in well-being, self-esteem empowerment and other areas of psychological health. What is more, whereas the effects of conventional programmes typically decrease sharply after three months, the effects of TM on total abstinence from tobacco, alcohol and illicit drugs ranged from 51 per cent to 89 per cent over an 18–22 month period.

Other conditions

Chronic pain can systematically erode quality of life. Although great strides are being made in traditional medicine to treat recurring pain, treatment often involves drugs or surgery, both of which can bring a trade-off of unwanted effects.

Pain can be made worse by certain emotional states such as anxiety. When you are anxious your threshold for pain decreases and the heightened perception of pain causes more anxiety. Meditation may be useful in breaking this vicious cycle.

While meditation may not eliminate pain, it can help people cope more effectively. In one study over half the participants suffering from fibromyalgia found pain symptoms improved when they meditated. Likewise, research with HIV-positive men found that meditation improved immune function as well as psychological well-being.

Today childbirth-preparation classes routinely teach pregnant women deep breathing exercises to minimise the pain and anxiety of labour. Few call it breath meditation, but that's what it is.

Cautions

There are few reports of adverse reactions to meditation. In general, the same guidelines apply here as would for *hypnotherapy*. Those who are not in touch with reality, who are strongly paranoid or who suffer from psychosis, should avoid meditation as it can make their condition worse.

Those with psychiatric conditions such as schizophrenia are probably at greatest risk of experiencing adverse effects and there is evidence to suggest that in these individuals meditation can bring on psychotic episodes. Meditation can also bring with it a temporary loss of sense of self – those with a poor sense of self may not benefit from it and those who enter into it intensely may feel an occasionally disturbing loss of self.

Meditation, although relaxing, can sometimes produce paradoxical effects such as an increase in tension, confusion, disorientation and anxiety.

People suffering from overwhelming anxiety should probably consider a course of counselling rather than meditation so that any insights gained will not be the cause of more anxiety, but instead will be gained in a supportive and supervised environment

There are around 50 centres in the UK that teach TM; you can go along for a free introductory session before signing up for training sessions. You can write to a freepost address for details. The Friends of the Western Buddhist Order (which has centres in Scotland and England) also run courses.

Chapter 15

Naturopathy

Commonly used for

Heart Disease • Arthritis • Digestive Complaints
• Auto-immune Diseases • Allergies
• Skin Conditions • Diabetes • Stress
• Chronic Infections • Pre-menstrual Syndrome • Fatigue

*• Requires a professional therapist • Some aspects
suitable for self-treatment*

While naturopathy is a relatively new therapy and very much a product of the West, its philosophy dates back to the 5th century BC and the time of the founder of modern medicine, Hippocrates, perhaps best known for saying, 'Let your food be your medicine.'

The term 'naturopathy' – a combination of the terms 'nature cure' and 'homeopathy' – emerged in the US in the early 1900s. The man credited with founding naturopathy, Benedict Lust, originally trained in the methods of the European nature cure movement but gradually added homeopathy, herbalism and manipulation to his repertoire, as well as setting rigorous training standards for the practice of this new, somewhat eclectic therapy.

While based on ancient principles, the therapeutic approach of naturopathy represents the essence of a broad, holistic attitude to health and disease. In naturopathic philosophy people are seen as an integral part of nature and the universe, and good health is dependent on maintaining internal harmony as well as with the wider environment. Naturopaths, for instance, believe that the world is governed by certain natural laws and that most disease is the direct result of ignorance and violation of these laws. Accordingly, good health can be maintained and healing will result if an individual engages in the following practices:

- Consuming natural, unrefined organically grown foods

- Getting adequate amounts of rest and exercise

- Living a moderately paced lifestyle

- Having constructive and creative thoughts and emotions

- Avoiding environmental toxins

- Maintaining the health and efficiency of the body's eliminatory system.

The body-machine

Almost as soon as Sir Isaac Newton formulated his explanation of the physical world, medical thought began to view the body as a machine in which various parts (lung, heart etc.) could be studied in isolation. This philosophy was known as mechanism. Mechanism is the philosophical foundation of today's conventional medicine and mechanists maintained that the only difference between life and non-life was the degree of complexity of the system.

According to mechanistic philosophy, the symptoms and the disease are the same thing – disruptions in the normal function of the body are caused by some 'offending agent'. If the physician can make the symptoms disappear then, by this theory, he has succeeded in making the disease disappear too. We now know that this is patently not true. For instance, a powerful painkiller such as morphine may well take away the pain, but it does not cure the disease. Similarly, a surgeon may remove a cancerous growth, but without attention to what caused the cancer in the first place, the chances of the growth returning and spreading are high.

These principles, which guided early practitioners, also hold true today. There is, of course, nothing remarkable about such advice – except perhaps the fact that so few of us follow it.

How does it work?

Naturopathy is a complete healthcare system. It is both a way of life and a concept of healing that makes use of natural remedies such as **herbal medicines**, hydrotherapy (using water both externally and internally), **massage**, manipulative therapies such as **osteopathy** and **homeopathy**, as well as providing advice on nutrition, exercise and other methods that may help to prevent and treat disease. In this respect it is the Western equivalent of ethnic therapies such as **Ayurveda** and **traditional Chinese medicine**. The practice of naturopathy is founded on six basic principles:

1. *First, do no harm.* A principle dating back to Hippocrates, and the guiding tenet of the Hippocratic oath which all doctors are expected to uphold. Naturopaths aim to choose remedies and natural therapeutics to safely treat illness without causing harmful side effects.

2. *Vis medicatrix naturae.* Otherwise known as the healing power of nature. While not strictly a form of energy medicine (like **homeopathy**), naturopaths believe in the fundamental ability of the body to heal itself given the opportunity and if 'obstacles to cure' are removed (quitting smoking, for instance, provides the lung tissues with the opportunity to use the healing power of nature to repair themselves).

3. *Treat the cause, not the effect.* For example, you don't have a headache because of an aspirin deficiency. Naturopaths seek out the underlying cause of the disease rather than trying to suppress the symptoms with treatment.

4. *Treat the whole person.* This means taking into account the emotional, mental and spiritual aspects of illness, as well as its physical manifestations.

5. *The physician is a teacher.* Part of the naturopath's job is to empower patients by educating them about healthy lifestyles. The

key to the success of naturopathic treatment is the high level of involvement that patients are expected to have in their own healing process.

6. *Prevention is the best cure.* The emphasis that naturopathy places on lifestyle is one of the ways in which it is most effective. Naturopaths can treat illness when it arises, but fundamental to its philosophy is the idea that if we don't create an environment where disease can develop, then good health is much easier to maintain and disease, should it strike, is likely to be much more responsive to treatment.

In applying these principles, the naturopathic practitioner will aim to fit the therapy to the person, working with their own constitutional and emotional strengths to obtain the best result.

Unconventional diets

Most recommendations for unconventional diets are made on the basis of theory, rather than actual research data. Naturopaths may recommend any number of different ways of eating, according to their diagnosis. However, apart from the withdrawal of all allergenic foods, which can be effective in relieving allergies and auto-immune disease such as arthritis (see **fasting & detox**), none of the diets below has anything other than anecdote to show that it works.

Hay diet – where proteins and carbohydrates are eaten separately

Raw food diet – avoiding all cooked foods

Stone age diet – avoiding grains, pulses and products of the agricultural revolution.

In addition, while there is some evidence to suggest considerable benefit of diets high in vegetables and fruits, particularly in preventing heart disease and certain types of cancer and in promoting longevity, there is little evidence to show that strict vegetarian, macrobiotic and vegan diets are universally 'better' than omnivorous ones. The key benefit is the inclusion of vegetables, not the exclusion of meats.

What the research says

Naturopathy can be used to treat all the conditions that can be seen in any typical general practice. Like many alternative therapies, it can be particularly successful at treating chronic conditions that have failed to respond to conventional methods. In addition, the naturo-pathic approach can work in a complementary capacity with conventional medicine. For example, a person suffering congestive heart failure and taking drugs such as digoxin or furosemide may benefit from the appropriate use of vitamin supplements such as thiamine, carnitine and coenzyme Q10.

While there is copious research to show that these supplements are of value in congestive heart failure, they are rarely prescribed by conventional physicians because they have not been educated in their use.

Similarly, there is evidence that disease-prevention programmes that involve the aspects of healthy living promoted by naturopaths can provide substantial benefits. In one study participation in wellness-oriented programmes has been found to reduce the number of days of disability (43 per cent in one study), the number of days spent in hospital (54 per cent in one study) and the amount of money spent on healthcare (up to 76 per cent in one study). Given this it is not surprising that the largest ever study into patient satisfaction, comparing natural therapies with conventional general practice care in the Netherlands (where naturopathy is fully integrated into the healthcare system) found that among the 3,782 people surveyed, those who consulted a natural health practitioner felt they had better results.

Research into naturopathy is limited and certainly none exists to evaluate the system as a whole. Elsewhere in this book the research data for components of nature cure such as *homeopathy*, *osteopathy*, *massage* and *herbal medicine* has been reviewed. While it is beyond the scope of this book to delve deeply into all the conditions which might respond to a naturopathic approach, below are some common conditions that may respond to the nutritional element of naturopathy.

Headaches

Headaches, particularly migraine, may respond well to the naturo-pathic approach of detecting allergies. Several well-conducted studies have shown that the removal of allergens from the diet can greatly reduce migraine symptoms anywhere from 30 to 93 per cent. The key foods that appear to trigger headaches are cow's milk, wheat, chocolate, eggs and the food additive benzoic acid.

The mineral magnesium is necessary to maintain the health of the vascular system. Because of this it is not surprising to find there is reasonable evidence to suggest that deficiencies in magnesium can result in both migraine and tension headaches. However, the evidence suggests that magnesium supplementation is only effective in migraine sufferers who are genuinely magnesium deficient.

Mega-dosing – too much of a good thing?

Nutritional therapy is an offshoot of naturopathy. However, in some parts of the world, particularly in America, this therapy, which involves treating disease and promoting health with the use of specific nutritional supplements, has become something of a monster. There is no doubt that many conditions – more than can be detailed in this book – respond to supplementation with vitamins, minerals, essential fatty acids, amino acids and other supplements. However, the tendency in nutritional therapy is to be too focused on this single aspect of care, to the exclusion of others.

While naturopaths sometimes use supplements as part of the nature cure, they are rarely used in isolation. Nor would the naturopath view disease in such a limited cause and effect way. What is more, many people use supplements as medicine, subscribing to the more-is-better philosophy. This may have its own drawbacks, since in the body levels of nutrients are very finely balanced. And while it is true that this balance can be affected by outside forces such as poor diet and stress and taking certain medications, mega-dosing with nutritional supplements could be viewed as an aggressive and ham-fisted approach to health. In the final analysis, in a body that is already not functioning optimally, such an approach may only serve to make the problems of deficiency and imbalance worse.

Benign prostatic hyperplasia

This condition, which is characterised by an enlargement of the prostate, can be the result of several lifestyle factors. Increased alcohol consumption is one thing that raises a man's risk. In a 17-year study in Hawaii involving 6,581 men, alcohol intake of at least 25 oz per month was strongly associated with an eventual diagnosis of BPH.

The nutritional approach may yield beneficial results. The mineral zinc, for instance, is involved in the metabolism of androgenic hormones and adequate zinc intake and absorption is necessary for the prostate to function properly. Studies show that zinc supplementation can reduce the size of the prostate.

Supplements of fatty acid complexes containing linoleic, linolenic and arachidonic acids can also improve BPH symptoms for some men. In one small study all 19 men showed a gradual decrease in the amount of urine left in the bladder after voiding. By the end of the study 12 of the 19 had no residual urine left after urinating.

Other conditions

Chronic health problems associated with exposure to environmental chemicals can be difficult to treat. Many conventional doctors are not trained to detect such problems, and even if they were, would not always know how best to proceed. Naturopathy, with its emphasis on detoxification, may be one way to approach the problem.

A 1997 review of the clinical records of 122 persons using naturopathic approaches to removing environmental toxins from the body showed that several benefits could be gained from a programme that included exercise, heat therapy, hydrotherapy, colonic irrigation, homeopathy, massage, counselling and nutritional supplements. In this review there were reductions in a wide range of symptoms including asthma, auto-immune disorders and multiple chemical sensitivities, fatigue, allergies, addiction and gastrointestinal and liver disorders. Each person was treated for a minimum of 15 sessions and 46.4 per cent of the participants rated their results as great, while 36.6 per cent reported moderate to good outcomes.

Cautions
Perhaps the most controversial aspect of naturopathic treatment is **fasting & detox**. It is important that fasts and special diets are properly supervised. As discussed in Chapter 8, fasting can be detrimental to those who are already very run down, can place a burden on the liver and kidneys by overloading them with the release of toxins and make an individual feel very unwell indeed. People taking conventional medications should also beware of practitioners who advise them to quit taking their medications. A recent (and admittedly uncommon) case in Canada, where a naturopath recommended that a 12-year-old diabetic girl use bath salts and herbs instead of insulin – a move which resulted in the girl's death three days later – should sound a note of caution to anyone using life-sustaining conventional medications. For other cautions please see under individual therapies.

What to expect
Your first consultation with a naturopath will take approximately an hour, during which time the therapist will take a full medical history. Subsequent sessions take approximately half an hour.

In practice, naturopaths advise on lifestyle changes, dietary changes or methods of purifying the body with occasional fasting, hydrotherapy treatments and exercise programmes in conjunction with specific remedies, acupuncture or specific herbal or homeopathic remedies. Many naturopaths are also trained in osteopathy (and vice versa) and this may feature in their treatment. The number of sessions you require will vary according to the type of condition you are trying to treat or what you are trying to achieve. Naturopathy is a gentle form of medicine that works slowly, so do not expect instant results.

Today, in the US naturopathic doctors are practitioners who have attended university pre-med courses and are then trained for a further four years as specialists in natural medicine. In the UK training does not require any background in medicine, but can still be very rigorous, requiring several years of study. Naturopathic training approaches the study of the body and its systems in the same way conventional medical training does and a naturopath will go about the business of diagnosis using techniques similar to those of a general practitioner, though the interpretation of what he or she finds may be very different.

Having said this, naturopathy is not a regulated profession in the UK and anyone can call themselves a naturopath or set up a naturopathic school and register of practitioners. To find a qualified practitioner look for one who is registered with the General Council and Register of Naturopaths – the only organisation that requires its members to have completed full-time training.

Chapter 16

Osteopathy & Chiropractic

Commonly used for

• Back Pain • Muscle and Joint Pain • Neck and Shoulder Pain •
Improving Posture • Low Energy • Oedema • Headaches •
• Bladder Problems • Morning Sickness • Poor Circulation •
• Indigestion and Heartburn

• Requires a professional therapist

Not every alternative therapy has its roots in the mysterious East. Both osteopathy and chiropractic emerged in the West a little over 100 years ago. Both evolved from the 'bone setters' of early America and began life with a somewhat mechanistic view of the body – though many practitioners in both disciplines now take a much more holistic approach than their rustic predecessors.

Osteopathy is a system of diagnosis and therapy which was devised by an American doctor, Andrew Still, in the late 1800s. Still was an engineer, so not surprisingly he developed an early interest in the body as a machine. He was also an army surgeon whose experience taught him just how brutal the conventional medicine of the day could be. Spurred on by the fact that three of his children died from spinal meningitis, he began to explore more compassionate ways of approaching the process of preventing disease and maintaining health.

213

Dr Still quickly became convinced that the body was a self-regulating, self-healing organism. He was among the first to stress the importance of the structure of the body in relation to its function. Good health, in his view, was the result of the joints being properly aligned and the spine played a vital role in supporting the whole structure of the body, linking not only joints but muscles as well. When any of these systems was out of alignment, he reasoned, illness was the likely result. Although radical for its time, Still's theory was not entirely new. The ancient Greeks and Romans also appreciated the role of the spine in our overall health and well-being and practitioners of **traditional Chinese medicine** and **Ayurveda** also believe in the benefits of gentle manipulation of body tissues.

Other practitioners such as William Garner Sutherland took Still's ideas and refined them further. Sutherland, in particular, is credited with proving – in spite of medical scepticism – that the body, even the bony skull, is in a constant dynamic state of motion and that our tissues, organs and bones have a unique pulse and are continuously expanding and contracting in a harmonious rhythmic impulse.

Osteopathy spread from America to Britain in the early 1900s. Today it is a flourishing and well-respected system of physical therapy. In the UK osteopathy has been accorded the status of a statutorily self-regulating profession, which means that patients are protected by law from untrained and unauthorised practitioners.

Although primarily viewed as a therapy for back and neck problems, osteopathy has a good track record in treating a wide range of other common problems. Today, a great many osteopaths see their role as encompassing more than just a mechanical cause and effect view of the body. Many are also trained in **naturopathy** and approach the treatment of their patients in a holistic way. Apart from joint manipulation, osteopaths believe that soft tissue manipulation can help improve the flow of vital energy in the body, in much the same way as **acupuncture** does.

Bowen technique

Tim Bowen was an industrial chemist who changed his profession to become an osteopath. But Bowen soon abandoned conventional osteopathic techniques and began to develop his own extremely gentle, very specific form of massage. Bowen's therapeutic technique was to move his thumbs and fingers across various tendons and muscles, applying only the sort of limited pressure that an eye might withstand. The moves took the form of a rolling action that, Bowen said, disturbed the muscle, creating 'energy' throughout the body. To concentrate the 'energy' in certain parts of the body, Bowen put *blockers* and *stoppers* at various points. His treatments, which rarely lasted more than 20 minutes, contained many frequent deliberate pauses to allow the body to respond to the information gradually. Bowen's patients typically reported a significant response within 48 hours, though such reports have never been confirmed through any formal research. To find a Bowen practitioner contact the Bowen Association UK.

Chiropractic

The first documented chiropractic adjustment was performed in 1895. A janitor in the building where the founder of chiropractic, Daniel David Palmer, worked had been deaf for 17 years. He lost his hearing when, while stooping down to pick something up, he felt something give way in his back and immediately became deaf. Palmer reasoned that the deafness was due to this back injury and could be restored by reversing the process. A relatively simple adjustment to a misaligned vertebra in the janitor's neck restored his hearing completely. Within two years Palmer had founded the first Chiropractic School and Cure.

Chiropractic places even more emphasis on the spine than osteopathy. Chiropractors will sometimes use X-rays and other conventional diagnostic tools to help them reach a diagnosis and will generally treat all perceived disorders through spinal manipulation. The treatment is more robust than in osteopathy and can involve sharp, thrusting movements. Chiropractic aims to put things back in place: to adjust bad posture, restore function of the spinal and pelvic joints and correct any interference with the nervous system which has been caused by deviation in the spinal and pelvic alignment.

In common with osteopathy, most people go to a chiropractor because of back and neck pain. As a therapy it also has a good track record for easing headache pain. Individuals who have sustained an injury from a fall or car accident, even if it was long ago, also report a reduction in pain with chiropractic treatment.

Also, like osteopathy, there can be a wide range of practice among chiropractors. Some prefer to work just on the spine, whereas others take a more holistic view of the body, believing that simply focusing on the mechanics of the spine is missing the original aim of the therapy. These latter therapists will treat the spine and extremities and give counsel on diet and lifestyle in order to treat the whole person. Some liken their practice to that of the homeopath, believing that information on the mental, emotional and spiritual symptoms is necessary to make a more comprehensive diagnosis of the individual's needs. Not all chiropractors take this view, however, so it might be worth spending some time talking to individual therapists to find out what their philosophy of health is, and whether this resonates with yours. Chiropractic is a statutorily self-regulating profession in the UK.

Gentle chiropractic

McTimoney Chiropractic is a particularly gentle whole-body manipulative technique. Developed by John McTimoney, it uses a very light touch to correct the alignment of bones and other joints of the body to restore nerve function, alleviate pain and promote better overall health. Unlike regular chiropractic, it can safely be used on babies, indeed McTimoney practitioners believe that chiropractic care should begin at birth. McTimoney-Corley chiropractic is a further variation on the technique. To contact a practitioner get in touch with the McTimoney Chiropractic Association.

How does it work?

Little research has ever been done to determine specifically how osteopathy or chiropractic work, but several theories prevail.

What the manipulative therapies call homeostatic forces, practitioners of energy or ethnic medicines might call life energy, the vital force, *qi* or *prana* – it is the governing, life-giving principle of the body that maintains balance throughout the entire system.

From the manipulative therapist's point of view, the musculoskeletal system is important because it is connected to the autonomic nervous system, which permeates the entire body and connects all the muscles, tendons and internal organs, and whose function depends partly on the unhindered flow of nerve impulses and blood.

The autonomic nervous system, which is comprised of the sympathetic and parasympathetic systems, is responsible for maintaining homeostasis, the dynamic balance of the body. There is evidence to show that when the body is exposed to toxins, when there is disease or trauma, the sympathetic nervous system (the body's first line in maintaining homeostasis and which is involved in the control of, among other things, heart rate, breathing, digestion and elimination) can become over-stimulated. This can result in a range of disorders such as hormonal imbalance, digestive disorders, breathing difficulties, high blood pressure and elevated blood sugar.

In addition, we now know that nerves don't just transport electrical impulses; they also transport fats, proteins and other essential cell substances, a fact that goes some way towards explaining why the proper functioning of the nervous system is so central to our continued good health. Working through the spine can restore sympathetic nervous function to normal, and in so doing may exert a healing effect on many parts of the body.

Increased knowledge of the interconnectedness of the musculoskeletal and nervous systems has even moved some doctors to suggest that conventional medicine could increase its understanding of the back and its problems by adopting a chiropractic/osteopathic understanding of back pain. In this way the back then becomes part of a whole, complex structure that includes the spine, hips, pelvis, ribs and their surrounding muscles and ligaments and other supporting tissues, as well as the organs contained within those bony structures. Dysfunction or displacement of any of these parts of the structure can eventually lead to backache.

Both osteopathy and chiropractic use similar techniques, working with bones, muscles and connective tissue. The high velocity thrust is one well-known technique – a short, sharp motion, usually applied to the spine. This is the technique that produces that distressing 'crack' that has come to be associated particularly with chiropractic. More gentle techniques are also applied to soft tissues, as are methods intended to increase the range of motion in a particular joint.

In addition to soft tissue manipulation, gentle mobilisation of the joints and sometimes more forceful movement of the joints, osteopaths can also work through the head to treat a number of disorders. This is called cranial osteopathy. Comparing the skills of a cranial osteopath to osteopathy in the rest of the body is rather like comparing the skills of a watchmaker to those of a car manufacturer. Cranial work is very precise and gentle, providing maximum benefit with minimum input. This is what makes it particularly suitable for babies. By gently manipulating specific areas of the skull and upper neck, your practitioner will be able to feel the pulse, or energy, of the membranes, cerebrospinal fluid and brain (which are quite different from the pulse of the blood) and use these to make a diagnosis and as a guide to appropriate treatment.

What the research says
While both osteopathy and chiropractic were originally viewed as complete systems of healthcare, today they tend to be used for very specific problems or as adjuncts to conventional care. In general, chiropractic has benefited from more research than osteopathy. Even so, making sense of the results is difficult because most studies are small and because conventional researchers do not always differentiate, in their thinking or their writing, between chiropractic, osteopathy and physiotherapy.

Likewise, guidelines for the referral of patients to physiotherapy or spinal manipulation do not differentiate between these different types of therapy. This lack of a precise, common language may be at the root of continuing disagreements over which type of physical therapy is best for which type of problem. Medical research has not helped to clarify the issue; indeed, researchers have been found to deliberately misuse terms such as 'chiropractic' in their research, especially if the result is negative!

In one important paper, published in the *Journal of Manipulative and Physiological Therapies* in 1995, the ways in which this sort of bias creeps into back pain research were highlighted. In a review of studies on adverse effects of spinal manipulation, the researchers found that when there was an adverse effect, it was more often attributed to 'chiropractic' (often regardless of whether the original paper actually focused on chiropractic). When there was no adverse effect, the therapy was usually referred to as 'spinal manipulation'. As the reviewers noted, 'In many cases, this is not accidental; the authors had access to original reports that identified the practitioner involved as a non-chiropractor.'

Another problem, common to many types of alternative therapy, is the quality of the studies which can be pretty marginal. Indeed one review of 36 randomised clinical trials comparing spinal manipulation to other treatments concluded that out of a possible 100 points (indicating the highest quality studies) the highest score achieved by studies of spinal manipulation was 60. Nevertheless, the review showed a significant number of positive results for spinal manipulation, which clearly justified more and better research into the field.

Back pain

This is by far the most common reason why people seek the help of an osteopath or chiropractor and there is reasonable evidence that it can help. In 1990 a study, conducted by the Medical Research Council in the UK, compared conventional hospital treatment with chiropractic for 741 men and women suffering from low back pain. After three years, improvement in the chiropractic group was 29 per cent greater than in the hospital group. Five years later the scientists reviewed the progress of the group and found firm evidence for the benefits of chiropractic over the longer term.

In another trial, osteopathic spinal manipulation was compared with the use of pain-relieving drugs in 178 people with chronic low back pain. Individuals in both groups improved over the 12-week study period, suggesting that osteopathy was as effective as the drugs. But as the authors pointed out, osteopathy had the advantage of producing no unpleasant side effects (such as stomach upsets) sometimes associated with the use of analgesics, anti-inflammatory agents and muscle relaxants.

The problem with bi-peds

It has been argued that the human animal is poorly adapted to its upright posture. In bi-peds – that is, two-footed animals – the discs and joints of the spine have become weight bearing, but they were originally intended to be slung underneath a horizontal back. The stomach and the pelvic contents, including the diaphragm, sag easily which can contribute to health problems such as constipation, hernia and hypertension. In our upright position, the heart and much of the circulatory system must work against gravity and the air passage of the lungs must drain upwards by coughing and sneezing.

Adding insult to injury, we don't use our bodies in a healthy way. We sit at desks all day, performing small, repetitive movements over long periods of time. Women, in particular, wear restrictive clothing and high heels that prevent free movement. Certain body states such as obesity, pregnancy, and emotional stress which makes the muscles tense up, only add further strain, affecting almost every area of the body.

These are just a few reasons why, when an osteopath or chiropractor treats your aching back, they may not be simply treating your aching back.

Headaches

Chiropractic research suggests that chronic headaches may be the result of neck injury or strain (which can sometimes occur even without the sufferer knowing it) that can be addressed through spinal adjustment. When an Australian researcher conducted a study of 105 people, each suffering from regular, sustained headaches, he found that 80 per cent of those treated with nine short sessions of chiropractic manipulation reported sustained benefits two years after treatment.

In another study of 53 subjects suffering from chronic headache conducted in Denmark in 1997, half were randomised into receiving spinal manipulation or laser treatment combined with deep friction massage twice weekly for three weeks. The use of analgesic decreased by 36 per cent in the spinal manipulation group, but was unchanged in the massage group; the number of headaches per day decreased by 69 per cent in the manipulation group, compared with 36 per cent in the massage group; and headache intensity decreased by 36 per cent in the manipulation group, compared with a 17 per cent decrease in the massage group.

In yet another study in New Zealand, 85 volunteers suffering from migraine were randomly allocated either spinal manipulation performed by a physiotherapist, spinal manipulation performed by a chiropractor or mobilisation performed by a medical practitioner or physiotherapist. No difference was found between the groups in terms of reducing frequency, duration or disability of attacks, but the chiropractic patients did report a greater reduction in the pain associated with their attacks.

Similar results have been found elsewhere. In the US in 1995 a group of 150 subjects with chronic tension headaches were randomly assigned to receive either 10–30 mg of the antidepressant/sedative amitriptyline at bedtime for six weeks, or chiropractic treatment twice a week for six weeks. Results showed that while both groups improved at similar rates at first, at follow-up four weeks after treatment ceased, chiropractic management was more effective than the drugs for reducing pain and improving overall health. More than 80 per cent of the drug group reported side effects such as drowsiness, dry mouth and weight gain, as opposed to around 4 per cent in the manipulation group who reported neck soreness and stiffness.

Even amidst reasonable evidence that spinal manipulation can aid headache pain, some researchers are miserly with their praise. For instance, a review of 30 years of research up to 1996 found 134 references to chiropractic in the treatment of neck pain and headache in the existing literature. Analysis of these showed that spinal manipulation compared favourably with muscle relaxants, providing somewhat better relief after three weeks of treatment. The authors, who were conventional scientists, rather grudgingly concluded that spinal manipulation 'probably' provided short-term benefits for some individuals and had only a small complication rate.

Respiratory problems

In individuals with respiratory problems neither osteopathy nor chiropractic can be considered a primary therapy. However anecdotal evidence suggests they may be useful adjuncts to other types of therapy.

For instance, US research has recently concluded that elderly people hospitalised with pneumonia make better recoveries if they are given osteopathic treatment. This was after randomly assigning 58 older people with acute pneumonia to receive either standardised osteopathic manipulative treatment or simple light touch. Those who received the osteopathy recovered much more quickly and required shorter courses of antibiotics than those who did not.

Chiropractic has had less success in this area. A small trial compared sham chiropractic with the real thing twice weekly over a four-week period in individuals hospitalised with asthma. No significant differences were found in improvement between the two groups.

Other conditions

People hospitalised for a variety of conditions – including heart problems, gastrointestinal conditions and even psychosis – may derive benefit that goes beyond just the musculoskeletal system from regular osteopathic treatment. In one 1998 survey of 133 hospitals in the US that offer osteopathic treatment, researchers found that those receiving osteopathy generally had shorter hospital stays and reported a greater sense of well-being.

A small number of trials have shown that chiropractic may be of benefit in treating menstrual cramps. In one that compared sham techniques with chiropractic, the real thing was found to be twice as effective at alleviating pain and discomfort.

Children may also benefit from manipulative therapies. Osteopathy is increasingly being used on babies who had a difficult birth and/or

OSTEOPATHY & CHIROPRACTIC

who are colicky or fussy, often with very good results. One trial of 316 infants found that chiropractic treatment also improved symptoms of colic for 94 per cent of the babies observed.

Another small study comparing sham with genuine chiropractic found that chiropractic adjustment helped to improve bed-wetting, but not significantly more than the sham treatment.

Finally, some reports say that children with ADD and/or hyperactivity may be helped with a cranial osteopathic approach, as may those who have been labelled developmentally delayed. However this is an anecdotal and theoretical possibility rather than a proven benefit.

Cautions

Chiropractic, more than osteopathy, has been the subject of several legal cases in which overly forceful movements were alleged to have caused damage to the spine. Because individual practitioners can vary in their approaches, be selective about who you choose as your therapist. Forceful manipulation is rarely appropriate and positively undesirable in certain individuals such as children, pregnant women and the elderly.

Chiropractic should be avoided in cases of infectious diseases, where the patient has an aneurysm or where there is narrowing of the vertebral artery and in those with a tumour, bone infection or fracture.

Osteopathy is usually contraindicated in those who have cancer and is unlikely to be helpful in diseases of emotional or psychological or nutritional origin. More energetic techniques such as the thrust are contraindicated in those with fractures at the site of the thrust, with severe rheumatoid arthritis and severe pain at the site.

While the manipulative therapies can be considered primary therapies for conditions such as backache, in other conditions such as hypertension, respiratory disorders or ulcers they would take on a more complementary role.

What to expect

Most people consult an osteopath or chiropractor when they are in pain. However, you do not need to be in pain to consult either. It is reasonable to consult them for advice and reassurance or as part of a holistic approach to health maintenance.

During your initial appointment your practitioner will take a full case history including information about your lifestyle, work, diet and any medical conditions you have suffered from.

You may occasionally be asked to undress down to your underwear – your practitioner will want to see how you stand, checking spinal curves and posture and how your weight is distributed. You may be asked to move your arms, bend your legs or bend forward so that your practitioner can judge the range of movement in your joints. Your sitting posture will also be observed. Once all this is done, your practitioner will have a good picture of what parts of your body need treatment.

Subsequent sessions will involve different techniques. The osteopath may use soft tissue manipulations, joint mobilisation techniques or friction to improve local circulation and occasionally a high velocity thrust to mobilise a very stubborn joint. The chiropractor will check the condition of your neck and spine and make adjustments and/or work to bring greater mobility to the joints according to his or her diagnosis.

Whether you choose osteopathy or chiropractic, sessions usually last half an hour and treatment may be weekly, bi-monthly or monthly, depending on what is appropriate to your condition.

Both osteopaths and chiropractors go through lengthy and rigorous training and you can generally be assured of the competence of a practitioner if you choose one belonging to any of the following organisations.

Since 1999 all osteopaths must be registered with the General Osteopathic Council. Those who are not are not fully qualified and should not be practising. To find a qualified osteopath you can contact the Council directly. You can also get in touch with the British Osteopathic Association, who can help you find find a local practitioner.

If you are looking for a chiropractor, you can ask to be referred by your NHS GP or you can contact the British Chiropractic Association, the Scottish Chiropractic Association, the McTimoney Chiropractic Association or the British Association for Applied Chiropractic (McTimoney-Corley).

Chapter 17

Placebo

Commonly used for

Pain Relief • Depression • Anxiety • Allergies
• Heart Problems • Mild Hypertension
• Digestive Problems • Skin Disorders

• May be administered by a doctor • Important part of self-help

There is a cure for a significant number of ailments – all in fact except the most chronic and fatal diseases – which has no adverse effects, which is as effective and in some cases more so than many modern synthesised drugs and 'natural' remedies, but which many scientists refuse to validate. It is called the placebo.

A placebo is a substance with no (known) medicinal properties which causes a patient to improve because of his or her belief that it will work. When used in drug or other research, a placebo is administered to a 'control group' – a group of individuals who are receiving non-medical treatment who can be compared to another group, which is receiving genuine, usually experimental treatment. The goal of such research is to prove that the experimental treatment is better than taking or doing nothing. However, this is often not the case. When those in the control group experience the same or even better outcomes than those in the experimental group, this is known as the 'placebo effect'. When applied as a procedure (as in trials with ultrasound, surgical procedures, acupuncture or biofeedback) a placebo is known as a sham treatment.

The placebo effect is particularly significant for those interested in wellness because it reminds us of the power of suggestion and belief – an innate power that can change the way the body functions, and one that is normally only attributed to man-made drugs. Placebos also provide a broad platform from which to construct broader questions about relationships – between the body and the mind, but also between the practitioner and the patient – and how influential these are on health and illness.

Conventional medicines, having been tested in medical trials, are supposed to be free from any association with the placebo effect. Yet many scientific trials completely ignore the complexities of the placebo and the possible placebo effect that the simple act of prescribing a remedy or treatment can have on a patient.

For instance, when a doctor can see no clear pattern to an illness he may throw something in the general direction of the patient's symptoms, if only to reassure the patient that he is doing his best. Even if it is the wrong remedy, the fact of doing something to help may inspire the patient to recover.

Across the country, in fact throughout the world, the over-use of the wrong drugs and procedures in this haphazard way may be concealing a widespread placebo effect – the very thing which serious scientists aim to eliminate when conducting medical trials. The over-use of antibiotics is a good example. Many doctors continue to prescribe antibiotics for colds and flu, even though these conditions are caused by viruses and cannot be cured with antibiotics (which only work against bacteria). Nevertheless, many people report feeling better after having taken these drugs, and often request them the next time they fall ill with the same complaint.

With this in mind it can be difficult to say categorically how much of any drug's efficacy is down to a genuine pharmacological effect and how much is down to the mutual belief (by doctor and patient) that it might do some good.

For instance, in 1996 psychologist Dr Guy Sapirstein from the University of Connecticut addressed the American Psychological Association's annual convention and dropped the bombshell that, after analysing 39 studies of depressed individuals from 1974 to 1995, he believed that the placebo effect accounted for half the improvements in depressed persons taking antidepressants.

Dr Sapirstein found that many of the self-reported improvements in depressed people could not be traced to their pharmacological effect, and concluded that only 27 per cent of the response was due to medication alone (what he called a true pharmacological effect); 50 per cent was due to the psychological impact of administering the medication (or the placebo effect); and 23 per cent was due to other 'non-specific factors'. His conclusions were later published in the APA's journal, *Prevention & Treatment*.

If his observations are correct, this means that even when an individual is taking a 'proven' drug, the placebo effect may significantly outweigh the effect of the drug. 'If we take these results and say that improvement is due to what the patients think,' commented Sapirstein, 'then how people think and its effect on how they feel are more powerful than the chemical substance.'

The prescribing physician also has a role to play in the placebo effect. For instance, a study reported in the *New England Journal of Medicine* in 1979 found that when a doctor enthusiastically supports a treatment, the placebo response could be greater than 80 per cent. Similar studies have shown that the effectiveness of the placebo is increased when both practitioner and patient believe that the treatment will work and nearly 40 per cent of the time, under these circumstances, it will. This appears to be true even when the physician tells the patient he or she is receiving a placebo – as long as the physician also provides reassurance that he feels it will help. Conversely, when given by a non-caring physician, evidence shows that both drugs and placebos are less effective.

The placebo effect has been noted in just about every research situation in which placebos are used and this has led some clinicians to argue that there is no such thing as a true placebo. Instead, they believe that any substance that we put into the body, which was not there before, will cause a reaction, sometimes beneficial, and that this might account for what is commonly known as the placebo effect.

But the debate on what it is, how it works, when it works, whether it's ethical and whether there is a difference between 'true' and 'perceived' placebo effects, ignores the facts – placebo and sham treatments can improve and even cure between 30 and 70 per cent of those to whom they are administered.

Accentuating the negative

Much of the conventional research into placebos has an interesting bias to it – trying to expose the gullibility of patients and what doctors see as the frailties of the human psyche. How different the attitude of alternative and integrative practitioners is!

For instance, according to Andrew Weill MD, a well-known alternative practitioner in the US: 'As a practitioner of mind/body medicine, I consider the placebo response my greatest ally. I view it as a pure healing response from within and want to encourage it as much as I can.'

Renowned physician Leo Galland goes further: 'Three hundred years after the scientific revolution, the placebo is still the strongest force in medicine and for the majority of patients the major determinant of the outcome of healthcare.'

Not surprisingly, an important factor in maintaining health and even reducing mortality is a person's confidence in and understanding of what is happening to them. Because of the negative connotations of the words 'placebo effect', it has been suggested that when talking to patients about the placebo effect, the term could be replaced by 'remembered wellness'.

So why is 'placebo' such a dirty word among conventional physicians? Placebo is derived from the Latin verb *placere*, to please. Placebos were used throughout the 19th century in blind assessments of medical treatments. These blind assessments were created to test controversial or experimental medical treatments of the time, such as mesmerism or homeopathy, and involved using a blindfold or withholding information from the patients so that they would remain unaware of the exact nature of the treatment they were being given. According to some medical historians, from the early 1800s until as late as the Second World War placebos, usually in the form of sugar pills or saline injections, were prescribed regularly to up to 80 per cent of patients. Doctors used placebos to appease patients for whom they had no effective treatment or for those patients whom they considered demanding or difficult (though interestingly, according to data in the *Annals of Internal Medicine* in 1979, anxious patients are the ones least likely to respond to such treatments).

The desire to take medicine or receive relief from a healer is one of the features that distinguishes humans from other living things. It is evident in the ancient written and pictorial records of every culture going back well over 6,000 years. For centuries, common medical treatment included things that we would consider unscientific, even barbaric, today. Standard treatments for a variety of conditions included bleeding, cupping, leeches, maggots, enemas, plasters, purging, catharsis, and even incantations to rid the body of evil spirits.

Egyptian physicians prescribed crocodile dung, and similar outlandish treatments were common in other parts of the world. Roving lay practitioners sold various forms of cure-all pills and potions made from substances that had no known therapeutic benefit (and were sometimes even poisonous). Wise women in villages would prescribe herbs and other natural substances for which there was no proof save centuries of anecdote. For many years this was medicine.

As our knowledge of the human body expanded and medicine became more sophisticated and more powerful, such practices became denigrated as quackery.

This arrogance displayed by the new scientific medicine men, however, completely ignored the fact that the use of these remedies persisted for so long because people perceived them as helpful. Nevertheless, doctors began to associate in their minds outmoded practices, the efficacy of which they could not explain, with a placebo effect, and quackery and placebo soon became synonymous.

Why then is the placebo included here in a book about alternative therapies? Because placebo is the most alternative and daring therapy of all. Indeed, one review published in *Anthropology Quarterly* in 2000 which focused on the cultural variations in the placebo effect in treating ulcers, anxiety and blood pressure concluded: 'Placebo healing is the ultimate and inescapable "complementary medicine".'

How does it work?

Medical science consigns to a kind of 'placebo dustbin' any healing effect that it cannot explain or feels it cannot measure. Because the placebo's usefulness has yet to be fully explained or fully scientifically explored, many alternative therapies that are difficult to explain in the conventional sense – such as homeopathy – are maligned as 'just placebos'.

Many scientists believe placebos work by exerting a systemic effect, such as releasing natural morphine-like substances that circulate throughout the body. While this may be true, placebos can also have extremely specific effects. In one famous anecdote 13 people extremely sensitive to poison ivy were rubbed on one arm with a harmless leaf and told it was poison ivy. The other arm was rubbed with poison ivy and they were told it was harmless. All 13 developed a rash where they were rubbed by the harmless leaf, while only two reacted to the poison ivy leaf.

Another theory is that placebos somehow stimulate the secretion of small brain peptide messengers, like endorphins, that have strong effects on mood and sensitivity to pain. Although there are no measurements to confirm this, support comes from the observation that placebo pain relief can be diminished by the administration of naloxone, a drug that blocks opiate effects and also reduces the analgesic response to acupuncture.

Stimulation of endorphin secretion alone, however, would not explain all the wide-ranging benefits of placebos. The common denominator appears to be the belief, faith and/or expectation of a favourable outcome.

In addition, stress can contribute to or aggravate the course of almost any illness. Placebos can provide a sense of control for some, which can reduce stress and create a more positive outlook. What is more, the resultant expectation of a positive outcome may translate into genuine benefits.

Finally, there is what is called the 'caring effect' – though some argue this is not a true placebo effect. Some doctors believe there is no difference between placebo and no treatment. Others believe that placebo barely differs from what Professors Julian Tudor Hart and Paul Dieppe, writing in the *Lancet* in 1996, called 'caring effects'. Caring effects, they suggest, are a form of active treatment, the effect of which can be measured.

For instance caring about, as well as for, people with chronic arthritis can reduce pain and substantially improve mobility – reducing the individual's need for pain-relieving drugs and also the cost of treatment (both in financial terms and in terms of potential adverse effects). After an observational study suggested that twice-weekly telephone contact helped people with osteoarthritis, a controlled trial was done to assess the effectiveness of monthly telephone contact for one year. People with symptomatic osteoarthritis fared better than those who had no support, showing significant improvements in pain, physical disability and psychological disability. Other studies show that a regular telephone call may be as beneficial to health and mood as clinic visits, particularly for the elderly.

Randomised trials of emotional support given to women in labour have been shown to reduce Caesarean rates, and labouring women who have good emotional support are also less likely to need pain-relieving drugs. Likewise, extra time spent with an anaesthetist before an operation discussing pain and pain relief can lessen post-surgical pain and shorten hospital stays; and a patient whose doctor has taken the time to talk about headache pain, its nature and its relief, is likely to respond better to whatever treatment is offered.

Such discussions are becoming increasingly rare in the cause and effect cattle market of today's clinics and hospitals. But as Tudor Hart and Dieppe so eloquently pleaded: 'To account for clinical improvement solely by placebo effects (as simplistic interpretations of controlled trials might easily do) is an insult to the importance of caring. It diverts attention from the fundamental need always to provide optimum caring as a necessary basis for technical intervention. These are caring effects, and so they should be called.'

The colour of healing

Prescribing something that has no known benefit – but doing it with care and attention – may be the most potent medicine of all. But many factors can influence the power of placebos, including their size, shape, and especially colour. While not all trials agree, red, yellow and orange placebos are perceived as energising and therefore better for depression, while blue, purple and green have a tranquillising effect and are preferred for anxiety disorders.

The type of placebo given also has a perceived effect. For instance, larger capsules tend to be viewed as stronger. Injections may produce larger effects than do pills and two placebo capsules can have a more pronounced effect than one.

Placebos have also been associated with various adverse effects such as drowsiness, headaches, nervousness, insomnia, nausea, dry mouth and constipation. In heart patients placebos have been known to cause an increase in heartbeat (tachycardia).

What the research says

Clearly some people who get better with placebos (as well as standard therapies) would have done so on their own because so many of the disorders we suffer from are self-limiting – that is, they heal naturally after a limited period of time. Placebos also seem to be most effective in conditions where symptoms are somewhat subjective and where the severity of the condition can fluctuate over time – conditions like pain, depression, mild hypertension, anxiety disorders, depression, mood changes, hay fever and cough, acne, menstrual and menopausal symptoms.

The strength of the placebo effect can also depend on how compliant the patient is – those who are highly compliant (who take at least 80 per cent of the placebo) are likely to have a better outcome than those who are less compliant (taking less than 80 per cent). Placebos are also more beneficial in certain types of individuals. Those who respond well to placebos also respond better to 'real' drugs. In contrast, those who respond poorly to placebos also show a poor response to active treatments. In these individuals the active treatment may work no better than the placebo.

Relieving pain
One area in which the placebo effect has clearly been demonstrated is pain relief. Almost any type of pain, from headache to heart pain to cancer pain, can be reduced by as much as 50 per cent by a placebo. For instance, even people with long-term back pain have shown both clinical and statistically significant improvement with placebo in between 20 and 40 per cent of cases.

In pain relief, placebos have demonstrated long-term benefits and responses to different doses that mimic active medicines. For instance, when varying doses of analgesic followed by an identical looking placebo are administered, the patient's response to the placebo is often equal to that experienced with the active drug.

Expectation of pain relief is also relevant to the amount of pain relief experienced. As an example, a placebo compared with morphine will provide much greater pain relief than if the placebo is compared with aspirin, because the expectation of relief is greater with morphine than with aspirin.

This is an important point which scientists often ignore. When a placebo is used in double-blind trials, the expectation that it (or the active medicine) will work is reduced – since both parties know that there is approximately a 50 per cent chance of the substance being inert.

Italian researchers at the University of Torino have conducted several experiments in the role that expectation plays in the placebo effect. In these studies of pain relief the researchers have found that giving a placebo, but telling the patient it is a powerful painkiller, can both produce effective pain relief and reduce the amount of genuine painkilling medication the patient uses.

Healing ulcers

For years people with ulcers were given medication to reduce stomach acid. Indeed, for a long time antacids were the only treatment available. Then in the 1970s a new miracle drug, Tagamet (cimetidine), was developed. Instead of neutralising stomach acid Tagamet slowed the production of acid by the cells in the lining of the stomach. When Tagamet first came on the market there were several trials comparing it to placebo. Individually, these studies didn't show much about the effectiveness of Tagamet over placebo. But taken as a whole, some interesting findings emerged. Between 10 and 90 per cent of those taking a placebo improved, but on average 48 per cent of people improved on the placebo, compared to 76 per cent of those taking the active drug. The fact that we now know that ulcers are caused by a bacterium, *Helicobacter pylori*, and not excess acid makes these findings even more intriguing.

Surgical placebo

The placebo effect is not limited to medicines, but can appear with any kind of medical procedure. Indeed in his book, *Doctors, Patients and Placebos*, H.M. Spiro comments that 'sceptics have long noted that an operation, particularly a new one, seems to bring benefit for several years, until it is re-evaluated and then often abandoned'. In other words, the belief in the greater efficacy of the new procedure is often very influential in its perceived success. He also noted that the experience of surgery and the symbol of the scar must themselves be important sources of pain relief, something which has been confirmed by other scientists.

In a trial to test the value of a surgical procedure to treat angina pectoris, the placebo procedure consisted of anaesthetising the patient and only cutting his skin. Amazingly, the fictitiously treated patients showed an 80 per cent improvement, while among those actually operated upon only 40 per cent improved. In this study clinically significant improvement in angina symptoms was maintained for as long as one year after the sham surgery.

In addition, one review of 2,504 operations for lumbar disc disease found that after simple exploratory surgery 37 per cent of patients reported complete relief from sciatica and 43 per cent of those without slipped or ruptured discs were free from all back pain. These figures compare favourably with reviews of common spinal surgery techniques as well as several other procedures.

Reducing drug dosages

There is also evidence to suggest the placebo effect could allow patients to gradually reduce the dosages needed to treat their condition. This is a genuine benefit as lower doses mean less risk of those on long-term treatment developing drug-related side effects. This is a new field of study, but Dr Robert Ader, director of the Division of Behavioral and Psychosocial Medicine at the University of Rochester School of Medicine, and his colleague, the immunologist Dr Nicholas Cohen, have conducted an animal experiment which has led them to suggest that the placebo effect is 'a learned response available to anybody under appropriate circumstances'.

In their study, a group of animals was given a combination of a drug that reduces antibody production and the artificial sweetener saccharine. Later the group was divided into two: one given the immuno-suppressant only, the other given saccharine only. Both groups were later found to have reduced antibody levels, suggesting the rats' bodies had learned to associate saccharine with antibody reduction. The researchers suggest patients could similarly train themselves to get the same effect using smaller doses of drugs.

The nocebo effect

If a patient is given a placebo he or she believes to be harmful to their health in some way, he or she may develop symptoms appropriate to this belief. This is known as the nocebo effect. Like placebo, it does not require the physical giving of a substance or the performing of a procedure. Any physician who shows an inability to care and/or who interferes with the beliefs and value systems of his or her patients can conjure up the nocebo effect.

Cautions

Human response to pain and discomfort is extremely sensitive to environment and psychological factors. Generally speaking, coping skills and life attitudes make the difference between an ailment that is relatively easy to bear and one which becomes a terrible burden. The placebo effect is testimony to the value of positive suggestion, the harnessing of the psyche and the fortifying of one's coping skills – attributes used to good effect in **hypnosis**, **meditation** and even **spiritual healing**.

Some ethical objections have been raised about the risk of withholding medication from patients when studying placebo. This is not an area that has been fully explored. However, in a large review published in the *Archives of General Psychiatry* in 2000, scientists looked at both symptom reductions and suicide rates among depressed patients who were given placebo, and compared it to those who took conventional antidepressants. The rates were nearly identical in both groups for both measurements, suggesting that giving a placebo did not cause undue harm.

There is also a difference between knowingly deceiving someone by giving him or her an inert substance and telling them it is active, and using something so many physicians sorely lack – people skills – to harness the positive power of suggestion. Many objectors do not acknowledge this difference.

Whatever we call it, placebo has long been one of the physician's most potent assets and should not be belittled or ridiculed. Neither should it be used cynically by those who do not have faith in their own skills or in their patients' innate ability to heal themselves. Unlike many other conventional treatments, it is safe and inexpensive, and has withstood the test of time.

Chapter 18

Spiritual Healing

Commonly used for

Recovery from Surgery • Heart Health • Protection from Disease
• Depression • Pain Relief • Improved Immunity
• Stress Relief • Longevity

• *Suitable for self-help*

A t one time or another most of us have tried to send 'good vibes' to loved ones in distress. In its simplest form this is a type of spiritual healing. In its more complex form, for instance in days gone by, what we now call spiritual healing was simply medicine and involved a shaman who may have used ritual, dance, music, even mind-altering drugs to help him direct healing energy to those in need.

Spiritual healing is a difficult concept to grasp for anyone who does not believe in things beyond that which their senses can perceive. Yet many reputable scientists suggest that there are energies in the universe that bind us all together and organise our being – spiritually, psychologically and biologically. Different cultures have given different names to this universal energy.

The Chinese call it *qi*, the Japanese call it *anma*, and Hindus call it *prana*. Hippocrates called it the *viz medicatrix naturae*. In the West we have given it similarly exotic names. Psychiatrist Wilhelm Reich believed it was *orgone energy*, Franz Mesmer, the father of hypnotism, *animal magnetism* and scientist Karl von Reichenbach, *odic force*. In world religions this force is given various other names (God, Supreme Being, Allah, Buddha) and in quantum physics it is known as the *zero point field*.

In the context of spiritual healing, 'spiritual' doesn't necessarily mean belonging to an organised religion or practising the rituals and styles of prayer that belong to that religion. Generally speaking, religion implies a sect and traditions, as well as belief systems about the nature of God. Spirituality is a more abstract concept, implying the individual's capacity for recognising and experiencing an intangible presence or higher power that orders life and makes it feel meaningful.

It is the channelling of this universal energy from its spiritual source to someone in need that is generally referred to as spiritual healing. Tapping into this energy for our own benefits or for the benefit of someone else was for many years considered a noble art. Today, however, several things stand in the way of spiritual healing being taken seriously. For many years scientists have worked hard to remove spirituality and belief from their theories about what sustains life. Many doctors consider the concept of a universal force archaic and unsubstantiated, and believe that while medicine may once have been a mixture of science and art, it is now strictly a science (an ironic point of view, given that so much modern medicine relies on the patient's faith in the doctor's ability to heal; see **placebo** for more).

The powerful influence that drug companies have on individual practitioners, medical institutions and even medical researchers, has led to a disproportionate belief in the healing power of drugs. The rise in private health insurance, which generally only allows access to conventional treatments that can be packaged and priced, also mitigates against the freely available power of divine energy.

Healers see mind, body and spirit as interconnected – what affects one necessarily affects the others, and all three must work in harmony to maintain good health. The practice of spiritual healing, which uses the power of the spirit to balance and heal the whole person, takes several forms. The two most common are distance healing, where a person or a group of persons (known as 'intercessors') pray for another person's welfare, and therapeutic touch, which paradoxically often doesn't include touch at all but simple close contact or 'stroking' the space around the body. In addition, prayer for one's self rather than for others can be used as a form of self-help.

Evidence of the benefits of religious faith are often used to support the idea that spiritual healing works – though the two, although linked, are not entirely the same thing. In order to gain some kind of scientific foothold, spiritual healing has generally tried to distance itself from religious faith healing. The former, say proponents, is an active process where one person channels divine energy towards another. The latter has more to do with harnessing the power of belief and convincing a person that they have the ability to heal themselves. Nevertheless, it may be that for spiritual healing to work, all those involved – intercessor/healer and recipient – need to have faith that the process will work. What is more, faith must be a meaningful concept to those involved.

For instance, at Harvard University Dr Herbert Benson, author of *Beyond the Relaxation Response*, has conducted scientific experiments to determine the efficacy of prayer or mantra. He studied Christians and Jews who prayed regularly and taught some participants to meditate using the word 'one' or any other phrase they felt comfortable with. In another group he asked Catholics to use their mantra phrases such as, 'Hail Mary, full of grace' or to use the Jesus Prayer. Jews used the peace greeting, 'Shalom' or 'Echad', meaning one. Protestants used the first line of the Lord's Prayer, 'Our father who art in heaven' or the opening of the twenty-third psalm, 'The Lord is my shepherd'.

Initially, all these mantras worked equally well in invoking a relaxation response and stimulating the healthful physiological changes in the body. But as the study went on, Benson found that those who used the word 'one' or a similar simple phrase that had no particular spiritual meaning for them did not stick with the programme, whereas those who used prayer-based mantras continued because of their belief.

This may be an important piece of information for Westerners who dabble with exotic religions. The practice of spiritual materialism – the collecting (and often abandoning) of different rituals of spirituality like so many lipsticks or sports shoes – may ultimately end in disappointment because it is a form of greed rather than devotion.

To try and separate spirituality from religion, believers in spiritual healing often cite experiments in distance healing involving non-human subjects. Such studies often show remarkable results, according to Larry Dossey MD, an outspoken proponent of spiritual healing and co-chair of the Panel on Mind-Body Interventions of the Office of Alternative Medicine at the US National Institutes of Health. In his own reviews of over 100 experiments on the effects of prayer/visualisation, most published in parapsychological literature, more than half showed an effect on everything from seed germination to wound-healing.

Among the most well known of these are experiments with mice in the 1960s which showed that wounded animals healed much more quickly when a healer held his hands over them for 15 minutes twice a day.

Other experiments have shown that the growth of plants and fungi can be significantly affected by healing. Human cells too have been subjected to the power of spiritual healing. In one study a healer was able to prolong the life of red blood cells in a weak salt solution (a medium that would normally cause them to burst) by up to four times. According to the experimenters, the chance of this happening naturally was about 100,000 to 1.

How does it work?
Believers in distance healing and therapeutic touch are not sure how it works, though several theories abound. Some say it involves sending some kind of subtle, as yet unidentified energy to the person in need. Others say quantum physics and the theory of the zero point field – which postulates that everything in the universe, including human beings, are made from the same energy, highly organised sub-atomic particles that are able to co-operate and communicate with each other – may play a role.

The other kind of prayer, in which sick people pray for their own recovery, is somewhat easier for scientists to understand. Given the way that meditation can restore health – for instance, by lowering blood pressure and stress – it's not difficult to see how prayer, which is both meditative and relaxing, might bring about the same effects.

Prayer, like **meditation**, may induce a sense of calm and so inhibit the secretion of stress hormones such as epinephrine, and norepinephrine, released by the adrenal glands in response to stress. Continuous high levels of these fight-or-flight chemicals can compromise the immune system, increasing the risk of developing any number of illnesses, including heart disease, stroke, peptic ulcers and inflammatory bowel disorder (IBS).

Religion, of course, is a facet of spirituality and research has shown that religious people of all faiths are less depressed, have healthier immune systems and are less prone to addictions than the non-religious. However, it is important to acknowledge that those with religious convictions may also take better care of themselves. They may eat better, smoke and drink less, have more social support and a greater sense of community, and this will have a knock-on effect on good health.

Prayer, like **placebo**, may also harness the power of belief. Results of studies show that the more a person believes that prayer will work to heal them, the more likely it is that it will. Likewise a healer's belief that prayer will heal is also influential.

Therapeutic touch

Practitioners of therapeutic touch believe that everyone has an innate healing mechanism, an energy field that flows around the body, mind and spirit to keep them in perfect order. Unfortunately, stress, an inadequate diet, a negative attitude and other adverse factors can block this healing mechanism, preventing it from functioning correctly. When this happens we get ill. Spiritual healing in the form of therapeutic touch provides one way of nudging a person's individual healing mechanism back into action. When healers lay their hands on a person, or as is more common 'stroke' the space around the body, they act as a conductor or channel for healing energy which they believe has the 'intelligence' to go where it is needed.

During a treatment, which may last anywhere from five to 30 minutes or longer, the healer will 'scan' your body, with his hands hovering just above you, in order to take a reading of your body's energy levels and to locate areas of low or blocked energy. Some may concentrate on using the *chakras* – the seven main energy centres of the body, according to Vedic medicine.

Throughout the therapy you may feel heat coming from the healer's hands, although some people report feeling a draught, a tingling sensation, pins and needles or a feeling of light-headedness. Some healers also use additional healing tools such as visualisation or meditation. Afterwards, most people report feeling relaxed and peaceful, although some feel thirsty or sleepy. Leave a few days or a week between sessions to give the healing time to work.

What the research says

Given that medical science has tried to stringently separate itself from God and faith, there is an astonishing amount of research into the effect of spirituality on health. More than a thousand studies have sought to explore the 'faith factor' and what it means to health and healing.

Most of the available evidence shows that prayer is most effective as a complementary, rather than a primary therapy. Nevertheless, there is reasonable proof that prayer has a healing effect. One analysis of 23 studies involving more than 3,000 individuals concluded that more than half demonstrated that prayer had significant effects. In this review therapeutic touch appeared to show the most promise.

Naysayers point out that no study has ever proven the ability of prayer to stop a person from dying from conditions such as heart disease and cancer. They note, and fairly, that the quality of the studies done into spiritual healing can be very uneven and often do not follow people long enough to make sweeping statements about its effectiveness. This, however, appears to be missing the point.

Scientific research by its very nature requires a measurable endpoint – usually focusing on quantity rather than quality of life. Even Larry Dossey has warned that holistic practitioners should not over-extend the power of spirituality. We will all die eventually. Short-term studies do show that prayer can have an effect on longevity (see below), but perhaps more importantly prayer may be a beneficial way to improve the quality of life for those in need. Even researchers who are sceptical have been moved to say that the occasionally remarkable results of studies into spiritual healing are interesting enough to warrant further and more serious investigation.

High blood pressure and heart problems

In one of the most widely publicised studies of the effect of intercessory prayer, cardiologist Randolph Byrd studied 393 men and women admitted to the coronary care unit at San Francisco General Hospital and receiving conventional medical care there. Some were prayed for by home prayer groups, others were not, and because the study was 'blinded' neither the doctors, nurses nor the patients knew who would be the objects of prayer.

The results were surprising and dramatic. The men and women whose medical care was supplemented with prayer fared better overall than their counterparts who received medical care but nothing more. The prayed-for people, for instance, were significantly less likely to require antibiotics, significantly less likely to develop pulmonary oedema (where the lungs fill with fluid because the heart cannot pump properly), and significantly less likely to require mechanical assistance with breathing. They were also less likely to die during the course of the study, though the difference between the groups was small.

Another study in the *Archives of Internal Medicine* in 1999 examined the health outcomes of nearly 1,000 heart patients newly admitted to hospital – all with serious heart conditions. Without their knowledge the people were randomly divided into two groups. For four weeks five volunteers who believed in God and in the healing power of prayer prayed daily 'for a speedy recovery with no complications' for half the patients. The other half were not assigned anyone to pray for them.

When comparing the groups, using a comprehensive list of adverse health conditions common to cardiac patients, the researchers concluded that the prayed for group fared 11 per cent better – a statistically significant figure suggesting that prayer can be a useful adjunct to the care of heart patients.

Recovery from surgery

A study at the University of Michigan in 1997 analysed two questionnaires completed by 151 heart patients. The questionnaires looked at symptoms of depression, general distress, healthcare practice after surgery, perceived social support and chronic conditions other than cardiac disease. An amazing 85 per cent of the sample practised complementary health approaches, in particular prayer, exercise and lifestyle diet modification. The study concluded that those who pursued complementary approaches after surgery, especially prayer and exercise, experienced a significantly improved psychological recovery.

Depression often accompanies hospitalisation, and researchers at the Center for the Study of Religion/Spirituality in Medicine, Duke University, Durham, North Carolina, have conducted several studies into the ability of prayer to alleviate this problem. In one, involving 850 men aged 65 years and older, what was termed 'religious coping' – in other words employing strategies such as prayer to deal with depression – was not only common but related to significantly less depression among the hospitalised men. Another study from the same centre showed that depressed individuals who had a strong religious faith recovered 70 per cent faster from depression than those with a weaker faith.

Longevity

While not strictly proof of the efficacy of spiritual healing, the overall conclusion of studies into faith have found that people who practise religion appear to live longer. In one large analysis in 1999 of a nationally representative sample of 21,204 US adults, those who regularly attended religious services outlived those who did not attend church. People who went to church more than once a week lived on average to 62.9 years compared to 55.3 for those who did not. Those who attended once a week and those who went less than once a week had an average lifespan of 61.9 and 59.7 years respectively. Other studies have found similar results.

An earlier study of 91,909 people in one Maryland county in the US found that those who attended religious services weekly were less likely to die during the study period than those who did not. The figures were startling with attendees 53 per cent less likely to die from coronary diseases, 74 per cent less likely to die from cirrhosis (liver disease) and 53 per cent less likely to commit suicide – figures very similar to those for people who regularly engage in **meditation**.

Belonging to a religious collective may also have a protective effect. A study published in the *American Journal of Public Health* in 1996 of people living in kibbutz communities showed that in every age group those belonging to a religious community were about half as likely to die as their non-religious counterparts during the 16 years of the study.

Conversely, loss of faith can shorten life. Researchers at Bowling Green State University in Ohio questioned 596 hospitalised patients over the age of 55 about how they were using religion to cope with the stress of illness. The vast majority were of Christian faith.

Some expressed negative religious feelings included feeling 'abandoned or punished by God' or 'questioning God's love'. Feelings of doubt and anger towards one's faith are natural and normal when dealing with serious illness. But by the end of the 14-month study period those who said they felt 'unloved by God' and 'attributed their illness to the devil' were found to have a 19 to 28 per cent increased risk of dying within two years.

Improved immunity
Because of its associations with relaxation and focused awareness, spirituality may also have a beneficial effect on the immune system. One 1997 trial, for instance, found that therapeutic touch could improve the immunity of stressed out individuals.

According to another published in the same year those who regularly attend church have a measurably healthier immune system than those who do not. The researchers looked at a range of biological indicators of immune function including levels of interleukin-6 (IL-6, a protein released by the body during an immune response) in elderly adults. Regulation of IL-6 tends to be impaired in elderly adults and high levels are linked to stress and depression and the development of conditions such as osteoporosis. In this study attendees were around 50 per cent less likely to have high levels of IL-6.

Other conditions

A study of the mental health of both intercessors and recipients found that prayer had a healing effect on both, including better self-esteem, less anxiety and depression and that the intercessors experienced even greater improvement than the recipients. Similarly, a number of studies have associated a deep religious faith with an ability to cope more effectively with breast and other types of cancer.

In one Australian study of people with cancer of the colon or rectum, 715 patients were compared with 727 people without cancer. The researchers found that the respondents who saw themselves as most religious were less likely to have cancer than those who were not as religious. In other words, self-perceived 'religiousness' was a statistically significant protective factor against the disease.

Another interesting finding in this study was that self-reported or perceived religiousness was associated with average survival times of 62 months. In contrast, those who reported themselves as 'non-religious' had a median survival time of only 52 months.

One small study found that in-person intercessory prayer helped relieve symptoms of rheumatoid arthritis. Distance prayer did not have the same beneficial effect.

According to conventional researchers the efficacy of any therapy, the outcome of which can be influenced by the person administering the treatment, can be difficult to assess accurately. This, of course, ignores the fact that individual physicians' attitudes can also influence, for good or ill, the outcome of a particular study or therapy. Research into therapeutic touch, while not as abundant as that into spiritual healing, is accumulating.

For instance, a small, single-blind, randomised trial has shown that osteoarthritis sufferers can benefit from therapeutic touch. Twenty-five people with osteoarthritis of the knee received either therapeutic touch, mock therapeutic touch or standard care. The main outcomes studied were pain, general well-being and health status. Those in the therapeutic touch group had significantly decreased pain and improved function, compared to those receiving mock therapeutic touch or standard care.

Cautions

There has been a great deal of debate recently about trials involving distance healing and some important ethical points have been raised. For example, how can ethics committees (whose job it is to make sure that trial participants fully understand the purpose, potential risks and benefits of the trial) approve trials in which a person with an illness is unaware that he or she is being prayed for and has not consented to such treatment. In the early days of researching spiritual healing, this might not have seemed like a rational concern. But if prayer really is powerful medicine, then researchers must seek permission, and ethics committees must insist that permission is sought before conducting such experiments.

It is important to acknowledge that some people subconsciously prefer to be ill, some people (for a variety of reasons that we may not understand) need to be ill, and some people who are ill prefer to die. Prayer must not be used to interfere with someone else's life. Without the patient's permission intercessory prayer could be viewed as a form of spiritual assault – something which is clearly not acceptable.

More practical concerns should also be addressed. While study into spiritual healing suggests that recipients may use fewer medications, this should not be taken to mean that prayer and therapeutic touch could be substituted for medication. Discontinuing medication for conditions such as diabetes, epilepsy and hypertension may result in an occasionally drastic worsening of the condition.

It's also wise to remain aware that in this field, as in all walks of life, there are charlatans who exploit the sick and vulnerable for profit. There is no formal training for spiritual healers and so individuals are advised to choose their practitioners with care. If you are interested but uncertain how to proceed, try contacting the Confederation of

Healing Organisations for advice. This is an umbrella group for several organisations concerned with healing, the largest of which is the National Federation of Spiritual Healers (whose register comprises 7,000 members of all faiths and denominations).

Chapter 19

Traditional Chinese Medicine

Commonly used for

Skin Diseases • Digestive Complaints • Menstrual Problems
• Respiratory Disorders • Allergies • Chronic Fatigue
• Boosting Immunity

• *Requires a professional therapist*

Traditional Chinese medicine is used to treat all the illnesses and conditions that Western medicine treats – but this is where the similarity ends. Whereas Western doctors look for a single cause of illness – usually a bacteria or virus, genetics or an injury – and a single cure, oriental practitioners believe that many factors can contribute to illness. Susceptibility, for instance, can be related to a person's constitutional type as well as environmental factors, and illness is caused, not by germs, but by damp, heat, wind or cold. Having determined the nature of the illness, a person must be treated according to this total picture or the cure will not be complete.

Western doctors are rarely interested in such a total picture of a patient. Instead, their training encourages them to see people as specific body parts or chemicals – lungs, joints, heart, hormones and so on. But to oriental practitioners the body is a whole and highly organised system both within itself and also as part of the wider environment. Because of this, while a Western doctor may diagnose a collection of symptoms as 'peptic ulcer', a Chinese practitioner may diagnose any number of separate conditions which may lead to a similar collection of symptoms, for instance: 'damp heat affecting the spleen'; 'deficient cold affecting the spleen'; 'excess cold dampness affecting the spleen and stomach'; 'disharmony of the liver invading the spleen'; or 'disharmony of congealed blood in the stomach'.

There are also differences between Western and oriental approaches to the way a body functions. In Chinese medicine the organs have much broader functions than are normally assigned to them by Western medicine. The kidney, for example, does not simply regulate water balance; it is a link between sources of energy and growth, the bones and brain, will power and memory.

In ancient China traditional medicine was practised as a complete system of healthcare. Today, particularly in the West, Chinese medicine, like **Ayurveda**, has become fragmented into its main component parts: **herbal medicine**, **acupuncture** and Chinese **massage** (known as *tui na*).

Tired and frustrated with the way conventional medicine works (or doesn't work), many individuals have turned to traditional Chinese medicine (TCM) as a more ancient, more holistic and particularly a more spiritual way of approaching health. In so doing they threaten to mystify traditional Chinese medicine and turn what is an entirely rational body of knowledge into a religious faith system (yet another thing that Chinese medicine has in common with Ayurveda). The language of traditional Chinese medicine may be different, even more poetic than we are used to hearing in connection with health matters. But underneath is an elegant and insightful system for defining disease and restoring health.

How does it work?
Every culture has its own traditional system of medicines and healthcare and its own theories about how these should be used and how they work. Often these theories involve a dynamic connection between the living human body, the earth and the universe.

The wider philosophies behind traditional Chinese medicine, and the way these are applied to healthcare, are complex. According to this philosophy, human energy, or *qi*, is influenced by outside phenomena in both heaven and earth. Each of us has an inherited amount of qi which we get from our parents – a reserve of energy we can call upon and which organises our bodily processes. Our personal qi can be nourished by food, exercise and other healthful practices, but can be depleted by a poor lifestyle – long-term lack of sleep, drinking, smoking, lack of exercise, poor diet and even, according to traditional texts, excessive sex.

Two fundamental concepts underpin Chinese thinking about human health in relation to our environment: *yin* and *yang* and the five elements.

Yin and yang According to the Chinese, the universe and everything in it is held together by what could be called the tension of opposites. Male and female, light and dark, hot and cold – these are necessary, interrelated opposites that give our world its dynamism, its movement and flow. In Chinese philosophy yin is usually given to represent those things that are inactive, cold, internal, dark and descending. Yang represents things that are active, hot, external, bright and ascending. In TCM the human body, since it is a part of the universe, is also governed by this tension of opposites. Physiological functions of the body, internal organs and the meridians – complex pathways that run throughout the body and conduct the flow of qi – can all be defined in terms of their yin or yang qualities, and as long as these remain in balance, good health is assured.

The fundamental aim of Chinese medicine is to diagnose the cause of the internal disease, or yin yang imbalance, within the body and by using the appropriate therapy or therapies, correct the imbalance and restore health.

The five elements The theory of the five elements is the Chinese way of explaining the relationship between the human body and its environment as well as the interrelationship between our internal organs, body fluids and other biological processes.

252

In Chinese philosophy the universe is governed by five basic elements: wood, fire, earth, water and metal. These five elements are completely interrelated and each is also necessary to support the others. The five element theory aligns all living and inanimate objects with one of these five dominant elements. In the body each of our internal organs resonates with the energy of one of these elements. The five elements are also linked in a specific sequence of circulating energy pathways that can be disrupted by many things including our emotional responses to outside events as well as environmental factors. An understanding of this sequence and its relationship with the five elements helps a practitioner reach a diagnosis.

All things in nature of course also have yin and yang qualities, and by further factoring this into the equation, the practitioner of Chinese medicine is able to draw in his mind a total picture of the complex relationship a person has with the universe, the balance of the relationship between our internal organs, body fluids and qi, and how these affect an individual's health.

The idea of five elements or qualities is common throughout Chinese medicine. For instance, there are five main organs (spleen, liver, kidney, lungs and heart) and five main emotions (anger, joy, pensiveness, grief and fear). There are also five smells, sounds, colours and tissues all corresponding to the five elements.

What's in the mix?

The Chinese rarely use herbs singly. Instead they are used in complex combinations which are made to balance disturbances in damp, heat, dark, light and so on. Typically, Chinese mixtures contain between six and 16 herbs. Medicinal herbs are combined to increase positive health benefits while minimising negative ones. One way to think of these mixtures is in terms of chiefs, deputies, assistants or envoys. The chief provides the main therapeutic action, and the deputies enhance the action of the chiefs. The assistants treat accompanying symptoms or moderate the harshness of other herbs and the envoys have a harmonising effect or guide the formula to a certain area of the body or acupuncture channel.

Chinese herbs are also classified according to five flavours: pungent, sweet, sour, bitter or salty. They also have five qi attributes (hot, cold, warm, cool or neutral) as well as four directions (ascending, floating, descending, sinking). The combination of these attributes gives a herb its individual quality. In order to restore balance in the qi and in the blood, Chinese herbal medicine is applied according to the principle of opposites. So if the patient is 'hot' and 'dry', a 'cold' and 'damp' remedy will be used.

What the research says

Traditional Chinese medicine, like **Ayurveda** and **naturopathy**, is a total system of healthcare and prevention, but it has never been evaluated as such. Research into TCM invariably examines its components such as **acupuncture** or **acupressure** or the use of Chinese herbs or herbal mixtures.

Research into Chinese herbal medicine is still relatively scarce. What there is often comes from China and is universally positive, suggesting a potential bias that makes it difficult to know which herbs are really useful and which ones are not. Other research is carried out on animals or in test tubes, useful only to a degree since it can be difficult to predict from such experiments just how a herb will perform once in the human system. In spite of this, some herbs associated with Chinese medicine have shown some promise in specific health complaints.

Eczema

When most people think of the Western use of Chinese herbs they think of eczema. Success in treating this condition, especially in children, has had a great deal of publicity. Two well-conducted trials, under the auspices of the Royal Free Hospital in London, have shown that children with eczema experience a reduction in symptoms like itching after taking Chinese herbs. The main trial consisted of a group of 47 children with severe disabling atopic eczema unresponsive to conventional therapy.

Each was given either a mixture of ten Chinese herbs or a placebo. Not all the children completed the study, but among the 37 that did all showed some improvement and an impressive 60 per cent showed clinically significant improvements. The herbal treatment did not appear to alter blood chemistry and no laboratory abnormalities in the liver or kidneys were detected during treatment. A follow-up trial a year later showed that the improvement persisted even after discontinuing the herbs.

A second trial involving adults also produced improvement in a similar proportion of participants.

That's the good news. But, as with many Chinese herbal formulations, frequently these mixtures taste terrible. Often they require boiling and simmering and then consumption while still warm and these factors can lead to poor compliance on the part of the child and the parent (this often accounts for high levels of patient 'drop outs' in clinical trials). Also remedies on their own are not always successful unless other aspects of the child's life – such as the removal of dietary allergens – are changed.

Prostate cancer
PC-SPES is a traditional Chinese medicine consisting of eight herbs. Since it first became commercially available in 1996 scientists have been trying to understand more about how it works.

There is some evidence to show that supplements of PC-SPES cause a dramatic decrease in levels of prostate specific antigen (or PSA, high levels of which indicate a raised risk of prostate cancer) and inhibit the growth of prostate tumours in animals. Human research exists, but trials are usually too small to provide definitive conclusions.

In October 2000 researchers from Columbia University in New York divided 69 men into three groups: 43 who had received prior therapy and who had a hormone-sensitive disease, 22 who had hormone-resistant cancer and four who were already receiving PC-SPES as first therapy.

The men took 320 mg capsules of PC-SPES three times daily. After two months a significant proportion of men in each group had a decrease in PSA. Among the men with hormone-sensitive cancer, lower levels of PSA were observed in 82 per cent and this number was maintained at six months. Among the men with hormone-resistant cancer PSA decreased in 90 per cent and remained lower after six months in 74 per cent. Among the four men already receiving PC-SPES as a treatment, two showed a drop in PSA levels of more than 50 per cent.

But the study also noted uncomfortable side effects similar to those produced by conventional hormone therapies in some men: 43 per cent of all the men reported swollen, tender breasts, 7 per cent had hot flushes and 2 per cent had clots in their veins. This latter effect is most worrisome since it could mean an increased risk of stroke among some users.

Adverse effects like these have caused some researchers to look deeper into how PC-SPES works. For a long time PC-SPES was considered a non-estrogenic alternative and so unlikely to produce the adverse effects of conventional hormone treatments. However, a 1998 study that tested PC-SPES in the lab as well as on mice and men with prostate cancer showed that this may not be true. Laboratory analysis showed that PC-SPES contained unique estrogenic compounds. Animal testing further showed that the mixture exerted an estrogenic effect. In the human arm of the study, in all of the men with prostate cancer, PC-SPES was shown to decrease serum concentrations of testosterone as well as decreasing serum concentrations of PSA. All the men experienced breast tenderness and loss of libido, and one had venous thrombosis – adverse effects associated with estrogen activity.

Malaria

One Chinese herb, *Artemesia annua* (more commonly called wormwood or in Chinese, *quinghaosu*), has been shown to be particularly effective against a disease that threatens those living in and travelling to undeveloped countries – malaria. Drug resistance and major side effects have become major problems in treating malaria conventionally. This is why herbalists are so excited about the possibilities of this ancient herb.

Artemesia has been used in Chinese medicine for thousands of years to treat a variety of ailments. But only recently has its anti-malarial potential been recognised. In papers published in reputable Western journals it has been found to be as effective as quinine in preventing deaths from severe malaria. It also acts more rapidly than other anti-malarial medications and has no known toxicity, though individual responses can vary.

Irritable bowel syndrome

Irritable bowel syndrome affects around 10 to 20 per cent of people in the West. As yet there is no reliable conventional treatment for the disorder, though several alternative therapies claim success. In a well-designed study in 1998 involving 116 sufferers, individually prescribed Chinese herbal treatments offered significant improvement in symptoms.

Participants were randomly assigned to receive either individualised Chinese herbal preparations, a standard Chinese herbal formula or a placebo. Participants received five capsules three times daily for 16 weeks and were evaluated regularly by both a traditional Chinese herbalist and a gastroenterologist who were looking for improvement in both general well-being and in specific bowel symptoms.

The results showed that those taking the Chinese herbals experienced a significant reduction in the degree to which IBS interfered with their lives. Bowel symptoms were also diminished, a finding that was independently confirmed by the gastroenterologist. Surprisingly, the individually tailored herbs did not perform any better than the standard Chinese remedy during the trial. However, only those who took individualised herbal medicines maintained their improvement at follow-up 14 weeks after the completion of the trial.

Hepatitis B

Hepatitis B virus infection is a serious worldwide health problem. The virus affects the liver and if left untreated can be fatal. Many Chinese herbal combinations are purported to protect, nourish and repair the liver, but research in this area is patchy. In one review in 2001 that combined the results of all the known trials into Chinese herbs and hepatitis B, only the compound *Fuzheng tang* had a significant positive effect in clearing the virus from the blood of those with chronic hepatitis infection. In another review published at the same time, involving hepatitis B carriers, the herbal compound *Jianpi wenshen* recipe showed a significant antiviral activity against the virus.

Menstrual irregularities and menopause

Dang gui, the root of the herb *Angelica sinensis*, is the number one herb for generalised female complaints in traditional Chinese medicine. It has an estrogenic effect and is mainly used to regulate menstruation (particularly painful periods). But because women with menstrual problems may also have a greater tendency towards menopausal symptoms, many have turned to dang gui as a way of replacing estrogen without having to take conventional estrogen replacements (and thus exposing themselves to increased risks of breast and other estrogen-dependent cancers). Dang gui is also sometimes used to relieve symptoms associated with pregnancy.

Amazingly, given that dang gui is such an old herb and has been so widely recommended to women, few studies are available to prove its effectiveness. There is, for instance, little to suggest that dang gui can really aid menstrual problems. And while once thought to be a panacea for treating menopause, dang gui's popularity has diminished in recent years as it has become apparent that plant estrogens can exert just as powerful an effect on the body as synthetic ones. Indeed, dang gui's efficacy in regulating hot flushes is thought to be due to its estrogenic effects and its ability to regulate blood vessels.

Studies into the use of dang gui in menopause show little promise. In one at the Kaiser Permanente Medical Care Program of Northern California in 1997, 71 post-menopausal women complaining of night sweats or hot flushes were randomly given dang gui or a placebo three times a day for 24 weeks. At the end of the study researchers found no differences between the two groups of women.

In light of the paucity of studies, it might be worth bearing in mind the adverse effects of ginseng, another estrogenic herb sometimes used in TCM. Cases have been reported of abnormal bleeding in post-menopausal women who took this natural alternative.

What's in a name?

Some people love the mystery of taking medicines that have exotic-sounding names. Others are more reticent. However, many of the most popular Chinese herbal ingredients are not as alien as they seem and are also common to Western and other herbal traditions. The chart below gives both the traditional Chinese and Western names of some Chinese herbs. You may already be using them for certain conditions without realising it.

Chinese name	Western name	Commonly used for
Dang gui	*Angelica sinensis*	Used for menstrual disorders and irregularities. Dang gui is an estrogenic herb which is why it is sometimes included in menopause formulas.
Yi zhi ren	**Black cardamom** *Alpinia oxyphylla*	Also used in ***Ayurveda***, this is a warming spice often found in spicy herb teas (and of course curries) used to treat digestive disorders.
Ma huang	*Ephedra sinica*	For colds and flu, fever, chills, headache, oedema, bronchial asthma and aching joints and bones. Alkaloids of this herb are used in commercial cold and flu remedies in the UK but are now banned from commercial products in the US because use increases the risk of stroke.
Ren shen	**Panax ginseng**	As detailed in the ***Herbal Medicine*** section this herb is used to provide short-term energy and reduce stress.
Wu wei zi	**Schisandra fruit** *Schisandra chinensis*	Popular additive to herbal fruit-based drinks. In ***Chinese Medicine*** it is used for coughs, wheezing and asthma, and to support the kidneys and lift the spirit.

Huan qin	**Skullcap root** *Acutellaria biacalensis*	Skullcap is also used in Western herbal medicine. Its primary function is to remove heat from the body and so it is used in any condition where fever is present.
Gan cao	**Liquorice root** *Glycyrrhiza glabra*	Used to boost energy, relieve bronchial conditions and aid digestion. See ***Herbal Medicine*** for more.
Shan zha	**Hawthorn berry** *Crataegus pinnatifida*	In the West this fruit is used to treat high blood pressure. In ***Chinese Medicine*** it is a digestive, blood purifier and anti-diarrhetic.
Huo ma ren	**Cannibis seeds/ Hemp** *Cannibis sativa*	Used for a variety of things in the West. Most recently the seeds (which can be used in cooking) have been found to be high in omega 3 fatty acids. The Chinese believe it lubricates the intestines, eases constipation and helps rehydrate the body.
Gui zhi	**Cinnamon** *Cinnamonum cassia*	Another warming spice often used to treat rheumatic conditions. Also used in ***Ayurveda***.
Chen pi	**Tangerine peel** *Citrus reticulata*	Tonic used to rejuvenate the spleen and for abdominal bloating wind, nausea and vomiting. Candied citrus peel is used in Western cooking.
Xing ren	**Apricot kernel** *Prunus armenica*	Primarily used to treat coughing and wheezing. The Italians make sweet biscuits from ground apricot kernels.
Da huang	**Rhubarb root and stalk** *Rheum palmatum*	A purgative used in cases of jaundice, constipation and cystitis and some menstrual conditions. Also used in Western ***Herbal Medicine***.

Cautions

Almost more than any other type of alternative therapy, the use of Chinese herbal preparations has been associated with a high number of adverse effects – especially irreversible liver and kidney damage and allergies.

Because Chinese medicine uses a different language to describe health and healing and the properties of the herbs it employs, other problems associated with TCM herbs, such as hormone imbalance and hypertension, have been slower to come to light in the West.

Given that there is no universal language of healing, potential users would be well advised to find out exactly what is in the mixture they have been advised to take and to do a bit of homework on its potential effects in the body.

As a general rule, do not try to self-treat with Chinese herbal medicines. To an untrained Westerner one Chinese name can look much like another and it is very easy to get the wrong remedy and use it in the wrong way.

When marketed as dietary supplements Chinese herbs do not come under the same regulations as they would as medicines. It is hardly surprising then that there have been reports of contaminated products, Western drug adulterants used as additives, accidental substitutions of patented herb products by commercial manuacturers (usually in the West) as well as inappropriate use of the herb. These can all plague the casual user and end up causing very poor health indeed.

In addition, many practitioners mix their own herbs, and as such these herbs do not need to be licensed. If you are given a herbal mixture ask your practitioner to write down exactly what is in it. No reputable practitioner should refuse to do this. The same applies to patented pills which often come in their original Chinese packaging. If you experience any adverse effect from the mixture, stop taking it and contact your therapist immediately.

The Chinese herb Ma huang has a reputation (largely unproved) of increasing energy levels, improving your sex life and reducing asthmatic symptoms. Not surprising since Ma huang contains an adrenaline-like substance, ephidrine, which speeds up the heart and excites the nervous system.

According to a recent review, more than 800 adverse reactions to ephedrine have been reported to the FDA since 1993, including strokes (particularly in women), heart attacks and seizures. Most recently kidney stones were added to the potential risks of taking large regular doses of this drug.

What to expect

As with most alternative therapies, the first consultation with a Chinese herbalist usually involves a lengthy process of history-taking. You will be asked about your symptoms, your family and medical history, lifestyle and diet. You will be asked about your bowel movements, what kind of stresses you are under and how you react to things like changes in temperature and weather.

Your practitioner will perform a physical examination which will involve looking at your eyes, tongue and hair and perhaps noting how you smell and listening to the sound of your voice. Your pulses (in Chinese medicine there is more than one) will usually be taken, often at both wrists.

Having diagnosed your condition, your practitioner may prescribe a mixture of herbs for you to take. Often these have very specific preparation instructions that can involve boiling and reboiling. It is important to follow these carefully to get the most benefit from the mixture. You may be prescribed patented pills on their own or in addition to herbal brews. *Acupuncture* may also be recommended. The length of therapy will vary depending on the condition being treated.

The training and experience of a practitioner can often make a substantial difference to the success, as well as the rate of adverse effects, experienced with Chinese herbs. Generally speaking there are three types of practitioners: those who have trained in China (where training is quite rigorous); those who have trained partly in China and partly in the UK or elsewhere in the West; and those who have not trained at all. Chinese herbalists are not regulated in the UK, which means that anyone with a handful of herbs and a cash register can set up shop and claim to be a practitioner of Chinese herbal medicine. Unfortunately many do just that.

Without some knowledge of Chinese medicine and which schools here and abroad are reputable, it is frankly impossible for most consumers to tell a good practitioner from a bad one.

To be on the safe side you might try choosing a practitioner who is registered with the Register of Chinese Herbal Medicine. Members of this organisation must have a minimum of five years' training including three years in Western medicine. No other organisations of this type exist to register practitioners of Chinese herbal medicine, and while it is true that many highly trained professionals do not belong to the RCHM, if any of their members are in your area, you can consult them with confidence.

Chapter 20

Urine Therapy

Commonly used for

Emergency Rehydration in Drought Conditions
• Nourishment during Fasting • Boosting Immunity
• Beauty Treatments • Allergies

• Suitable for self-treatment

You'll never find a cheaper more easily accessible therapy than this. You don't need a prescription for it, it appears to be non-toxic, has no adverse effects and anyone can administer it to themselves in doses that they themselves determine. The more diplomatic (or perhaps squeamish) call it autotherapy or autour-therapy, but to the more plain speaking it's simply urine therapy.

While the common perception is that urine is simply human waste, there is a strong body of opinion that believes that it is, in fact, the perfect medicine. Anecdotes from practitioners suggest that drinking urine can promote increased energy, better health and a rediscovery of the joy of living. However, there is no scientific proof of any of this – nor is there ever likely to be.

In Ayurvedic tradition this therapy was called *amaroli*. Originally amaroli was simply one element in the spiritual practice of yogis and rishis, not a form of medical treatment, and because it was not practised by the general populace, amaroli eventually fell into disuse for many years. But re-emerging interest in Eastern traditions, especially in **Ayurveda** and **yoga**, has brought with it curiosity about the benefits of urine therapy.

The usual argument against urine therapy is that it is somehow 'dirty'. This is patently not true. The function of the kidneys is to regulate the balance of essential elements in the blood, not to filter out toxic waste – that's the liver's function. In healthy people urine is a sterile substance containing not waste products but a variety of pre-assimilated nutrients. Around 95 per cent of urine is water, 2.5 per cent is urea and the remaining 2.5 per cent is a mixture of minerals, salt, hormones and enzymes.

Be that as it may, many would maintain that drinking your own is not entirely 'natural'. There is no other species in the entire animal kingdom that drinks its own urine. Animals may roll in it and use it to mark their territory, but they do not drink it.

Whether drinking urine is therapeutic or not, the disgust with which urine therapy is met seems somewhat irrational. The Age of Reason elevated the mind to a superior position, while at the same time encouraging a completely irrational revulsion against anything to do with the deep inner workings of the human body. At the very least the acceptance of one's own urine as 'clean' (whether we choose to drink it or not) might be a first psychological step towards breaking down unhealthy barriers between body and mind.

How does it work?
Taken internally, urine is reputed to be a nourishing drink (particularly during fasting). It can be used as a gargle, an enema and a vaginal douche, as ear or eye drops and a nasal wash. Externally, its uses include massaging, rubbing, footbaths, compresses and hair and scalp massage.

Proponents of urine therapy claim that urine is a kind of in-house pharmacy and that rubbed on to the skin or drunk it can purify the blood and tissues, provide useful nutrients and also send the body a subtle signal about whether it is in or out of balance. This last point, if true, may have quite profound implications for health. Sometimes called 'oral auto-immunisation', it is said to be the result of the body's reaction to minute particles in the urine. These minute particles are mainly antibodies which upon re-ingestion may help the body to fight disease. This could be why urine therapy is said to have a beneficial effect on everything from colds and toothaches to tuberculosis and asthma, minor skin rashes and eczema, psoriasis and even skin cancer.

In addition, for some, using their own body processes to heal themselves can provide a psychological boost and a sense of control that has a knock-on effect on physical health.

What the research says

The problem is that most of what we know about urine therapy is based on the accounts of motivated individuals who say it made them feel better, or therapists who report that it made their patients feel better. However, there has never been any research into the benefits of drinking one's own urine.

Designing proper research for urine therapy would be a scientific nightmare. For instance, even if one could find a large enough group of people motivated to drink their own urine for long periods of time, the trial could never be randomised or blinded (since the object is to drink your own urine), nor could it be placebo controlled (once you have drunk your own urine you will know its individual taste). There may also be something psychologically different about people who are comfortable drinking their own urine that could influence the outcome of any trial. These problems, along with the conviction among enthusiasts that belief is a large part of the process of healing, means that urine therapy may never be properly evaluated.

However, in 1991 scientific study did shed some light on a potential benefit of drinking urine. Australian researchers, seeking to discover a biological basis for urine drinking, found that urine contains large quantities of the hormone melatonin. Melatonin is released by the brain's pineal gland during the night and is involved in setting the body's daily rhythms. It can also dull pain and make people feel sleepy.

The traditional practice of amaroli consists of rising very early in the morning (4 a.m.) and drinking one's own mid-stream urine. Urinary melatonin levels are high at this time. The researchers speculated that melatonin may induce a slight state of tranquillity by slowing brainwave activity. It can also fool the body into thinking it has had more sleep than it has, and may reduce the pain of sitting for long periods during meditation. They suggested that drinking one's own early morning urine may provide a melatonin supplement that enhances the user's subsequent meditation and visualisation practice. They also acknowledge that synthetic melatonin may represent a more acceptable experimental tool for such purposes.

While some would argue that the medical profession doesn't promote the use of urine therapy because there is no money in it, this argument only goes so far. Many modern medicines are synthesised from urine. For instance, Urokinase, made by the US company Enzymes of America and used to unclog arteries, is made from men's urine collected from the 10,000 portable outhouses owned by its subsidiary firm PortaJohn.

The fertility drug Pergonal is produced from the urine of post-menopausal women in Italy, Spain, Brazil and Argentina. Its manufacturer's yearly earnings from this product are in the region of £570 ($855) million and women pay up to £935 ($1,400) per month for the treatment.

In addition, the HRT supplement Premarin is made from the urine of pregnant mares (in fact, its name is derived from *Pregnant Mares' Urine*). This, however, begs the question, wouldn't women benefit more from a product made from the urine of pregnant women?

Urea is a powerful antibacterial and antiviral. Products that contain urea include Ureaphil, a diuretic; Urofollitrophin, also a fertility drug; Ureic, a cream for skin problems; and Panafil, ointment for skin ulcers, burns and infected wounds. Carbamide is the name for synthesised urea as found in Murine eye drops.

Urea and cancer

Many proponents of urine-drinking believe that a daily dose will prevent cancer. The notion that human urine might have anti-cancer properties has been around since the Second World War. However, it was never seriously investigated until the late 1950s, when Dr Evangelos D. Danopoulos, professor of medicine at the Medical School of Athens University and a specialist in optic oncology, began to explore the uses of urea in preventing various types of cancer.

Urea, he found, appears to disrupt the water system on the surface of cancer cells – which treat water differently than do normal cells – thus interfering with some of the metabolism necessary for cells to replicate and spread.

In one of his many studies involving 46 patients with cancer in or around the eye (a difficult condition to treat), Dr Danopoulos discovered that treatment with surgery and local urea injections was successful in 100 per cent of cases. In another study of nine people with cancer of the mucous membrane inside the eyelid, eight out of the nine given local applications of urea were cured.

In other small studies 18 patients with liver cancer given urea survived 26.5 months – five times longer than expected, as did 28 liver cancer patients, 17 of whom had cancer that had spread.

Such studies, while encouraging and often paraded by urine enthusiasts as proof of urine's cancer-busting ability, cannot really be considered proof of urine's efficacy. Studies using high concentrations of urea do not reflect what a person might get in a glass full of their own urine. Urine contains only a small amount of urea and this becomes further diluted once returned to the body.

While urea (the end product of protein metabolism) is utilised in many bodily functions, it is unlikely that any person could be diagnosed as being deficient in this substance or in need of supplementation. Few scientists have followed up Dr Danopoulos's findings in this particular area and indeed he was pilloried by his colleagues and lost his position at the university shortly after publishing his research.

Cautions

There are many things we do not know about urine therapy. We can analyse urine for its content and know scientifically what the urine of a healthy person is likely to contain. We can produce purified drugs made from the constituents of human and animal urine.

But what we cannot say is whether the small amounts of vitamins, minerals, hormones and other substances may have effects which we have not considered in our rush to find yet another 'natural' means to better health. Could it be possible, for example, that minute amounts of chemicals in urine could cause homeopathic reactions that we cannot yet foresee? There is a reaction, well known to practitioners of urine therapy, when the body goes through a period of crisis, shaking, nausea, vomiting and tiredness. This is generally considered a 'good' sign, a sign that the body is healing itself – but how do we know this is the case?

Equally, we have not given much thought to the fact that the original practitioners of amaroli were men. What different reactions might there be for women – whose hormonal system adjusts itself anew daily to meet the demands of the reproductive cycle – who drink their own urine and thus consume more of these excreted hormones? For some it may prove helpful; for others it may cause debilitating side effects.

We must also pause to consider the pitfalls in Western individuals wantonly appropriating Eastern practices. Amaroli developed out of a culture which was largely rural and poverty stricken and where the diets were largely vegetarian. It is unlikely that the yogis ingested any of the toxic chemicals in the form of pesticides, synthetic hormones, artificial food additives and preservatives as well as prescription and over-the-counter drugs which we in the West consume daily, often in vast quantities. Because of our high-pressure lifestyle, Westerners may also be excreting more stress hormones in their urine. Is re-ingesting these things via our own urine really a healthy alternative? Enthusiasts cannot have it both ways: urine therapy cannot be both powerful medicine and completely benign.

As a rule, it is generally not recommended to combine urine therapy with the use of prescribed chemical, allopathic medicines, recreational drugs or even over-the-counter remedies; and this prohibition should also extend to those taking herbal remedies. The combination may be dangerous to your health. If you wish to try urine therapy and are taking any form of allopathic medicine, begin with external applications only until you are free of all medication, if possible.

If it is not possible or safe to stop the use of certain medicines, start by taking a few drops of urine internally or use a homeopathic tincture or gently rub fresh urine into the accupressure points in your ears. Keep a careful watch on how your body is responding to the treatment. When suffering from a serious illness it is generally advisable to consult an experienced Ayurvedic practitioner about the best way to proceed. Urine therapy might help you – but as with any form of 'natural' medicine, it is advisable to weigh both the pros and cons before you begin.

How to use urine therapeutically

Proponents of urine therapy believe that urine can be beneficial no matter how it is used. If you wish to try urine therapy for yourself, consider some of the following applications:

Internally

Drinking – morning urine is best. Take the mid-stream sample and start with a few drops, building up to one glass a day. Considered a tonic and a preventative.

Fasting – drink all the urine you pass, except for the evenings, otherwise you might experience difficulty falling asleep. You can also take some extra water. During fasting the taste of urine is said to become almost neutral. Fasting on urine and water is supposed to cleanse the blood and aid the removal of toxins.

Gargle – for sore throats, colds and possibly toothache.

Enemas – used to cleanse the colon and provide a direct immune stimulant.

Vaginal douche – thought to be helpful in yeast infections and other types of inflammation.

Ear and eyedrops – for ear infections, conjunctivitis, glaucoma. When using on the eyes, dilute the urine with some water.

Nasal rinse/neti – to alleviate sinusitis and other nose problems. A potential preventative for colds and flu.

Externally

Massaging/rubbing – you can use either fresh or old urine. Old urine (4 to 8 days) is generally more effective, but it often has a very strong smell. Massaging the whole body is considered an important complement to fasting. You can leave the urine on or wash it off after an hour or so, with just water or with a mild, natural soap. Fresh urine as an aftershave is supposed to soothe the skin and leave it soft, but it may also help other kinds of skin problems including itching, sunburns, eczema, psoriasis and acne.

Rubbed into acupressure points – gentle massaging of urine into acupressure points (e.g. on the ears) may be useful when reactions to taking urine in other forms are otherwise too strong, for instance, with very heavy allergic reaction.

Footbaths – for any skin and nail problems of the feet (athlete's foot, ringworm etc.).

Compress – when rubbing is not appropriate, this is another way of applying urine on the skin.

Hair and scalp massage – reputed to leave the hair soft and clean and, some say, stimulates new hair growth.

Chapter 21

Yoga

Commonly used for

Flexibility • Posture • Vitality • Relaxation • Digestive Function
• Respiratory Disorders • Muscle Tone • Circulation
• Backache/Sciatica • Constipation • Depression
• High Blood Pressure • PMS • Joint and Nerve Pain

• Requires professional instruction • Suitable for self-help

Imagine feeling a sense of balance and harmony as you move through your day. This is how practitioners of the ancient art of yoga say they feel.

A form of body movement developed over the centuries, yoga is a unique way to increase the body's supply of energy. Most leisure centres and gyms now include yoga as part of their regular routine and classes are often among the most popular on offer. Yoga is an integral part of **Ayurveda** and Ayurvedic physicians often advise their patients to practise postures, breathing exercises and meditation.

While many people take up yoga as a form of exercise, to call it 'exercise' is somewhat misleading since the practice of yoga stems from a philosophy that takes a bigger view of health and well-being. In common with **osteopathy** and **chiropractic**, yoga emphasises the importance of the spine in relation to our health. Indeed, maintaining a strong, supple spine is seen as an important way to promote good general health.

The term yoga has come to encompass many different styles and philosophies. However, in the West the form of yoga which we are most familiar with is known as Hatha yoga. Although historically yoga was developed by men for men, there is some evidence that in prehistoric cultures women may have used the postures that were later adopted by the yogis. In recent times women have shown an unprecedented interest in yoga and their influence has revolutionised the approach which some practitioners take (something seen most clearly in the antenatal yoga classes that are on offer for pregnant women, where yoga postures have been adapted to help women labour more easily).

While some forms of yoga seek to master the body and control the breath, others seek to work with the body and with the breath to establish a state of harmony in the body. While some forms of yoga seek (or so it seems) to defy gravity and may use forceful movements to attain certain postures, others work with gravity allowing the body to adapt gradually to the postures and feel a greater sense of connection with the earth. What this means is that there are very few 'pure' types of yoga being practised throughout the West. Instead, there is an abundance of eclectic teachers who mix and match styles to create their own individual type of yoga. If one type of class does not suit you, it is likely there will be others that do.

How does it work?

Many physicians who are otherwise sceptical about alternative therapies are often surprisingly passionate about the benefits of yoga. Such views are supported by a number of clinical studies confirming its benefits, which can include lowered blood pressure and relief from stress and anxiety, as well as from physical complaints such as arthritis and asthma.

In general, however, yoga is not used to create health or to cure disease. Instead, its aim is to create an environment, internally and externally, in which the individual can come to his or her own state of dynamic balance. Good health is not static and how we feel physically and emotionally will vary from day to day. The practice of yoga reinforces the interdependence of body and mind, allowing the individual to meet these daily changes with greater ease.

For many devotees, yoga becomes a philosophy that offers guidance and insight into every aspect of life – the spiritual, the mental, the emotional and the physical. It provides instruction on how to live and interact with others, and even what to eat; many serious practitioners, for instance, are strict vegetarians. However, if you wish to practise yoga, there is no need to take on the whole lifestyle unless you want to. Yoga is equally satisfying as a form of physical therapy, and you will still derive great benefit from engaging in a regular routine at this basic level.

The practice of yoga includes postures, breathing practices, progressive, deep relaxation and sometimes **meditation**. The most immediate benefit you will find from taking up yoga is relaxation. We live in an age of anxiety. In everyday living most of our tensions are pushed to the back of our minds where they become a part of the great, shadowy unconscious. Because we keep them hidden, we often describe ourselves as becoming tired, depressed or anxious for 'no good reason'. Even if you cannot locate the cause of your stress, you will certainly become quickly aware of the effect it has on your body, e.g. insomnia, poor digestion, headaches, tight muscles and a lack of basic vitality. Through the practice of yoga you may find new insights to your problems and a gradual release of long-held anxiety and tension.

The postures

The body postures, known as *asanas*, involve stretching movements that help strengthen, tone and balance the body and mind. They were originally used by the Indian philosophers to improve physical stamina and postural alignment, enabling them to sit in a balanced and still way for long periods of meditation.

More recently it has emerged that the postures used in yoga can also rejuvenate the body at a very deep level. The way this is achieved is complex but includes three basic beneficial actions:

* increasing circulation to the brain, spine and specific organs and glands while also providing a massaging and/or stimulating action on certain areas of the body (see also **massage**)

- deep breathing and visualising specific areas of the body can help to send an extra supply of blood and oxygen to them (similar to techniques used in **meditation** and **biofeedback**)

- the nerves from the spinal column branch out to all the organs and glands; by increasing the spine's flexibility, the postures ensure a healthy central nervous system with a good connection to all parts of the body (see **osteopathy** and **chiropractic**).

Breathing

Many types of yoga use specially developed breathing techniques, known as *pranayamas*. Like the postures, yogic breathing techniques are designed to calm the mind and improve the flow or *prana*, or vital energy (see **Ayurveda**). There are two main uses of breathing practices in yoga:

- aligning the movement into and out of the postures with breathing; so, for example, some movements are done with the outbreath and others on an inbreath

- pranayama is both cleansing and revitalising; often it involves specific breathing practices which encompass more than just breathing in and out, and include the ideas of life force, energy and vitality.

The Western way of breathing is often shallow and gasps sharply at the inbreath. In yoga, breathing practices help the breathing to be slower and more rhythmic. Some teachers emphasise the importance of breathing out, maintaining that a full outbreath will improve the circulation of various bodily fluids, increase energy and enable wastes and toxins to be removed more easily.

Focused awareness and relaxation

Most yoga sessions include a period of relaxation with focused awareness, usually at the beginning or end of each session. Some people use this time to get in touch with themselves; others focus on affirmations or visualisations.

The reflective aspect of yoga is important since the asanas and pranayamas also involve a focused attention and work on the mind as well as the physical body. This is particularly helpful in this computer and video age where we are all so used to assimilating things quickly, and on a superficial level, that the spiritual 'muscle' of concentration has become very flabby.

In more advanced yoga sessions there may also be a period of **meditation**. In the yogic sense meditation is different from contemplation or visualisation. Meditation in yoga involves sitting in an upright, still posture and clearing the mind of activity by focusing on one simple object. The object for meditation can be a simple image, a sound (sometimes called a mantra) or the natural rhythm of the breath. It can be quite a challenge to be quiet and still when our lives are so full of constant stimulation, but it can also be a relief and a welcome respite. The process of meditation, in which we continually let go of any thoughts that arrive, brings us closer to being centred and peaceful.

What the research says

Since the early 1970s there have been more than a thousand studies into yoga and meditation. Overall, these show that people who practise yoga have reduced anxiety, are more resistant to stress, and have lower blood pressure, more efficient heart function, better respiratory function and improved physical fitness. Yoga is being assessed for its potential in treating illnesses such as multiple sclerosis, cerebral palsy, osteoporosis, rheumatoid arthritis and postnatal depression.

Although yoga has been shown at least anecdotally to be beneficial in a variety of specific conditions, its primary emphasis is upon general well-being. Yoga employs a broad holistic approach that focuses on teaching people a new lifestyle, as well as new ways of thinking and of being in the world. By attending to practices for improving, regaining and retaining general good health, a person is likely to find that some more specific difficulties tend to disappear.

Most studies into yoga are observational and lack a control group – that is, a group of comparable individuals not practising yoga – so it can be difficult to know whether in some cases yoga is significantly better than other relaxing therapies or simply doing nothing. In addition, most are published in Indian medical journals and, like the studies of TCM published in Chinese journals, tend to be positive. Because of this it can be hard to sort the myth from the medicine. Nevertheless, there is general agreement on some basic ways in which yoga can be therapeutic.

Respiratory problems

Perhaps the most widely researched benefits of yoga practice are those that affect the respiratory system. Many studies have shown that practising yoga improves respiratory function and can lessen the severity and duration of asthma attacks.

This is largely because of the emphasis that yoga places on correct breathing and the importance of the outbreath. Studies conducted at yoga institutions in India have reported impressive success in improving asthma. With the increasing concern about the widely used orally administered bronchodilators and the increasing death rate from asthma, this non-invasive approach has appeal since even small gains in respiratory function can mean significant improvement in breathing function for asthmatics.

At the Northern Colorado Allergy Asthma Clinic in the US, a controlled clinical study of university students (19 to 52 years old) with asthma concluded that yoga techniques seem beneficial as a complement to the medical management of asthma. Using a set of asanas, pranayama and meditation, the yoga group practised three times a week for 16 weeks. At the end of that time the subjects in the yoga group reported a significant degree of relaxation, positive attitude and better yoga exercise tolerance – even though objective tests showed no difference in lung function. There was also a tendency towards less use of inhalers.

Other studies have confirmed the beneficial effects of yoga for patients with respiratory problems. For instance, in a study at City Hospital in Nottingham, yoga was found particularly useful at reducing the frequency of asthma attacks. In a study of 40 adolescent asthmatics yoga training (which included the more rarely prescribed cleansing methods of induced vomiting and diarrhoea and rinsing the nose and throat with a saline wash) resulted in a significantly increased lung function and a reduced need for medication.

In an Indian study in 1895, 53 people with asthma were taught yoga postures and breathing exercises. The researchers found that, compared to another group who continued to take conventional medications, those who practised these exercises for 65 minutes each day had a significant improvement in their symptoms.

In 1982 researchers followed 570 asthma sufferers for three to 54 months after receiving training in yoga. Results showed that those

Health conditions benefited by yoga

Yoga has been shown to produce many subjective benefits for those who practise it. The table below is a summary of a British survey of 3,000 individuals with health problems who were prescribed yoga as an alternative form of therapy.

Ailment	Reported cases	% claiming benefit
Back pain	1,142	98
Arthritis	589	90
Anxiety	838	94
Migraine	464	80
Insomnia	542	82
Nerve/muscle disease	112	96
Menstrual problems	317	68
Premenstrual tension	848	77
Menopausal symptoms	247	83
Hypertension	150	84
Heart disease	50	94
Asthma/bronchitis	226	88
Duodenal ulcers	40	90
Haemorrhoids	391	88
Obesity	240	74
Diabetes	10	80
Cancer	29	90
Tobacco addiction	219	74
Alcoholism	26	100

Source: *Yoga Biomedical Trust Survey, 1983–4*

who practised yoga regularly experienced the greatest improvement in their condition and on average 69 per cent felt able to stop using their asthma medication.

Heart disease

The relaxation and exercise components of yoga have a major role to play in the treatment and prevention of high blood pressure (hypertension) and atherosclerosis because of their ability to reduce blood pressure, stress and anxiety, as well as improving self-confidence and muscular strength.

Several studies, for instance, have found that the practice of yoga can lower blood pressure significantly in a relatively short period of time.

One study in 1973 tested the effects of yoga and biofeedback as a combined relaxation therapy to reduce hypertension. After three months of practising yoga and biofeedback, five of 20 patients were able to stop using antihypertensive drugs and drug use was reduced by 33 per cent to 60 per cent in seven others. Blood pressure was lowered in four additional patients, with little or no change in the remaining four. Researchers suggest that yoga may work by reducing sympathetic reactions to stress, which are said to cause the increase of neurohormones that induce hypertension.

Two years later the same author studied a combination of biofeedback and yogic breathing or a relaxation technique in 34 people and found the combination to lower blood pressure and reduce the need for medication in people suffering from high blood pressure. Thirty-four patients with hypertension were randomised to practise both yoga and biofeedback or general relaxation.

In the yoga group, blood pressure dropped on average from 168/100 to 141/84 mm Hg compared to the relaxation group where the average drop was from 169/101 to 160/96. The untreated group were then given yoga training, at which point their blood pressure also fell to levels similar to those of the other group. Another study indicated that yoga, combined with a low-fat vegetarian diet, could produce similar results after just three months of practice.

Another study of 93 people at risk of coronary heart disease showed that yoga could lower blood fat levels and therefore the risk of atherosclerosis. The study divided participants into two groups. Both groups were given instruction on how to modify their lifestyles to reduce their risk of heart disease, but only one group was given instruction in yoga and asked to practise at home. After 14 weeks levels of HDL cholesterol remained unchanged but the yoga group had significantly lower LDL cholesterol levels. LDL is considered a risk factor for heart disease, while HDL cholesterol is not.

The heart benefits of yoga are not limited to those already suffering from cardiovascular disease; studies conducted with healthy subjects have also demonstrated significant results. One involved 40 male physical education teachers who all had an average of 8.9 years of regular physical activity prior to the study. However, following three months of a comprehensive daily yoga practice, there was a significant overall reduction in systolic and diastolic blood pressure, heart rate and respiratory rate, and body weight, in addition to a better response to stress.

Diabetes

People with non-insulin dependent diabetes mellitus (NIDDM) may also find that yoga helps to control their condition. In one small study of 21 people with NIDDM, participants were divided into two groups. All continued to take their medication and follow a special diet, but half also practised yoga 2–3 times a week. After three months the yoga group were able to reduce their medication and reported feeling better and more in control of themselves.

Another study of 149 persons with NIDDM found that 104 had lowered blood sugar and needed less oral anti-diabetes medication after regularly practising yoga. Because the participants were placed on a vegetarian diet during the study, however, the effect of yoga practice alone on blood sugar levels cannot be determined.

Mood and vitality

Mental health and physical energy are difficult to quantify, but virtually everyone who participates in yoga over a period of time reports a positive effect on outlook and energy level. A British study published in the *Journal of the Royal Society of Medicine* in 1993 included 71 healthy volunteers aged 21 to 76 and compared the effects of relaxation, visualisation and yoga on participants' mood and vitality. Researchers found that a 30-minute programme of yogic stretching and breathing exercises was simple to learn and resulted in a 'markedly invigorating' effect on perceptions of both mental and physical energy and improved mood.

The yoga group also reported a significantly greater increase in mental and physical energy and feelings of alertness and enthusiasm than the other group. In contrast, relaxation was found to make people more sleepy and sluggish after a session. Visualisation, too, made participants more sluggish and less content than those in the yoga group.

Other conditions

Studies into yogic breathing practices make interesting reading. For instance, the practice of breathing through one nostril at a time has been shown through electroencephalographic or EEG readings (which measure brainwave activity) to selectively stimulate the opposite hemisphere of the brain. The right side of the brain is generally considered to be the seat of creativity, while the left side is where logic and thought originate. Some postulate that using this form of pranayama it may be possible to temporarily increase the function in either side of the brain, though studies in this area have produced inconsistent results.

Another EEG study found that after practising a particular type of yogic cleansing breath, *kapalabhati* – which involves short, sharp outbreaths – subjects showed a decrease in faster alpha and beta brainwaves and so a relative increase in the slower theta brainwaves which are produced as part of our relaxation response.

While it has been suggested that yoga may help control epileptic seizures, there is little evidence to show that this is the case. Only one small well-conducted study involving 32 people has been performed and while those in the yoga group remained seizure free for longer and had a reduction in seizure frequency, more studies would be necessary before making any recommendations.

Traditional yogic texts describe benefits for arthritis and painful joints and study in this area is encouraging but limited. In the first randomised trial of yoga for arthritis, symptoms such as pain, tenderness and finger range of motion was shown to improve after eight weeks of yoga training. One careful study published in the *Journal of the American Medical Association* in 1998 also concluded that regular yoga was more effective at relieving carpal tunnel syndrome in elderly individuals than the standard treatment of wrist splints.

Regular yoga practice has also been shown to be of benefit in pain management and motor control, and one study into yoga and mentally handicapped children found that yoga helped to produce a highly significant improvement in IQ and social adaptation.

Cautions

There are very few contraindications for yoga. Indeed, because yoga involves minimal impact, it might be particularly valuable for older adults. If you are suffering from low blood pressure, postures which involve standing motionless for extended periods of time can make the condition worse.

If you have never practised before, it is probably best to begin at an elementary level with an experienced teacher. While there are many excellent books on yoga, these are no substitute for expert instruction. It is not advisable to begin a yoga programme on your own as you can easily end up doing the postures wrong (and thus not getting their full benefit) or stretching too far or in the wrong way and doing yourself an injury. There are no advantages to pushing your body beyond its limits.

Pregnant women, many of whom are taking up yoga for the first time, should also take care. To make sure you get the most benefit out of the experience, always go to a class which is specially designed for pregnant women. There are many different schools of yoga and many different approaches. Some such as power yoga and its close relative, ashtanga yoga, are not suitable for pregnant women (and indeed are not suitable for beginners or those who have not exercised for a long time).

If you are pregnant, make sure that you let your teacher know and also tell her how far along you are, whether you suffer from symphysis pubis dysfunction and also whether you have any pregnancy-related conditions such as pelvic pain or blood pressure fluctuations. This information is important since there are certain postures that are not appropriate during pregnancy.

What to expect

Your yoga class will last between one and two hours and will usually involve a small group of five to 15 people. What you are expected to bring along depends on the teacher. Many already have special yoga mats and occasionally belts available for their students to use, whereas some require you to bring your own. It is important that you wear loose, comfortable clothing to encourage freedom of movement. Socks are better than tights since they can be removed to give you more stability during standing postures.

Yoga sessions usually involve warming-up exercises at the beginning and a period of relaxation at the end. In between, your instructor will usually provide a varied programme of standing and floor postures and breathing exercises which you can also practise at home.

You should not feel any strain or pain in any of the postures. If you do, or if you begin to feel light-headed or uncomfortable in any way, come out of the posture. Yoga is not a competition – though in a very few classes it can feel that way. You are not there to see how much longer you can hold a posture or how much more flexible you can be than the person on the mat next to you. The only person you are doing it for is yourself, so know your limits and respect them.

You can find qualified yoga teachers through the British Wheel of Yoga and the Iyengar Yoga Institute.

Part III

Appendices

Appendix 1

What Type of Therapy?

Read through the descriptions of the therapies in this book and you will notice that there is a lot of cross-over between them. Massage, for instance, works on many levels and has links with biofeedback, meditation and spiritual healing. Traditional ethnic therapies such as Ayurveda and Chinese medicine are aligned with the Western practice of naturopathy. The use of flower essences is similar to that of homeopathy, and so it goes on. The chart on p. 288 gives a brief overview of some of the most common therapies and the levels at which they may be beneficial. By understanding what each therapy involves you can, to some extent, fine-tune your choice of therapy to suit your needs.

	Manipulation & massage	Movement & whole body	Psychological	Subtle energy	Biochemical	Sensory
Acupressure	✓			✓		
Acupuncture	✓			✓		
Aromatherapy	✓				✓	✓
Ayurvedic medicine	✓	✓		✓	✓	
Biofeedback			✓			✓
Bowen technique	✓			✓		✓
Chiropractic	✓					✓
Colour healing			✓	✓		✓
Counselling/ Psychotherapy			✓			
Fasting & detox			✓		✓	
Flower remedies			✓	✓	✓	
Herbalism					✓	
Homeopathy				✓	✓	
Massage therapy	✓	✓		✓		✓
Meditation			✓			✓
Metamorphic technique	✓			✓		
Naturopathy	✓	✓			✓	
Nutritional medicine					✓	
Osteopathy	✓			✓		✓
Placebo			✓			
Rebirthing			✓			
Reflexology	✓			✓		✓
Shiatsu	✓			✓		✓
Spiritual healing	✓		✓	✓		
Stress management			✓			
Traditional Chinese medicine	✓			✓	✓	
Yoga		✓		✓		✓

Appendix 2

Drug-Herb Interactions

The importance of careful history-taking by the practitioner, and full disclosure by the patient seeking alternative care, has been highlighted in several recent reviews of the potential interactions of herbal preparations with conventional drugs.

Some practitioners do not ask, and some patients do not volunteer that they are taking other drugs, which may either be potentiated by or whose action might be in some way interfered with by herbal remedies.

However, several such interactions between commonly used drugs and herbal remedies are well documented. While the following table is not intended to be comprehensive, it includes drug interactions with some of the most commonly used herbal remedies.

Herb	Avoid taking with	Reasons
Aloe	• Digoxin • Diuretics • Steroids • Laxatives	• Taken with other potassium wasting medications such as steroids, diuretics, digoxin and commercial laxatives, it may lead to a dangerous decrease in serum potassium levels and a concomitant decrease in heart function. • Aloe is a strong purgative that can enhance the effect of other purgatives. ⊃

Herb	Avoid taking with	Reasons
Camomile	• Antiplatelets and anticoagulants (e.g. warfarin, heparin, aspirin and other NSAIDs, COX-2 inhibitotrs)	• Camomile contains coumarin constituents which may increase the potential for uncontrolled bleeding.
Echinacea	• Corticosteroids (e.g. decadron, prednisone) and immuno-suppressives (e.g. cyclosporin) • Alcohol • Liver dysfunction	• As it is an immuno-stimulant it should also not be given concomitantly with immuno-suppressants (e.g. corticosteroids and cyclosporin). • Has the potential to cause liver toxicity especially if used with other known liver toxic drugs such as anabolic steroids, amiodarone methotrexate and ketoconazole.
Ephedra	• Caffeine and over-the-counter stimulants such as phenylpro-panolamine or pseudoephedrine • Oxytocin • Digoxin • Corticosteroids (e.g. dexamethasone) • Bronchodilators (e.g. theophylline) • Diabetes medications	• The risks of ephedra (ephidrine, ma huang), found in some decongestants, weight-loss products and athletic performance enhancers, outweighs any possible benefits. It can for instance double your risk of stroke. • Taking ephedra with other stimulants can increase the risk of high blood pressure, nervousness, irregular heartbeat, or even heart attack or stroke. • Potentiates the hypertensive effects of oxytocin. • Potentiates the effect of digoxin. • Reduces the effectiveness of dexamethasone. • Can raise blood glucose levels.
Feverfew	• NSAIDs • Warfarin	• NSAIDS may negate the effectiveness of this herb. May alter bleeding time and should not be used with warfarin.

Herb	Avoid taking with	Reasons
Garlic	• Diabetes medications • Anticoagulants and antiplatelet drugs	• Garlic's active ingredients at medicinal levels may interfere with blood sugar-lowering medications, enhance the effects of anticoagulants and hypoglycemic drugs, and increase the risk of bleeding with antiplatelet drugs. • Should not be used with warfarin sulphate as it may alter bleeding time.
Ginkgo	• Anticoagulant drugs like warfarin (coumarin), aspirin and other NSAIDs, vitamin E or any medications that thin the blood • MAO inhibitors • Thiazide diuretics	• Ginkgo thins the blood. Taking it with other blood-thinning agents could increase your risk of excessive bleeding or even stroke. • May increase the effects of MAO inhibitors. • May increase blood pressure when used with thiazide diuretics.
Ginseng (Panax and Siberian)	• Warfarin (coumarin) • Digoxin • Antipsychotics • MAO inhibitors • Caffeine • Hormone therapy • Diabetes medications and insulin • Stimulant drugs	• Ginseng may decrease the effectiveness of warfarin or reverse the drug's effects. • Similarly it may interfere with digoxin. • It might interfere with antipsychotic drugs by interfering with neurotransmitters. Can cause headache, tremulousness and manic episodes in patients treated with phenelzine sulphate. • May interfere with MAO inhibitors, possibly causing insomnia, headache, tremors or hyperactivity. • May potentiate the effect of estrogens and corticosteroids. • Use with caution with diabetes medications and insulin because ginseng has a hypoglycemic effect. • Can increase the stimulant effect of caffeine and can lead to hypertension.

Herb	Avoid taking with	Reasons
Goldenseal	• Sedatives (e.g. benzodiazepines, barbiturates, non-benzodiazepines) • Alcohol • Heparin • Antihypertensives • Digoxin	• Increases the effect of sedatives. • Decreases heparin's anticoagulant effect. • Interferes with the action of antihypertensives, may cause both increases and decreases in blood pressure. • Interferes with digoxin activity.
Guarana	• Bronchodilators (e.g. theophyline and xanthine derivatives) • Stimulants	• Enhances the effects of theophyline and xanthine so may cause changes in blood pressure, nervousness, insomnia and headaches. • Guarana's main ingredient is caffeine and so it may potentiate the effect of other widely available stimulants.
Hawthorn	• Digoxin	• Interferes with digoxin activity.
Kava-Kava	• Alcohol • Anti-Parkinson's medications • Antipsychotics • Sedatives and anti-depressants (barbiturates, alcohol benzodiazepines)	• Can add to the effects of substances that depress the central nervous system, causing over-sedation. • May cause tremors, muscle spasms, or abnormal movements that may decrease the effectiveness of anti-Parkinson's medications. • Similar problems may be experienced if used with antipsychotic medications. • Kava-kava can increase the effects of antidepressants.
Liquorice	• Diuretics (e.g. spironlactone) • Digoxin • Antihypertensives	• Can reduce the effectiveness of diuretics. • May also increase potassium loss when used with diuretics and drugs like digoxin. • It can also interfere with the action of digoxin and with digoxin monitoring.

Herb	Avoid taking with	Reasons
Liquorice (*cont.*)		• Can interfere with anti-hypertensives causing an increase in blood pressure, and also increase sodium chloride and water retention.
St John's wort	• Antidepressants (e.g. MAO inhibitors and SSRIs) • Digoxin • Indinavir • Oral contraceptives	• May potenitate the actions of MAO inhibitors and SSRIs. • May decrease the effectiveness of digoxin. • Can render HIV medications such as indinavir ineffective. • Tannic acids present in the herb also have the ability to inhibit the absorption of iron.
Saw palmetto	• Antidepressants, sedatives, narcotics • Immuno-suppressants (e.g. cyclosporin, indinavir) • Digoxin • Anticonvulsants • Antihypertensives (e.g. reserpine)	• Interacts with antidepressants either increasing or decreasing their effectiveness. • Can decrease the drug-induced sleep time of barbiturates and narcotics. • Decreases effectiveness of immuno-suppressants. • Reduces the therapeutic effects of digoxin. • Can also lead to a reduced seizure threshold. • Reduces the effectiveness of reserpine. • Also contains tannic acids which may inhibit the absorption of iron.
Valerian	• Alcohol • Barbiturates • Benzodiazepines • Sedatives • Sleeping Pills	• Like kava-kava, valerian may add to the effects of sedatives, especially benzodiazepines like valium and barbiturates and alcohol.

Appendix 3

Helpful Organisations

GENERAL

**Institute for Complementary
Medicine** *and* **The British
Register of Complementary
Practitioners (BRCP)**
PO Box 194
London
SE16 7QZ
Tel: 020 7237 5165
www.icmedicine.co.uk

**British Complementary Medicine
Association (BCMA)**
Kensington House
33 Imperial Square
Cheltenham
Gloucestershire
GL50 1QZ
Tel: 01242 519911

ACUPRESSURE
Shiatsu Society
Eastlands Court
St Peters Road
Rugby
CV21 3QP
Tel: 01788 555051
www.shiatsu.org

ACUPUNCTURE
**British Acupuncture Council and
Register**
Park House
63 Jeddo Road
London
W12 9HQ
Tel: 020 8735 0400
www.acupuncture.org.uk

**British Medical Acupuncture
Society**
12 Marbury House
High Whitley
WA4 4JA
Tel: 01925 730727
www.medical-acupuncture.co.uk

AROMATHERAPY
**International Federation of
Aromatherapists**
182 Chiswick High Road
London
W4 1PP
Tel: 020 8742 2605
www.int-fed-aromatherapy.co.uk

**Aromatherapy Organisations
Council**
PO Box 19
London

SE 25 6WF
Tel: 020 8251 7912

International Society of Professional Aromatherapists (ISPA)

ISPA House
82 Ashby Road
Hinckley
Leicestershire
LE10 1SN
Tel: 01455 637987

AYURVEDA

Ayurvedic Medical Association UK

1079 Garratt Lane
Tooting Broadway
London
SW17 0LN
Tel: 020 8682 3876

Maharishi Ayur-Veda Health Centre

24 Linhope Street
London
NW1 6HT
Tel: 020 7724 6267

The Golden Dome

Woodley Park
Skelmersdale
WN8 6UQ
Tel: 01695 51008

Other areas phone:
0700 298783
www.maharishi.co.uk

BOWEN TECHNIQUE

Bowen Association (UK)

PO Box 4358

Dorchester
Dorset
DT2 7XX
Tel: 01305 849421

Bowen Technique European Register

Homeley
Bow Street
Somerset
TA10 9PQ
Tel: 01373 461 873

CHIROPRACTIC

British Association for Applied Chiropractic (McTimoney-Corley)

The Old Post Office
Cherry Streeet
Stratton Audley
Nr Bicester
OX27 9BA
Tel: 01869 277111

British Chiropractic Association

Blagrave House
17 Blagrave Street
Reading
Berkshire
RG1 1QB
Tel: 01189 505 950
www.chiropractic-uk.co.uk

McTimoney Chiropractic Association

21 High Street
Eynsham
Oxfordshire
OX8 1HE
Tel: 01865 880974

**Scottish Chiropractic
 Association**
16 Jenny Moore's Road
St Boswell's
Roxburghshire
TD6 0AL
Tel: 01835 824026

ENVIRONMENTAL MEDICINE
**British Society of Allergy,
 Environmental and
 Nutritional Medicine**
PO Box 7
Knighton
Powys
LD8 2WF
Tel: 01547 550380 (Answerphone)
0906 3020010 (Premium line)
www.bsaenm.org.uk

FLOWER REMEDIES
Dr Edward Bach Centre
Mount Vernon
Bakers Lane
Sotwell
Oxfordshire
OX10 0PZ
Tel: 01491 834678
http://www.bachcentre.com

Flower & Gem Remedy Association
Suite 1 Castle Farm
Clifton Road
Deddington
Banbury
Oxfordshire
OX15 0TP
Tel: 01869 337349

HERBALISM
**British Herbal Medicine
 Association**

Field House
Lye Hole Lane
Redhill
Bristol
BS18 7TB
Tel: 01934 862994
www.exeter.ac.uk/phytonet/bhma.
 html

The Herb Society
Sulgrave Manor
Sulgrave
Banbury
OX17 2SD
Tel: 01295 768899
http://dspace.dial.pipex.com/
 herbsociety

**National Institute of Medical
 Herbalists**
56 Longbrook Street
Exeter
Devon
EX4 6AH
Tel: 01392 426022
www.nimh.org.uk

**International Register of
 Consultant Herbalists and
 Homeopaths**
32 King Edward Road
Swansea
SA1 4LL
Tel: 01792 655886

HOMEOPATHY
**British Homeopathic
 Association/ Faculty of
 Homeopathy**
15 Clerkenwell Close
London
EC1R 0AA

Tel: 020 7566 7800
www.trusthomeopathy.org.uk

The Institute of Homoeopathy
23 Berkeley Road
Bishopston
Bristol
BS7 8HF
Tel: 0117 944 5147
www.hominf.org.uk

Society of Homoeopaths
2 Artizan Road
Northampton
NN1 4HU
Tel: 01604 621400

HYPNOTHERAPY
British Hypnotherapy Association
67 Upper Berkley Street
London
W1H 7DH
Tel: 202 7723 4443

British Society of Medical and Dental Hypnosis
17 Keppel View Road
Kimberworth
Rotherham
S. Yorkshire
S61 2AR
Tel: 07000 560309
www.bsmdh.org

Scotland:
PO Box 1007
Glasgow
G31 2LE
Tel: 0141 556 1606

National School of Hypnosis and Psychotherapy
The Central Register of Advanced
  Hypnotherapists

28 Finsbury Park Road
London
N4 2JX
Tel: 020 7359 6691

MASSAGE
British Federation of Massage Practitioners
78 Meadow Street
Preston
PR1 1TS
Tel: 01772 881063

Hale Clinic
7 Park Crescent
London
W1N 3HE
Tel: 0171 6310156
(for marma and tui na massage)

Massage Therapy Institute of Great Britain
PO Box 2726
London
NW2 4NR
Tel: 0181 208 1607

MEDITATION
Friends of the Western Buddhist Order London
Buddhist Centre
51 Roman Road
London
E2 OHU
Tel: 0845 4584716
www.ibc.org.uk

Transcendental Meditation UK
Tel: 08705 413733
www.transcendental-meditation.
  org.uk

METAMORPHIC TECHNIQUE
Metamorphic Association
67 Ritherdon Road
London
SW17 8QE
Tel: 020 8672 5951

NATUROPATHY
General Council and Register of
Naturopaths
Goswell House
2 Goswell Road
Somerset
BA16 0JG
Tel: 01458 840072
www.naturopathy.org.uk

NUTRITION
British Association of
Nutritional Therapists
27 Old Gloucester Street
London
WC1N 3XX
Tel: 0870 606 1284

Society for Promotion of
Nutritional Therapy
PO Box 47
Heathfield
East Sussex
TN21 8ZX
Tel: 01435 867007
http://freespace.virgin.net/nutrition
    .therapy/links/uk

Institute for Optimum Nutrition
13 Blades Court
Deodar Road
London
SW15 2NU
Tel: 0181 877 9993

OSTEOPATHY
British Osteopathic Association
Langham House West
Mill Street
Luton
Bedfordshire
LU1 2NA
Tel. 01582 488455
www.osteopathy.org

General Osteopathic Council
Osteopathy House
176 Tower Bridge Road
London
EC1R 0AA
Tel: 020 7566 7800
www.osteopathy.org.uk

The British College of
Naturopathy and
Osteopathy
Lief House
3 Sumpter Close
120–122 Finchley Road
London
NW3 5HR
Tel: 020 7435 6464
www.bcno.ac.uk

REFLEXOLOGY
Association of Reflexologists
27 Old Gloucester Street
London
WC1 3XX
Tel: 0870 567 3320
www.reflexology.org/aor
www.aor.org.uk

British Reflexology Association
Monks Orchard
Whitbourne

Worcester
WR6 5RB
Tel: 01886 822017

**British School of Reflex Zone
Therapy of the Feet**
23 Marsh Hall
Talisman Way
Wembley Park
London
HA9 8JJ
Tel: 020 8904 4825

SHIATSU
Shiatsu Society
Eastlands Court
St Peters Road
Rugby
CV21 3QP
Tel: 01788 555051
www.shiatsu.org

SPIRITUAL HEALING
**Confederation of Healing
Organisations**
Suite J
113 High Street
Berkhamsted
Hertfordshire
HP4 2DJ
Tel: 01442 870660

**National Federation of
Spiritual Healers**
Old Manor Farm Studio
Church Street
Sunbury-on-Thames
TW16 6RG
Tel: 01932 783164
www.nfsh.org.uk

TRADITIONAL CHINESE MEDICINE
**Register of Chinese Herbal
Medicine**
11–15 Betterton Street
London
WC2H 9BP
Tel: 020 7470 8740
www.rchm.co.uk

YOGA
British Wheel of Yoga
25 Jermyn Street
Sleaford
Lincolnshire
NG34 7RU
Tel: 01529 306 851
www.bwy.org.uk

Iyengar Yoga Institute
223a Randolph Avenue
London
W9 1NL
Tel: 020 7624 3080
www.iyi.org.uk

**Scottish Yoga Teachers'
Association**
26 Buckingham Terrace
Edinburgh
EH4 3AE
Tel: 0131 343 3553
www.yogascotland.org.uk

Yoga for Health Foundation
Ickwell Bury
Ickwell Green
Biggleswade
SG18 9EF
Tel: 01767 627271
www.yogaforhealthfoundation.co.uk

References

Chapter 1. Santé

A prospective study of walking as compared with vigorous exercise in the prevention of coronary heart disease in women, Manson JE *et al, N Engl J Med* 1999; 26: 650–8.

Alternative Medicine – the Definitive Guide, The Burton Goldberg Group, Tiburon, CA: Future Medicine Publishing, Inc.

Cleaning Yourself to Death – How Safe is Your Home?, Thomas P, Dublin: Newleaf 2001.

Comparison of lifestyle and structures interventions to increase physical activity and cardiorespiratory fitness: a randomized trial, Dunn AL *et al, JAMA* 1999; 281: 327–34.

Personality, coping style, emotions and cancer: towards an integrative model, Temoshok L, Cancer Surveys 1987; 6: 545–67.

Power Healing, Galland L, New York: Random House 1997.

Psychological concomitants of cancer: current state of research, Greer S and Silberfarb PM, *Psychological Med* 1982; 12: 567–8.

Stress and cancer: The state of the art, Bahnson C, *Psychosomatics* 1980; 21: 975–80.

The Handbook of Complementary Medicine, Fulder S, London: Century 1989.

Trends in alternative medicine use in the United States, 1990–1997, Eisenberg DM *et al, JAMA* 1998; 280: 1569–75.

Users and practitioners of complementary medicine, Zollman C and Vickers A, *BMJ* 1999; 319: 836–8.

What is complementary medicine? Zollman C and Vickers A, *BMJ* 1999; 319: 693–6.

Chapter 2. Becoming Your Own Health Expert

6-year experience of prenatal diagnosis in an unselected population in Oxford, UK, Boyd PA *et al, Lancet* 1998; 352: 1577–81; see also Commentary, Prenatal ultrasonography: first do no harm?, *Lancet* 1998; 352: 1568–9.

Complications of laparoscopic cholecystectomy: a national survey of 4,292 hospitals and an analysis of 77,604 cases, Deziel DJ *et al, Am J Surg* 1993; 165: 9–14.

Effect of d-Sotalol on mortality in patients with left ventricular dysfunction after recent and remote myocardial infarction. The SWORD Investigators. Survival with oral d-Sotalol, Waldo AL *et al, Lancet,* 1996; 348: 7–12.

Frequent nut consumption and the risk of coronary heart disease in women: prospective cohort study, Hu FB *et al, BMJ* 1998; 317: 1341–5.

Laparoscopic appendicectomy, Lomax D, *Lancet,* 1993; 342: 1247.

Measuring blood pressure: which arm?, Panayiotou BN, *JAMA* 1995; 274: 1343.

Nut consumption and risk of coronary heart disease: a review of epidemiologic evidence, *Curr Atheroscler Rep* 1999; 1: 204–9.

Problems in clinical trials go far beyond misconduct, Nowak R, *Science* 1994; 264: 1538–41.

Phytoestrogens – hormone heaven or hormone havoc?, Thomas, P, *What Doctors Don't Tell You* 2000; 11(5): 1–4.

Recording diastolic blood pressure in pregnancy, Brown MA and Whitworth JA, *BMJ* 1991; 303: 120–1.

Routine diagnostic testing [No authors listed], *Lancet*, 1989; 2: 1190–1.

Social connections and mortality from all causes and from cardiovascular disease: prospective evidence from eastern Finland, Kaplan GA *et al*, *Am J Epidemiol* 1988; 128: 370–80.

Social networks, host resistance, and mortality: a nine-year follow-up study of Alameda County residents, Berkman LF and Syme SL, *Am J Epidemiol* 1979; 109: 186–204.

Specificity of antenatal ultrasound in the Yorkshire Region: a prospective study of 2,261 ultrasound detected anomalies, Brand IR *et al*, *Br J Obstet Gynaecol* 1994; 101: 392–7.

The Healing Power of Illness, Dethlefsen T, London: HarperCollins 1997.

The Hidden Meaning of Illness – Disease as a Symbol and Metaphor, Trowbridge B, Virginia Beach, VA: A.R.E. Press 1996.

What Doctors Don't Tell You – The Truth about the Dangers of Modern Medicine, McTaggart L, London: HarperCollins 1996.

Women and Health Research, Institute of Medicine, London: National Academy Press 1994.

Your Body Speaks Your Mind, Shapiro D, London: Piatkus 1996.

Chapter 3. Avoiding Disappointment

Can it work? Does it work? Is it worth it?, Haynes B, *BMJ* 1999; 652–3.

Essentials of Complementary and Alternative Medicine, Jonas WB and Levin JS (eds), Baltimore, MD: Lippincott, Williams and Wilkins 1999.

Patient outcomes to alternative medicine therapies as measured by the SP-36 – preliminary report, Farr CH and White R, Townsend Lett Docs 1999; 186: 24–5.

Use of alternative medicine by women with early-stage breast cancer, Burstein HJ *et al*, *N Eng J Med* 1999; 340: 1733–9; 1758–9.

Chapter 4. Acupuncture

A controlled trial of the treatment of migraine by acupuncture, Vincent CA, *Clin J Pain* 1989; 5: 305–12.

A meta-analysis of acupuncture for chronic pain, Patel M *et al*, *Int J Epidemiol* 1989; 18: 900–06.

Acupuncture and chronic pain: a criteria based meta-analysis, ter Reit G *et al*, *J Clin Epidemiol* 1990; 43: 1191–9.

Acupuncture and insomnia, Montakab H, *Forsch Komp Med* 1999; 6: S29–S31.

Acupuncture and the relief of pain, Eadie MJ, *Med J Austral* 1990; 153: 180–1.

Acupuncture compared with placebo in post-herpetic pain, Lewith GT *et al*, *Pain* 1983; 17: 361–8.

Acupuncture for back pain: a meta-analysis of randomized controlled trials, Ernst E and White AR, *Arch Intern Med* 1998; 158: 2235–41.

Acupuncture for chronic low back pain: diagnosis and treatment patterns among acupuncturists evaluating the same patient, Kalauokalani D *et al*, *South Med J* 2001; 94: 486–92.

Acupuncture for idiopathic headache, Melchart D *et al*, Cochrane Database Syst Rev 2001; 1: CD001218.

Acupuncture for induction of labour, Smith, CA, Crowther CA, Cochrane Database Syst Rev 2001; 1: CD002962.

Acupuncture for recurrent headaches: a systematic review of randomized controlled trials, Melchart D et al, Cephalalgia 1999; 19: 779–86.

Acupuncture for the management of primary dysmenorrhea, Helms JM, Ob Gyn 1987 69: 51–6.

Acupuncture in the treatment of stroke patients in the subacute stage: a randomised, controlled study, Sallstrom S et al, Comp Ther Med 1996; 4:193–7.

Acupuncture – Its Place in Western Medical Science, Lewith G, Merlin 1989.

Acupuncture treatment of severe knee osteoarthritis, A long term study, Christensen BV et al, Acta Anaesthesiol Scand 1992; 36: 519–25.

Acupuncture, NIH Consensus Development Panel on Acupuncture, JAMA 1998; 280: 1518–24.

Acupuncture: a review of its history, theories and indications, Ceniceros S and Brown GR, South Med J 1998; 91: 1121–5.

Acupuncture: context and critique, Millman B, Ann Rev Med 1977; 28: 223–36.

Adverse events following acupuncture: prospective survey of 32,000 consultations with doctors and physiotherapists, White A et al, BMJ 2001; 323: 467–8.

Adverse events related to acupuncture, Yamashita H et al, JAMA 1998; 280: 1653–4.

Can acupuncture have specific effects on health? A systematic review of acupuncture antiemesis trials, Vickers AJ, J Royal Soc Med 1996; 89: 303–11.

Can sensory stimulation improve the functional outcome in stroke patients? Johansson K et al, Neurology 1993; 43: 2189–92.

Controlled trial of acupuncture for severe recidivist alcoholism, Bullock M et al, Lancet 1989, 1: 1435–9.

Effect of electroacupuncture on chronic pain conditions in general medical practice – a four years study, Cheung J, Am J Chin Med 1985; 13: 33–8.

Effects of acupuncture treatment on daily life activities and quality of life: a controlled, prospective, and randomized study of acute stroke patients, Gosman-Hedstrom G et al, Stroke 1998; 29: 2100–8.

Effects of electro-acupuncture on anovulation in women with polycystic ovary syndrome, Stener-Victorin E et al, Acta Ob Gyn Scand 2000; 79: 180–8.

Efficacy of acupuncture on osteoarthritic pain, Gaw AC et al, N Eng J Med 1975; 69: 51–6.

Electroacupuncture and postoperative pain, Christensen PA et al, Br J Anaesthesia 1989; 62: 58–62.

How acupuncture can help addicts, Wen AH and Cheung SY, Drugs and Society 1973; 2: 18–20.

How safe is acupuncture? MacPherson H, Caduceus 1999; 42: 37–9.

Influence of acupuncture on duration of labour, Zeisler H et al, Gyn Ob Invest 1998; 46: 22–5.

Life threatening adverse reactions after acupuncture? A systematic review, Ernst E and White A, Pain 1997; 71: 123–6.

Moxibustion for correction of breech presentation: a randomized controlled trial, Cardini F and Weixin H, JAMA 1998; 280; 1580–4.

Muscle tenderness in tension headache treated with acupuncture or physiotherapy, Carlsson, J et al, Cephalalgia 1990; 10: 131–41.

NADA Newsletter Committee, National Acupuncture Detoxification Association Newsletter, 1 December 1992: 1–6.

National Institutes of Health Consensus Statement on Acupuncture, Washington DC, NIH Publication No. 1087, 1997.

National survey of access to complementary health care via general practice, Thomas K et al, Medical Care Research Unit, August 1995.

Neurochemical basis of acupuncture analgesia, Han J and Terenius L, Ann Rev Pharmacol Toxicol 1982; 22: 192–220.

On the evaluation of the clinical effects of acupuncture, Lewith G and Machin D, Pain 1983; 16: 111–27.

Pain and discomfort in primary dysmenorrhoea is reduced by preemptive acupuncture or low frequency TENS, Thomas M et al, Eur J Physical Med Rehab 1995; 4: 71–6.

Pain treatment of fibromyalgia by acupuncture, Sprott H et al, Rheumatol Int 1998; 18: 35–6.

Randomised trial of acupuncture compared with conventional massage and 'sham' laser acupuncture for treatment of chronic neck pain, Irnick D et al, BMJ 2001; 322:1574–8.

Real vs. sham laser acupuncture and microamps TENS to treat carpal tunnel syndrome and worksite wrist pain: pilot study, Naeser MA et al, Laser Surg Med Suppl 1996; 8: 7.

The acupuncture treatment of low back pain: a randomised controlled study, Coan RM, Am J Chin Med 1980; 8: 181–9.

The acupuncture treatment of neck pain: a randomized controlled study, Coan RM et al, Am J Chin Med 1982; 9: 326–32.

The role of acupuncture in controlling the gagging reflex using a review of ten cases, Fiske J and Dickinson C, Br Dent J 2001; 190: 611–13.

The treatment of tension headache by acupuncture: a controlled single case design with time series analysis, Vincent CA, J Psychosom Res 1990; 34: 553–61.

The Web That Has No Weaver, Kaptchuk TJ, London: Rider 1986.

The York acupuncture safety study: prospective survey of 34,000 treatments by traditional acupuncturists, MacPherson H et al, BMJ 2001; 323: 486–7.

Therapeutic acupuncture for chronic pain, Sodipo J, Pain 1979; 7: 359–65.

Towards a safer choice: The practice of traditional Chinese medicine in Australia, Bensoussan A and Myers SP, Faculty of Health, University of Western Sydney, MacArthur 1996.

Traditional Chinese acupuncture in tension-type headache, Tavola T et al, Pain 1992; 48: 325–9.

Chapter 5. Aromatherapy

A study of the changes in the bioactivity of essential oils used singly and as mixtures in aromatherapy, Lis-Balchin M et al, J Altern Comp Med 1997; 3: 249–56.

Allergic contact dermatitis to plant extracts in patients with cosmetic dermatitis, Thomson KF and Wilkinson SM, Br J Dermatol 2000, 142: 84–8.

An evaluation of aromatherapy in palliative care, Wilkinson S et al, Palliat Med 1999; 13: 409–17.

An evaluation of the use of massage and essential oils on the wellbeing of cancer patients, Corner J et al, Int J Palliative Nurs 1995; 1: 67–73.

Antimicrobial effects of tea tree oil and its major components on Staphylococcus aureus, Staph. Epidermis and propionbacterium acnes, Raman A et al, Lett Applied Microbiol 1995; 21: 242–5.

Aroma Science – The Chemistry and Bioactivity of Essential Oils, Lis-Balchin M, East Horsley, Surrey: Amberwood Publishing Ltd 1995.

Aroma: sedative effects of lavender after inhalation, Buchbauer G et al, J Biosciences 1991; 46: 1067–72.

Aromatherapy and massage in palliative care, Wilkinson S, *Int J Palliative Nursing* 1995; 1: 21–30.

Aromatherapy positively affects mood, EEG patterns of alertness and math computations, Diego MA *et al*, *Int J Neurosci* 1998; 96: 217–24.

Aromatherapy Workbook, Price S, London: Thorsons 1993.

Carrier Oils For Aromatherapy and Massage, Price L *et al*, Riverhead 2001.

Comparison of two topical preparations for the treatment of onychomycosis: Melaleuca alternafolia (tea tree) oil and clotrimazole, Buck DA *et al*, *J Fam Pract* 1994; 38: 601–5.

Effects of olfactory stimuli on urge reduction in smokers, Sayette MA and Parrott DJ, *Exp Clin Psychopharmacol* 1999; 7: 151–9.

Environmental exposure to polycyclic aromatic hydrocarbons and total suspended particulates in a Taiwanese temple, Lin TC *et al*, *Bull Environ Contam Toxicol* 2001; 67: 332–8.

Essential oils and 'aromatherapy': their modern role in healing, Lis-Balchin M, *J Royal Soc Health* 1997; 117: 324–9.

Essential plant oils and headache mechanisms, Gobel H *et al*, *Phytomed* 1995; 2: 93–102.

Eucalyptus oil poisoning in childhood: 41 cases in south-east Queensland, Webb NJ and Pitt WR, *J Paed Child Health* 1993; 29: 368–71.

Evaluation of the efficacy of 3% citronella candles and 5% citronella incense for protection against field populations of Aedes mosquitoes, Lindsay LR *et al*, *J Am Mosq Control Assoc* 1996; 12: 293–4.

Inhalation of vapor from black pepper extract reduces smoking withdrawal symptoms, Rose JE and Behm FM, *Drug and Alcohol Dependence* 1994; 34: 225–9.

Inhibiting effect of jasmine flowers on lactation, Abraham M *et al*, *Indian J Med Res* 1979; 69: 88–92.

Melaleuca oil poisoning, Jacobs MR and Hornfeldt CS, *Clin Toxicol* 1994; 32: 461–4.

Pennyroyal oil poisoning and hepatotoxicity, Sullivan JB *et al*, *JAMA* 1979; 242: 2873–4.

Pennyroyal poisoning: a fatal case, Vallance WB, *Lancet* 1955: 2: 850–1.

Perception of memory preneoplast trans by tumour inhibitors, Katadare M, *Cancer Lett* 1997; 111: 141–7.

Raloxifen, retinoids and lavender: 'me too' tamoxifen alternatives under study, Ziegler J, *J Natl Cancer Inst* 1996; 88: 1100–102.

Randomized trial of aromatherapy: successful treatment for alopecia areata, Hay IC *et al*, *Arch Dermatol* 1998; 134: 1349–52.

Repellency of volatile oils from plants against three mosquito vectors, Tawatsin A *et al*, *J Vector Ecol* 2001; 26: 76–82.

Replacement of drug treatment for insomnia by ambient odour, Stretch D *et al*, *Lancet* 1995; 346: 701.

Sensing an improvement: an experimental study to evaluate the use of aromatherapy, massage and periods of rest in an intensive care unit, Dunn C *et al*, *J Adv Nurs* 1995; 21: 34–40.

Suppression of purpureal lactation using jasmine flowers (Jasminum sambac), Shrivastav P *et al*, *Austral New Z J Ob Gyn* 1988; 28: 68–71.

Susceptibility of methicillin-resistant Staphylococcus aureus to the essential oils of Melaleuca alternafolia, Carson CF *et al*, *J Antimicrob Chemother* 1995; 35: 421–4.

Tea tree oil in the treatment of Tinea pedis, Tong MM *et al*, *Ausralas J Dermatol* 1992; 33: 145–9.

The Art of Aromatherapy, Tisserand R, Saffron Walden: Daniel 1989.

The effect of foot-bath with or without the essential oil of lavender on the autonomic nervous system: a randomized trial, Saeki Y, *Comp Ther Med* 2000; 8: 2–7.

The psychophysiological effects of aromatherapy massage following cardiac surgery, Stephenson C, *Comp Ther Med* 1994; 2: 27–35.

The role of lavender oil in relieving perineal discomfort following childbirth: a blind randomised clinical trial, Dale MJ *et al*, *J Advanced Nursing* 1994; 19: 89–96.

The use of aromatherapy in intrapartum midwifery practice – an observational study, Burns E *et al*, *Comp Ther Nurse Midwifery* 2000; 6: 33–4.

Tiger Balm as a treatment of tension headache: A clinical trial in general practice, Scattner P and Randerson D, *Austral Fam Physi* 1996; 25: 216–22.

Chapter 6. Ayurveda

A double-blind, placebo-controlled clinical study on the effects of Withania somnifera (Ashwagandha) and Panax ginseng extracts on psychomotor performance in healthy Indian volunteers, Karnick CR, *Indian Med* 1991; 3: 1–5.

Adaptogenic properties of six rasayana herbs used in Ayurvedic medicine, Rege NN *et al*, *Phytother Res* 1999; 13: 275–91.

An alternative medicine treatment for Parkinson's disease: results of a multicenter clinical trial, HP-200 in Parkinson's Disease Study Group, *J Altern Comp Med* 1995; 1: 249–55.

Antineoplastic properties of Maharishi-4 against DMBA-induced mammary tumours in rats, Sharma HM *et al*, *Pharmacol Biochem Behav* 1990; 35: 767–73.

Antistress activity of sitonindosides VII and VIII, new acylsterylglucosides from Withania somnifera, Battacharya SK *et al*, *Phytotherapy Res* 1987; 1: 32–7.

Ayurveda: a historical perspective and principles of the traditional healthcare system in India, Mishra L *et al*, *Altern Ther Health Med* 2001; 7: 36–42.

Compapharmacology investigation of ashwagandha and ginseng, Grandhi A *et al*, *J Ethnopharmacol* 1994; 44: 131–5.

Current status of ayurveda in phytomedicine, Dahanukar S and Thatte U, *Phytomedicine* 1997; 4: 359–68.

Effect of ashwagandha on the process of ageing in human volunteers, Kupparanjan K *et al*, *J Res Ayurveda and Sadai* 1980; 247–58.

Effect of Maharishi-4 and Maharishi-5 on inflammatory mediators with special reference to their free radical scavenging effect, Niwa Y, *Ind J Clin Pract* 1991; 1: 23–7.

Healthcare and disease management in Ayurveda, Mishra L *et al*, *Altern Ther Health Med* 2001; 7: 44–50.

A double-blind, placebo-controlled clinical study on the effects of withania somnifera (ashwagandha) and Panax ginseng extracts on psychomotor performance in healthy Indian volunteers, Karnick CR, *Indian Medicine* 1991; 3: 1–5.

Inhibitory effects of Maharishi-4 and Maharishi-5 on microsomal lipid peroxidation, Dwivedi C *et al*, *Pharmacol Biochem Behav* 1991; 39: 649–52.

Lead poisoning from Indian herbal medicine (Ayurveda), Dunbabin DW *et al*, *Med J Aust* 1992; 157: 835–6.

Maharishi amrit kalash (MAK) prevents human platelet aggregation, Sharma HM *et al*, *Clinica E Terapia Cardiovasculare* 1989; 8: 227–30.

Maharishi Ayur-Veda: guru's marketing scheme promises the world eternal 'perfect health', Skolnick A, *JAMA* 1991; 265; 2633–7.

Inhibition of low-density lipoprotein oxidation by oral herbal mixtures Maharishi Amrit Kalash-4 and Maharishi Amrit Kalash-5 in hyperlipidemic patients, Sundaram V *et al*, *Am J Med Sci* 1997; 314: 303–10.

WHAT WORKS, WHAT DOESN'T

Traditional remedies and food supplements, A 5-year toxicological study (1991–1995), Shaw D *et el, Drug Safety* 1997; 17: 342–56.

Chapter 7. Biofeedback

A comparison of EMG biofeedback and a credible pseudotherapy in treating tension headache, Holroyd KA *et al, J Behav Med* 1980; 3: 29–39.

Behavioral v. drug treatment for urge incontinence in older women, Burgio KL *et al, JAMA* 1998; 280: 1995–2000.

Behavioural method for the treatment of idiopathic scoliosis, Dworkin B *et al, Proc Natl Acad Sci* 1985; 82: 2493–7.

Biofeedback treatment of Raynaud's disease, Birger M *et al, Harefuah* 1997; 133: 362–4.

Biofeedback treatment of vascular headache, Blanchard EB and Andrasik F, in *Biofeedback: Studies in Clinical Efficacy*, Hatch JP *et al*, eds, New York: Plenum 1987: 1–79.

Biofeedback: a noninvasive treatment for incontinence after radical prostatectomy, Jackson J *et al, Urol Nurs* 1996; 16: 50–4.

Biofeedback and physiotherapy versus physiotherapy alone in the treatment of genuine stress urinary incontinence, Glavind K *et al, Int Urogyn J Pelvic Floor Dysfunction* 1996; 7: 339–43.

Biofeedback training in treatment of childhood constipation: a randomized controlled study, Van der Plas RN *et al, Lancet* 1996; 348: 776–8.

Brainwave signatures. An index reflective of the brain's functional neuroanatomy: Further findings on the effect of EEG sensorimotor rhythm biofeedback training on the neurologic precursors of learning disabilities, Tansey MA, *International Journal of Psychophysiology* 1985; 3: 85–99.

Change mechanisms associated with combined relaxation/EMG biofeedback training for chronic tension headache, Rokicki LA *et al, Appl Psychophysiol Biofeedback* 1997; 221: 21–41.

Computerised biofeedback games: a new method for teaching stress management and its use in irritable bowel syndrome, Leahy A *et al, J R Coll Physicians (Lond)* 1998; 32: 552–6.

Controlled trial of biofeedback in muscle contraction headache, Bruhn P *et al, Ann Neurol* 1979; 6: 34–6.

Effect of biofeedback-assisted relaxation on migraine headache and changes in cerebral blood flow velocity in the middle cerebral artery, McGrady A *et al, Headache* 1994; 34: 424–8.

Effect of thermal biofeedback-assisted relaxation training on blood circulation in the lower extremities of a population with diabetes, Rice BI and Schindler JV, *Diabetes Care* 1992; 15: 853–8.

Electroencephalographic biofeedback of SMR and beta for treatment of attention deficit disorders in a clinical setting, Lubar JO and Lubar JE, *Biofeedback and Self-Regulation* 1984; 9: 1–23.

Electromyographic biofeedback for neuromuscular reduction in the hemiplegic stroke patient: a meta-analysis, Schleenbaker RE and Manious AG III, *Arch Phys Med Rehab* 1993; 74: 1301–4.

EMG and EEG biofeedback training in the treatment of a 10 year old hyperactive boy with a developmental reading disorder, Tansey M and Bruner R, *Biofeedback and Self-Regulation* 1985; 4: 299–311.

Enhancing the effectiveness of relaxation-thermal biofeedback training with propranolol hydrochloride, Holroyd KA *et al, J Consult Clin Psychol* 1995; 63: 327–30.

REFERENCES

Evaluating the efficacy of a biofeedback intervention to reduce children's anxiety, Wenck LS *et al*, *J Clin Psychology* 1996; 52: 469–73.

Evaluation of the effectiveness of EEG neurofeedback training for ADHD in a clinical setting as measured by changes in T.O.V.A. scores, behavioral ratings, and WISC-R performance, Lubar JO *et al*, *Biofeedback and Self-Regulation* 1995; 20: 83–99.

Fifteen month follow-up with asthmatics utilising EMG/incentive inspirometer feedback, Peper E and Tibbetts V, *Biofeedback Self-Regul* 1992; 17: 143–51.

Long-term maintenance of improvements achieved with (abortive) pharmacological and nonpharmacological treatments for migraine: preliminary findings, Holroyd KA *et al*, *Biofeedback Self-Regul* 1989; 14: 301–8.

Non-invasive treatment of vascular and muscle contraction headache: a comparative longitudinal clinical study, Reich BA, *Headache* 1989; 29: 34–41.

Pelvic muscle exercise/biofeedback for urinary incontinence after prostatectomy: an education program, Mathewson-Chapman M, *J Cancer Educ* 1997; 12: 218–23.

Pharmacological versus non-pharmacological prophylaxis of recurrent migraine headache: a meta-analytic review of clinical trials, Holroyd KA and Penzien DB, *Pain* 1990; 42: 1–13.

Predicting differential response to EMG biofeedback and relaxation training: the role of cognitive structure, Hart JD, *J Clin Psychol* 1984; 40: 453–7.

Prospective, randomized trial comparing four biofeedback techniques for patients with constipation, Heyman S *et al*, *Dis Colon Rectum* 1999; 42: 1388–93.

Psychologic and behavioural aspects of chronic headache, Andrasik F, *Neurol Clinics* 1990; 8: 961–76.

Respiratory sinus arrhythmia versus neck/trapezium EMG and incentive inspirometry biofeedback for asthma: a pilot study, Lehrer P *et al*, *Appl Psychophysiol Biofeedback* 1997; 22: 95–109.

Righting the rhythms of reason: EEG biofeedback training as a therapeutic modality in a clinical office setting, Tansey M, *Medical Psychotherapy* 1990; 3: 57–68.

Temperature biofeedback and relaxation training in the treatment of migraine headaches, One-year follow-up, Silver BV *et al*, *Biofeedback Self-Regul* 1979; 4: 359–66.

Voluntary control of vascular tone by using skin-temperature biofeedback-relaxation in patients with advanced heart failure, Moser DK *et al*, *Alt Ther Health Med* 1997; 3: 51–9.

Chapter 8. Fasting & Detoxification

A fasting and vegetarian diet treatment trial on chronic inflammatory disorders, Lithell H *et al*, *Acta Derm Venereol* 1983; 63: 397–403.

A trial of fasting cure for PCB poisoned patients in Taiwan, Imamura M and Tung T, *Am J Ind Med* 1984; 5: 147–53.

An OTC Antidote: Activated Charcoal in Medical Applications, Cooney DO, New York: Marcel Dekker, Inc.

Association of acetaminophen hepatotoxicity with fasting and ethanol use, Whitcomn DC and Block GD, *JAMA* 1994; 272: 1845–50.

Atomic absorption spectrometry of nickel, copper, zinc and lead in sweat collected from healthy subjects during sauna bathing, Hohnadel DC *et al*, *Clin Chem* 1973; 19: 1288–92.

Attenuation of exercise-induced asthma by local hyperthermia (Letter to the editor), Nieminen MM, *Thorax* 1993; 48: 411

Attenuation of exercise-induced asthma by local hyperthermia, Johnston SI *et al*, *Thorax* 1992; 47: 592–7.

Clearing of toxic volatile hydrocarbons from humans, Rea WJ *et al*, *Bol Asoc Med P R* 1991; 83: 321–4.

Comparison of fasting, nasogastric suction and cimetidine in treatment of acute pancreatitis, Navarro S *et al*, *Digestion* 1984; 30: 224–30.

Contraindications and therapeutic results of fasting in obese patients, Duncan TG *et al*, *Ann NY Acad Sci* 1965, 131: 632–6.

Controlled trial of fasting and one-year vegetarian diet in rheumatoid arthritis, Kjeldsen-Kragh J *et al*, *Lancet* 1991; 338: 899–902.

Detection of drugs in sweat, Belabanova S and Schneider E, *Beitr Gerichtl Med* 1990; 48: 45–9.

Effects of fasting and lactovegetarian diet on rheumatoid arthritis, Skoldstam L *et al*, *Scand J Rheumatol* 1979; 8; 249–55.

Encyclopaedia of Natural Medicine, Murray M and Pizzorno J, London: Optima 1995.

Excretion of nitrogen compounds in sweat during a sauna, Czarnowski D and G'orski J, *Pol Tyg Lek* 1991; 46: 186–7.

Fasting and rheumatoid arthritis: a multicenter study, Kroker GA *et al*, *Clin Ecol* 1984, 3; 137–44.

Fasting, intestinal permeability, and rheumatoid arthritis, Skoldstam L and Magnusson KE, *Rheum Dis Clin N Am* 1991; 17: 363–71.

Gorging and plasma HDL-cholesterol – the Ramadan model, Maislos M *et al*, *Eur J Clin Nutr* 1998; 52: 127–30.

Hyperthermia deaths in Finland in 1970–1986, Kortelainen ML, *Am J Forensic Med Pathol* 1991; 12: 115–18.

Is atheroma a reversible lesion?, Gresham GA, *Atherosclerosis* 1976, 23; 379–91.

Maternal heat exposure and neural tube defects, Milunsky A *et al*, *JAMA* 1992; 268: 882–5.

Neurobehavioral dysfunction in fire men exposed to polychlorinated biphenyls (PCBs): possible improvement after detoxification, Kilburn KH *et al*, *Arch Environ Health* 1989; 44: 345–50.

PCB reduction and clinical improvement by detoxification: an unexploited approach?, Tretjak Z *et al*, *Hum Exp Toxicol* 1990; 9: 235–44.

Preplanned fasting in the treatment of mental disease: survey of the current Soviet literature, Boheme DL, *Schizophren Bull* 1977; 3: 288–96.

Review of Medical Physiology, 12th ed. Ganong WF, Los Altos: Lange Medical Publications 1985.

The Diseases of Infants and Children, Griffith JPC and Mitchell A, Philadelphia: W B Saunders 1938: 187.

The Grape Cure, Brandt J, Simi Valley, Calif: Benedict Lust 1971.

The sauna and pregnancy, Yaha-Eskeli K and Erkkola R, *Ann Clin Res* 1988; 20: 279–82.

The sauna and rheumatic diseases, Isomaki H, *Ann Clin Res* 1988; 20: 271–5.

Therapeutic heat, Lehmann JF and DeLateur BJ, in: Lehmann JF, ed. *Therapeutic Heat and Cold*, 3rd ed. Baltimore: Williams & Wilkins 1982: 404–551.

Vegetarian fasting of obese patients: a clinical and biochemical evaluation, Sorbris R *et al*, *Scand J Gastroenterol* 1982; 17: 417–24.

Chapter 9. Flower Essences

An ABC of alternative medicine: Bach flower remedies, Cate P, *Health Visitor* 1986; 59: 276–7.

Bach flower remedies, Mantle F, *Comp Ther Nurse Midwifery* 1997; 3: 142–4.

REFERENCES

Efficacy of Bach flower remedies in test anxiety: a double-blind placebo-controlled, randomised trial with partial crossover, Walach H *et al*, *J Anxiety Disord* 2001; 15: 359–66.

Flower essences: their use in hospitals and patient care, Balinski A, *Lamp* 1994/95; 51: 33–4.

Flower Remedies, Mansfield P, London: Vermillion 1997.

Illustrated Handbook of the Bach Flower Remedies, Chancellor PM, Saffron Walden: Daniel 1986.

The doctrine of signatures: a historical, philosophical, scientific view (II), Richardson-Boedler C, *Br Homeopath J* 2000; 89; 26–8.

The relationship between homeopathy and the Dr Bach system of flower remedies: a critical appraisal, van Haselen RA, *Br Homeopath J* 1999; 88: 121–7.

Use of Western Australian flower essences in the management of pain and stress in the hospital setting, Balinski AA, *Comp Ther Nurs Midwifery* 1998; 4: 111–17.

With Bach flower remedies life can take on deeper meaning, Fisher R, *Beginnings* 1993; 13: 1–4.

Chapter 10. Herbal Medicine

5,300 years ago, the Ice Man used natural laxatives and antibiotics, Capasso L, *Lancet*, 1998; 352: 1864.

ABC of complementary medicine: herbal medicine, Vickers A and Zolman C, *BMJ* 1999; 319: 1050–3.

Health promoting properties of common herbs, Craig WJ, *AM J Coiln Nutri* 1999; 70: 491S-9S.

Phytopharmaceuticals: mass-production, standardization and conservation, Murch SJ *et al*, *Scientific Rev Alt Med* 2000; 4: 39–43.

Safety issues with herbal medicine, Boullata JI *et al*, *Pharmacotherapy* 2000; 20: 257–69.

The New Holistic Herbal, Hoffman D, Shaftesbury: Element 1990.

The Scientific Validation of Herbal Medicine, Mowrey DB, New Canaan, Connecticut: Keats 1986.

Echinacea

A randomized controlled trial of the effect of fluid extract of Echinacea purpurea on the incidence and severity of colds and respiratory infections, Grimm W and Müller HH, *Am J Med* 1999; 106: 138–43.

Adverse reactions associated with Echinacea: the Australian experience, Mullins RJ and Heddle R, *Ann Allergy Asthma Immunol* 2002; 88: 42–51.

An alternative medicine study of herbal effects on the penetration of zona-free hamster oocytes and the integrity of sperm deoxyribonucleic acid, Ondrizek R *et al*, *Fertil Steril* 1999; 71: 517–22.

Benefit-risk assessment of the squeezed sap of the purple coneflower (Echinacea purpurea) for long-term oral immunostimulation, Parnham MJ, *Phytomed* 1996; 3: 95–102.

Echinacea for preventing and treating the common cold, Melchart D *et al*, Cochrane Database Syst Rev 2000; (2): CDE000530.

Echinacea for upper respiratory infection, Barrett B *et al*, *J Fam Pract* 1999; 48: 628–35.

Echinacea root extracts for the prevention of upper respiratory tract infections: a double-blind, placebo-controlled, randomized trial, Melchart D *et al*, *Arch Fam Med* 1998; 7: 541–5.

Echinaforce and other Echinacea fresh plant preparations in the treatment of the common cold. A randomized, placebo controlled, double-blind clinical trial, Brinkeborn RM *et al*, *Phytomedicine* 1999; 6: 1–6.

Echinagard treatment shortens the course of the common cold: a double-blind, placebo-controlled clinical trial, Hoheisel O *et al*, *Eur J Clin Res* 1997; 9: 261–8.

Efficacy of Echinacea purpurea in patients with a common cold. A placebo-controlled, randomised, double-blind clinical trial, Schulten B *et al*, *Arzneim Forsch* 2001; 51: 563–8.

Inhibition of human sperm motility by specific herbs used in alternative medicine, Ondrizek R *et al*, *J Assist Reprod Genet* 1999; 16: 87–91.

Placebo-controlled, double-blind study of Echinacea pallidae radix in upper respiratory tract infections, Dorn M *et al*, *Comp Ther Med* 1997; 5: 40–2.

Garlic

A scientific basis for the active principle of garlic (Allium sativum) and its use as a hypercholesteremic and antibacterial/antifungal agent, Reichenberg J, *J Jon Bastyr College Nat Med* 1982; 2: 28–32.

Activity of multiple resistant bacteria of garlic (Allium sativum) extract, Singh KV and Shukla NP, *Fitoterapia* 1983, 55: 313–15.

Allium sativum (garlic) – a natural antibiotic, Adetumbi M, Lau B, *Med Hypoth* 1983; 12: 227–37.

Allium sativum (garlic) inhibits lipid synthesis by Candida albicans, Adetumbi M *et al*, *Antimicrob Agents Chemother* 1986; 30: 499–501.

Antifungal activity in human urine and serum after ingestion of garlic (Allium sativum), Caporaso N *et al*, *Antimicrob Agents Chemother* 1983; 23: 700–2.

Antimicrobial effects of Allium Sativum L (garlic), Allium ampeloprasum L (elephant garlic) and Allium cepa L (onion) compounds and commercial garlic supplement products, Hughes BG and Lawson L, *Phytother Res* 1991; 5: 154–8.

Daily supplementation with aged garlic extract, but not raw garlic, protects low density lipoprotein against in vitro oxidation, Munday JA *et al*, *Atherosclerosis* 1999; 144: 399–404.

Effect of a garlic oil preparation on serum lipoproteins and cholesterol metabolism: a randomized controlled trial, Berthold HK *et al*, *JAMA* 1998; 279: 1900–2.

Effect of garlic on total serum cholesterol: a meta-analysis, Warshafsky S *et al*, *Ann Intern Med* 1993; 119: 599–605.

Efficacy of ajoene, an organosulphur derived from garlic, in the short-term therapy of Tinea pedis, Ledezma E *et al*, *Mycoses* 1996; 39: 393–5.

Evaluation of the in vitro antifungal activity of allicin, Yamada Y and Azuma K, *Antimicrob Agents Chemother* 1977; 11: 743–9.

Garlic powder and plasma lipids and lipoproteins: a multicenter, randomized, placebo-controlled trial, Isaacsohn JL *et al*, *Arch Intern Med* 1998; 158: 1189–94.

Garlic powder in the treatment of moderate hyperlipidemia: a controlled trial and meta-analysis, Neil LA *et al*, *J Royal Coll Physicians (Lond)* 1996; 30: 329–34.

Inhibition of Candida adhesion to buccal epithelial cells by an aqueous extract of Allium sativum (garlic), Ghannoum MA, *J Appl Bacteriol* 1990; 88: 163–9.

Isolation, purification, synthesis and kinetic activity of the anticandidal component of Allium sativum and a hypothesis for its mode of action, Barone F and Tansey M, *Mycologia* 1977; 69: 793–825.

Garlicin – fact or fiction?, Koch HP, *Phytother Res* 1993; 7: 278–80.

On the effect of garlic on plasma lipids and lipoproteins in mild hypercholesterolemia, Simons LA *et al*, *Atherosclerosis* 1995; 113: 219–25.

Sensitivity of heat-stressed yeasts to essential oils of plants, Conner DE and Beuchat LR, *Appl Environ Microbiol* 1984; 47: 229–33.

Sensitivity of yeasts isolated from cases of vaginitis to aqueous extracts of garlic, Sandhu DK *et al*, *Mykosen* 1980; 23: 691–8.

Studies on the anticandidal mode of action of Allium sativum (garlic), Ghannoum MA, *J Gen Microbiol* 1988; 134: 2917–24.

The antiatherosclerotic effect of Allium sativum, Koscielny J *et al*, *Atherosclerosis* 1999; 144: 237–49.

The antimicrobial activity of garlic and onion extract, Elnima E, *Pharmazie* 1983; 38: 747–8.

The chemistry of garlic and onions, Eric Block PhD, *Scientific American* 1985; 252: 114–19.

The inhibitory action of garlic (Allium sativum L.) on growth and respiration of some microorganisms, Tynecka Z and Gos Z, *Acta Microbiol Pol[B]* 1973; 5: 51–62.

Ginkgo biloba

Clinical and therapeutic effects of Ginkgo biloba extract (GBE) versus placebo in the treatment of psychorganic senile dementia of arteriosclerotic origin, Mancini M *et al*, *Gazzetta Medica Italiana* 1993; 152: 69–80.

Effects of ginkgolide PAF-acether antagonists on arterial thrombosis, Bourgain RH *et al*, *Adv Prost Leuko Res* 1987; 17: 815–17.

Ginkgo biloba extract inhibits oxygen species production generated by phorbol myristate acetate stimulated human leukocytes, Pincemail J *et al*, *Experientia* 1987; 43: 181–4.

Ginkgo biloba, Kleijnen J *et al*, *Lancet* 1992; 340: 1136–9.

Inhibition of the metabolism of platelet activating factor (PAF-acether) by three specific antagonists from Ginkgo biloba, Lamant V *et al*, *Biochem Pharmacol* 1987; 36: 2749–52.

Proof of the therapeutical effectiveness of a Ginkgo biloba special extract: Meta-analysis of 11 clinical trials in aged patients with cerebral insufficiency, Hopfenmuller W, *Arzneim Forsch* 1994; 44: 1005–13.

Proofs of involvement of PAF-acether in various immune disorders using DN5202i (ginkgolide B): A powerful PAF-acether antagonist from Ginkgo biloba, Braquet P, *L Adv Prost Thromb Leuko Res* 1988; 16: 179–98.

Protective effect of Ginkgo biloba extract (EGB 761) on free radical-induced changes in the electroretinogram of isolated rat retina, Dorylefaix MT *et al*, *Drugs Exp Clin Res* 1991; 17: 571–4.

Six month double-blind randomized clinical trial of Ginkgo biloba extracts versus placebo in two parallel groups in patients suffering from peripheral arterial insufficiency, Bauer U, *Arzneim Forsch* 1984; 34: 716–21.

The antiradical properties of Ginkgo biloba extract, in: Rokan (Ginkgo biloba), Pincemail J and Deby C, in Recent results in pharmacology and clinic, Fungfeld W.E. (ed.) New York, NY: Springer Verlag 1988; 71–82.

The efficacy of EGb 761 in patients with senile dementia of the Alzheimer type, a double-blind, placebo-controlled study on different levels of investigation, Hofferberth B, *Human Psychopharmacology* 1994; 9: 215–22.

Treatment of senile macular degeneration with Ginkgo biloba extract, A preliminary double-blind drug versus placebo study, Lebuisson DA *et al*, *Presse Med* 1986; 25: 1556–8.

St John's wort

Benefits and risks of the hypericum extract LI 160: drug monitoring study with 3,250 patients, Woelk H *et al*, *J Geriatr Psychiatry Neurol* 1994; 7(Suppl 1): S34–8.

Comparison of equivalence between the St John's wort extract LoHyp-57 and fluoxetine, Harrer G *et al*, *Arzneim Forsch* 1999; 49: 289–96.

Controlled clinical trials of Hypericum extracts in depressed patients – an overview, Volz HP, *Pharmacopsychiatry* 1997; 30(Suppl): 72–6.

Effectiveness and tolerance of the Hypericum extract LI 160 compared to maprotiline: A multicenter double-blind study, Harrer G *et al*, *J Geriatr Psychiatr Neurol* 1994; 7(Suppl 1): S24–S28; S44–S46.

Effectiveness and tolerance of the Hypericum extract LI 160 in comparison with imipramine: Randomized double-blind study with 135 outpatients, Vorbach EU *et al*, *J Geriatr Psychiatr Neurol* 1994; 7(Suppl 1): S19–S23.

Hypericum in the treatment of seasonal affective disorders, Martinez B *et al*, *J Geriatr Psychiatr Neurol* 1994; 7(Supp 1): S29–33.

Hypericum treatment of mild depressions with somatic symptoms, Hübner WD *et al*, *J Geriatr Psychiatr Neurol* 1994; 7(Suppl 1): S12–S14.

Johanniskraut-extrakt zur ambulanten therapie der depression, Schmidt U and Sommer H, *Fortschr Med* 1993; 111: 339–42.

LI 160, an extract of St John's wort, versus amitriptyline in mildly to moderately depressed outpatients – a controlled 6-week clinical trial, Wheatley D, *Pharmacopsychiatry* 1997; 30(Suppl): 77–80.

Multicenter double-blind study examining the antidepressant effectiveness of the Hypericum extract LI 160, Hänsgen KD *et al*, *J Geriatr Psychiatr Neurol* 1994; 7(Suppl 1): S15–S18.

Psychomotorische leistungsverbesserung; antidepressive therapie mit Johanniskraut, Schmidt U, *Therapiewoche* 1995; 2: 106–12.

St John's wort as an antidepressant, DeSmet PAGM and Nolen WA, *BMJ* 1996; 313: 241–2.

St John's wort for depression – an overview and meta-analysis of randomized clinical trials, Linde K *et al*, *BMJ* 1996; 313: 253–8.

St John's Wort, an antidepressant? A systemic, criteria-based review, Ernst E, *Phytomed* 1995; 2: 67–71.

Aloe

Aloe vera and wound healing, Davis RH *et al*, *J Am Podiatr Med Assoc* 1987; 77: 165–9.

Aloe vera, a natural approach for treating wounds, oedema and in diabetes, Davis RH *et al*, *J Am Podiatr Med Assoc* 1988; 78: 60–8.

Anti-inflammatory and wound healing properties of aloe vera, Udupa SL *et al*, *Fitoterapia* 1994; 65: 141–5.

Bacteriostatic property of aloe vera, Lorenzetti LJ *et al*, *J Pharm Sci* 1964; 53: 1287.

Beneficial effect of aloe on wound healing in an excisional wound model, Heggars JP *et al*, *J Air Complement Med* 1996; 2: 271–7.

Beneficial effects of aloe in wound healing, Heggars JP *et al*, *Phytother Res* 1993; 7: 48–52.

Effect of aloe vera on herpes simplex and herpes virus (strain zoster), Sims RM and Zimmermann ER, Aloe Vera of America Archives, Stabilized Aloe Vera 1971; 1: 239–40.

Immunoreactive lectins in leaf gel from aloe barbadensis Miller, Winters WD, *Phytother Res* 1993; 7: 23–5.

Management of psoriasis with aloe vera extract in a hydrophilic cream: a placebo controlled double blind study, Syed T *et al*, *Tropical Med Internat Health* 1996; 1: 505–9.

Report – The effect of aloe vera on mycotic organisms (fungi). Sims RM and Zimmermann ER, Aloe Vera of America Archives, Stabilized Aloe Vera 1971; 1: 237–8.

The stimulation of postdermabrasion wound healing with stabilised aloe vera gel-polyethylene oxide dressing, Fulton JE, *J Dermatol Surg Oncol* 1990; 16: 460–7.

The therapeutic efficacy of aloe vera cream dermaide aloe in thermal injuries. Two cases, Cera LM *et al*, *J Am Anita Hosp Assoc* 1980; 16: 768–72.

Treatment of experimental frostbite with pentoxifylline and aloe vera cream, Miller MB and Koltai PJ, *Arch Otolaryngol Head Neck Surg* 1995; 121: 678–80.

Panax Ginseng

A double-masked study of the effects of ginseng on cognitive functions, Sorensen H and Sonne J, *Curt Ther Res* 1996; 57: 959–68.

Clinical efficacy of Korean red ginseng for erectile dysfunction, Choi HK *et al*, *Int J Impot Res* 1995; 7: 181–6

Effect of ginseng on the performance of nurses on night duty, Hallstrom C *et al*, *Comp Med East West* 1982; 6: 277–82.

Failure of chronic ginseng supplementation to affect work performance and energy metabolism in healthy adult females, Riley D *et al*, *Nutr Res* 1996; 16: 1295–305.

Ginseng does not enhance psychological well being in healthy, young adults: results of a double-blind, placebo-controlled, randomized clinical trial, Cardinal BJ and Engels HJ, *J Am Diet Assoc* 2001; 101: 655–60.

Ginseng supplementation does not enhance healthy young adults' peak aerobic exercise performance, Allen JD *et al*, *J Am Coll Nutr* 1998; 17: 462–6.

Ginseng therapy in non-insulin-dependent diabetic patients, Sotaniemi EA *et al*, *Diabetes Care* 1995; 18: 1373–5.

Ginsenosides of various ginseng plants and selected products, Lui JHC *et al*, *Lloydia/J Natural Prod* 1980; 43: 340–6.

No ergogenic effect of ginseng ingestion, Morris AC *et al*, *Int J Sport Nutr* 1996; 6: 263–71.

No ergogenic effects of ginseng (Panax ginseng C.A. Meyer) during graded maximal aerobic exercise, Engels HJ and Wirth JC, *J Am Diet Assoc* 1997; 97: 1110–15.

Non-organ specific cancer prevention of ginseng: a prospective study in Korea, Yun Tand Choi SY, *Int J Epidemiol* 1998; 27: 359–64.

Pharmaton capsules in the treatment of functional fatigue: A double-blind study versus placebo evaluated by a new methodology, le Gal M *et al*, *Phytother Res* 1996; 10: 49–53.

Preventative effect of ginseng intake against various human cancers: a case-control study on 1,987 pairs, Yun TK and Choi SY, *Cancer Epidemiol Biomarker Prev* 1995; 4: 401–8.

The cognitive, subjective, and physical effects of a ginkgo biloba/panax ginseng combination in healthy volunteers with neurasthenic complaints, Wesnes KA *et al*, *Psychopharmacol Bull* 1997; 33: 677–83.

The memory enhancing effects of a Ginkgo biloba/Panax ginseng combination in healthy middle-aged volunteers, Wesnes KA *et al*, *Psychopharmacol* (Berl), 2000; 152: 353–61.

Variability in commercial ginseng products: an analysis of 25 preparations, Harkey MR *et al*, *Am J Clin Nutr* 2001; 73: 1101–6.

Siberian Ginseng
Effect of Eleutherococcus on the disease incidence among miners in the Arctic, Kalashnikov BN, in: Abstracts of the reports delivered at the 2nd all-union conference on human adaptation to different geographical, climatic and industrial conditions, Siberian Branch, USSR Academy of Medical Sciences, Novosibirsk 1977.

Eleutherococcus in the Prophylaxis of Influenza and Relapses of Essential Hypertension, Galanova LK, in: Adaptation and the adaptogens, Far Eastern Scientific Centre, USSR Academy of Sciences, Vladivostok 1977.

Eleutherococcus in the prophylaxis of influenza, essential hypertension, and ischaemic heart disease in the drivers of the VAP, Shchezin AK *et al*, in: New data on Eleutherococcus and other adaptogens. Far Eastern Research Centre, USSR Academy of Sciences, Vladivostock 1981.

Eleutherococcus prophylaxis of the disease incidence in the Arctic, Gagarin IA, in: Adaptation and the adaptogens. Far Eastern Scientific Centre, USSR Academy of Sciences, Vladivostok 1977.

Eleutherococcus, Brekhman II, Moscow: Vneshtorgizdat 1977.

Eleutherococcus: 20 years of research and clinical application. Abstract of the report made at the 1st international symposium on Eleutherococcus, Brekhman II, 29 May 1980, Hamburg.

Tentative data on the mass eleutherococcus prophylaxis of influenza at the main assembly line and metallurgical plant of the Volga automobile plant. Shchezin AK *et al*, in: Abstracts of the reports delivered at the 2nd all-union conference on human adaptation to different geographical, climatic and industrial conditions. Siberian Branch, USSR Academy of Medical Sciences, Novosibirsk 1977.

Feverfew
Amounts of feverfew in commercial preparations of the herb, Groenewegen WA and Heptinstall S, *Lancet* 1986; i: 44–5.

Efficacy of feverfew as prophylactic treatment of migraine. Johnson ES *et al*, *BMJ* 1985; 291: 569–73.

Feverfew (Tanacetum parthenium) as a prophylactic treatment for migraine: A double-blind placebo-controlled study, Palevitch D *et al*, *Phytother Res* 1997; 11: 508–11.

Herbal medicines in migraine prevention, de Weerdt CJ *et al*, *Phytomedicine* 1996; 3: 225–30.

Melatonin in feverfew and other medicinal plants, Murch SJ *et al*, *Lancet* 1997; 350: 1598–9.

Parthenolide content and bioactivity of feverfew (Tanacetum parthenium (L.) Schultz-Bip.). Estimation of commercial and authenticated feverfew products, Heptinstall S *et al*, *J Pharm Pharmacol* 1992; 44: 391–5.

Randomized double-blind placebo-controlled trial of feverfew in migraine prevention, Murphy JJ *et al*, *Lancet* 1988; ii: 189–92.

Goldenseal
Berberine in the treatment of diarrhoea of infancy and childhood, Sharda DC, *J Indian Med Assoc* 1970; 54: 22–4.

Effect of berberine hydrochloride on the bacteria of the alimentary canal, Biul Inst Roslin Leczniczych, Brzezinska-Jezowa L and Kaczmarek F, 1963; 9: 115–20.

Encyclopaedia of Common Natural Ingredients Used in Foods, Drugs and Cosmetics, 2nd edition. Leung AY and Foster S, New York: John Wiley and Sons 1996.

Goldenseal and the common cold: The antibiotic myth, Bergner P, *Medical Herbalism* 1997; 8: 1.

Natural Products in Canadian Pharmaceuticals IV Hydrastis Canadensis, Genest K and Hughes DW, *Can J Pharm Sci* 1969; 4: 41–5.

Randomized controlled trial of berberine sulfate therapy for diarrhoea due to enterotoxigenic Escherichia coli and Vibrio cholerae, Rabbani GH *et al*, *J Infect Dis* 1987;155: 979–84.

Liquorice

3-Monoglucuronyl-Glycyrrhetinic acid is a major metabolite that causes liquorice-induced pseudoaldosteronism, Kato H *et al*, *J Clin Endocrinol Metab* 1995; 80:1929–33.

Antimicrobial agents from higher plants: Antimicrobial isoflavonoids from glycyrrhiza glabre L var. typica, Mitscher L *et al*, *J Nat Products* 1980; 43: 259–69.

Clinical trial of deglycyrrhizinated liquorice in gastric ulcer, Turpie AG *et al*, *Gut* 1969; 10: 299–303.

Comparison between cimetidine and Caved-S in the treatment of gastric ulceration, and subsequent maintenance therapy, Morgan AG *et al*, *Gut* 1982; 23: 545–51.

Deglycyrrhizinated liquorice in duodenal ulcer, Tewari SN and Wilson AK, *Practitioner* 1972; 210: 820–5.

Deglycyrrhizinated liquorice in peptic ulcer, Glick L, *Lancet* 1982; ii: 817.

Effect of deglycyrrhizinated liquorice on gastric mucosal damage by aspirin, Rees WDW *et al*, *Scand J Gastroenterol* 1979; 14: 605–7.

Effect of prednisolone and glycyrrhizin on passive transfer of experimental allergic encephalomyelitis, Kutoyanagi T and Sata M, *Allergy* 1966; 15: 67–75.

Endoscopic controlled trial of four drug regimens in the treatment of chronic duodenal ulceration, Kassir ZA, *Irish Med J* 1985; 78: 153–6.

Glycyrrhizin, an active component of licorice roots, reduces morbidity and mortality of mice infected with lethal doses of influenza virus, Utsunomiya T *et al*, *Antimicrobial Agents Chemother* 1997; 41: 551–6.

Interferon induction by glycyrrhizin and glycyrrhetinic acid in mice, Abe N *et al*, *Microbiol Immunol* 1982; 26: 535–9.

Licorice as a liver herb, Bergner P, *Townsend Lett Docs* 1994; 137: 1326–7.

Licorice extract and its major polyphenol glabridin protect low-density lipoprotein against lipid peroxidation: In vitro and ex vivo studies in humans and in atherosclerotic lipoprotein E-deficient mice, Fuhrman B *et al*, *Am J Clin Nutr* 1997; 66: 267–75.

Licorice, More than just a flavor, Chandler RF, *Can Pharm J* 1985; 18: 420–4.

Potentiation of hydrocortisone activity in skin by glycyrrhetinic acid, Teelucksingh S *et al*, *Lancet* 1990; 355: 1060–3.

The influence of glycyrrhetinic acid on plasma cortosil and cortisone levels in healthy young volunteers, Mackenzie MA *et al*, *J Clin Endocrinol Metab* 1990; 70: 1637–43.

Topical carbonoxelone sodium in the management of herpes simplex infection, Partridge M and Poswillo D, *Br J Oral Macillofac Surg* 1984; 22: 138–45.

Saw Palmetto

A combination of Sabal and Urtica extracts vs. finasteride in BPH (stage I to II acc. to Alken): A comparison of therapeutic efficacy in a one-year double-blind study, Sökeland J and Albrecht J, *Urologe [A]* 1997; 36: 327–33.

Benign prostatic hyperplasia – Treatment with an extract from the fruit of Sabal serrulata. A drug monitoring study involving 1,334 patients, Vahlensieck VW *et al*, *Fortschr Med* 1993; 18: 323–6.

Comparison of phytotherapy (Permixon (r)) with finasteride in the treatment of benign prostatic hyperplasia: A randomized international study of 1,098 patients, Carraro JC et al, Prostate 1996; 29: 231–40.

Efficacy and safety of the extract of Serenoa repens in the treatment of benign prostatic hyperplasia: Therapeutic equivalence between twice and once daily dosage forms, Braeckman J et al, Phytotherapy Res 1997; 11: 558–63.

Efficacy of a combined Sabal-Urtica preparation in the treatment of benign prostatic hyperplasia, Metzker H et al, Urologe [B] 1996; 36: 292–300.

Long-term drug treatment of benign prostatic hyperplasia – results of a prospective 3-year multicenter study using Sabal extract IDS 89, Bach D and Ebeling L, Phytomed 1996; 3: 105–11.

Saw palmetto extracts for treatment of benign prostatic hyperplasia: a systematic review, Wilt TJ et al, JAMA 1998; 280: 1604–9.

Saw palmetto shown to shrink prostatic epithelium, Overmyer M, Urology Times 1999; 27: 1, 42.

The extract of Serenoa repens in the treatment of benign prostatic hyperplasia: A multicenter open study, Braeckman J, Curr Ther Res 1994; 55: 776–85.

Chapter 11. Homeopathy

A controlled evaluation of a homoeopathic preparation in the treatment of influenza-like syndromes, Ferley JP et al, Br J Clin Pharmacol 1989; 27: 329–35.

A meta-analysis of homoeopathic treatment of pollinosis with Galphimia glauca, Ludtke R and Wiesenauer M, Wien Med Wochenschr 1997; 147: 3232–7.

A randomized comparison of homoeopathic and standard care for the treatment of glue ear in children, Harrison H et al, Comp Ther Med 1999; 7: 132–5.

A randomized equivalence trial comparing the efficacy and safety of Luffa comp.-Heel nasal spray with cromolyn sodium spray in the treatment of seasonal allergic rhinitis, Weiser M et al, Forsch Komp Med 1999; 6: 142–8.

Are the clinical effects of homeopathy placebo effects? A meta-analysis of randomised placebo-controlled trials, Linde K et al, Lancet 1997; 350: 834–43.

Changes caused by succussion on NMR Patterns and bioassay of bradykinin triacetate (BKTA) succussions and dilution, Smith RB Jr and Boericke GW, J Am Inst Homeopathy 1968; 61: 197–212.

Classical homoeopathy versus conventional treatments: a systematic review, Ernst E, Perfusion 1999; 12: 13–15.

Clinical trials of homeopathy, Kleijnen P et al, BMJ 1991; 302: 316–23.

Do homeopathic medicines provoke adverse effects? A systematic review, Dantas F and Rampes H, Br Homeopath J 2000; 89 (Suppl 1): S 35–8.

Double-blind, placebo-controlled, randomized clinical trial of homoeopathic arnica C30 for pain and infection after total abdominal hysterectomy, Hart O et al, J Royal Soc Med 1997; 90: 73–8.

Double-blind randomized placebo-controlled study of homeopathic prophylaxis of migraine, Whitmarsh TE et al, Cephalalgia 1997; 17: 600–4.

Effect of homoeopathic medicines on daily burden of symptoms in children with recurrent upper respiratory tract infections, de Lange de Klerk ES et al, BMJ 1994; 309: 1329–32.

Effect of homoeopathic treatment on fibrositis (primary fibromyalgia), Fisher P et al, BMJ 1989; 299: 365–6.

Flow-cytometric analysis of basophil activation: inhibition by histamine at conventional and homeopathic concentrations, Brown V and Ennis M, Inflam Res 2001, 50 (Suppl 2): S47–8.

'High dilution' experiments a delusion, Maddox J et al, Nature 1988; 324: 287–90.

Homeopathy for chronic asthma, Linde K and Jobst KA, Cochrane Database Syst Rev 2000; (2): CD000353.

Homeopathic oscillococcinum for preventing and treating influenza and influenza-like symptoms, Vickers AJ and Smith C, Cochrane Database Syst Rev 2000; (2): CD 001957.

Homeopathic remedies for the treatment of osteoarthritis: a systematic review, Long L and Ernst E, Br Homeopath J 2001; 90: 37–43.

Homeopathic treatment of migraines: a randomized double-blind controlled study of 60 cases, Brigo B and Serpelloni G, Berlin J Res Hom 1991; 1: 98–106.

Homeopathy and conventional medicine: an outcomes study comparing effectiveness in a primary care setting, Riley DS et al, J Altern Comp Med 2001; 7: 149–59.

Homeopathy: Will its theory ever hold water?, Morgan P, Canadian Med Assn J 1992; 146: 1719–20.

Homoeopathic therapy in rheumatoid arthritis: evaluation by double-blind clinical therapeutic trial, Gibson RG et al, Br J Clin Pharmacol 1980; 9: 453–9.

Human basophil degranulation triggered by very dilute antiserum against IgE, Davenas E et al, Nature 1988; 333: 816–18.

In vitro immunological degranulation of human basophils is modulated by lung histamine and apis mellifica, Poitevain B et al, Br J Clin Pharmacol 1988; 25; 439–44.

Is evidence for homoeopathy reproducible?, Reilly D et al, Lancet 1994; 344: 1601–6.

Is homeopathy a placebo response? Controlled trial of homeopathic potency, with pollen in hay fever as model, Reilly D et al, Lancet 1986; 2: 881–6.

Patient benefit survey: Liverpool regional department of homoeopathic medicine, Richardson WR, Br Homeopath J 2001; 90: 158–62.

Patient benefit survey: Tunbridge Wells homeopathic hospital, Clover A, Br Homeopath J 2000; 89: 68–72.

Randomised controlled trial of homeopathy versus placebo in perennial allergic rhinitis with overview of four trial series, Taylor MA et al, BMJ 2000, 321: 471–6.

Randomized controlled trials of individualized homeopathy: a state-of-the art review, Linde K and Melchart D, J Alt Comp Ther 1998; 4: 371–88.

Salicylates and homeopathy in rheumatoid arthritis: preliminary observations, Gibson RG et al, Br J Clin Pharmacol 1978; 6: 391–5.

Superradiance: a new approach to coherent dynamical behaviors of condensed matter, del Guidice E and Preparata G, Frontier Perspectives, Fall/Winter 1990, Philadelphia: Temple University, Centre for Frontier Sciences.

Thanks for the memory: Experiments have backed what was once scientific 'heresy', Milgrom, L, Guardian, 15 March 2001.

The homoeopathic treatment of otitis media in children – comparison with conventional therapy, Friese KH et al, Int J Clin Pharmacol Ther 1997; 35: 296–301.

The long-term effects of homeopathic treatment of chronic headaches: 1 year follow up, Walach H et al, Cephalalgia 2000; 20: 835–7.

Treatment of acute childhood diarrhea with homeopathic medicine: a randomized clinical trial in Nicaragua, Jacobs J et al, Pediatrics 1994; 93: 719–25.

Two pilot controlled trials of arnica montana, Campbell A, Br Hom J 1978; 65: 8.

Vibrational Medicine, Gerber R, MD, Santa Fe, NM: Bear & Co 1988: 84.

Chapter 12. Hypnotherapy

Acupuncture and hypnotic suggestions in the treatment of non-organic male sexual dysfunction, Aydin S et al, Scand J Urol Nephrol 1997; 31: 271–4.

Autogenic training and self-hypnosis in the control of tension headache, Spinhoven P et al, Gen Hosp Psychiatry 1992; 14: 408–15.

Chronic asthma and improvement with relaxation induced hypnotherapy, Morrison JB, J Roy Soc Med 1989; 81: 701–4.

Clinical hypnotherapy/self-hypnosis for unspecified, chronic and episodic headache without migraine and other defined headaches in children and adolescents, Gysin T, Forsch Komp Med 1999; 6: 44–6.

Comparison of self-hypnosis and propranolol in the treatment of juvenile classic migraine, Olness K et al, Pediatrics 1987; 79: 593–7.

Controlled trial of hypnotherapy in relapse prevention of duodenal ulceration, Colgan SM et al, Lancet 1988; 1: 1299–300.

Controlled trial of hypnotherapy in the treatment of severe refractory irritable bowel syndrome, Whorwell PJ et al, Lancet 1984; 2: 1232–4.

Factors predicting hypnotic analgesia in clinical burn pain, Patterson DR et al, Int J Clin Exp Hypn 1997; (45): 377–95.

Hypnosis and conversion of the breech to the vertex presentation, Mehl L, Arch Fam Med 1994; 3: 881–7.

Hypnosis and self-hypnosis administered and taught by nurses for relief of chronic pain: a controlled clinical trial, Buchser E, Forsch Komp Med 1999; 6: 41–3.

Hypnosis in dermatology, Shenefelt, PD, Arch Dermatol 2000; 136: 393–9.

Hypnotic analgesia reduces R-III nociceptive reflex: further evidence concerning the multifactorial nature of hypnotic analgesia, Kiernan BD et al, Pain 1995; 60: 39–47.

Hypnotic analgesia: 1. Somatosensory event-related potential changes to noxious stimuli and 2. Transfer learning to reduce chronic low back pain, Crawford HJ et al, Int J Clin Exp Hypn 1998; 46: 92–132.

Improvement in bronchial hyper-responsiveness in patients with moderate asthma after treatment with a hypnotic technique: a randomised controlled trial, Ewer TC and Stewart DE, BMJ (Clin Res Ed) 1986; 293: 1129–32.

Individual and group hypnotherapy in treatment of refractory irritable bowel syndrome, Harvey RF et al, Lancet 1989; 1: 424–5.

Integration of behavioral and relaxation approaches into the treatment of chronic pain and insomnia, Richmond K et al, JAMA 1996; 276: 313–18.

Migraine and hypnotherapy, Anderson JA et al, Int J Clin Exp Hypn 1975; 23: 48–58.

Owls and larks in hypnosis: individual differences in hypnotic susceptibility relating to biological rhythms, Lippincott B, Am J Clin Hypn 1992; 34: 185–92.

Preoperative hypnosis reduces postoperative vomiting after surgery of the breasts: a prospective, randomised and blinded study, Enqvist B et al, Acta Anaesthesiol Scand 1997; 41: 1028–32.

Psychological approaches during conscious sedation. Hypnosis versus stress reducing strategies: a prospective randomized study, Faymonville ME et al, Pain 1997; 73: 361–7.

Psychoneuroimmunology. The interface between behavior, brain, and immunity, Maier SF et al, Am Psychol 1994; 49: 1004–7.

Self-hypnosis reduces anxiety following coronary artery bypass surgery: a prospective, randomized trial, Ashton C et al, J Caridiovasc Surg 1997; 38: 6975.

Self-hypnosis for management of chronic dyspnea in pediatric patients, Anbar RD, Pediatrics 2001; 107: E21.

Self-regulation of salivary immunoglobulin A by children, Olness K et al, Pediatrics 1989; 83: 66–71.

Significant developments in medical hypnosis during the past 25 years, Frankel FH, Int J Clin Exp Hypn 1987; 35: 231–47.

The effect of clinical hypnosis and relaxation techniques on the functioning of the immune system: new directions for psychoneuroimmunology research and practice, Horton-Hausknecht JR, *Forsch Komp Med* 1995; 2: 196–202.

The effects of hypnosis on the labor processes and birth outcomes of pregnant adolescents, Martin AA *et al*, *J Fam Pract* 2001; 50: 441–3.

The use of hypnosis in medicine: the possible pathways involved, Gonsalkorale WM, *Eur J Gastroenterol Hepatol* 1996; 8: 520–4.

Treatment of cervical headache with hypnosis, suggestive therapy, and relaxation techniques, Carasso RL *et al*, *Am J Clin Hypn* 1985; 27: 216–18.

Treatment of chronic tension-type headache with hypnotherapy: a single-blind time controlled study, Melis PM *et al*, *Headache* 1991; 31: 686–9.

Using hypnosis to accelerate the healing of bone fractures: a randomized controlled pilot study, Ginandes CS and Rosenthal DI, *Altern Ther Health Med* 1999; 5: 67–75.

When hypnosis causes trouble, Barber J, *Int J Clin Exp Hypn* 1998; 46: 157–70.

Chapter 13. Massage

An exploratory study of reflexological treatment for headache, Launso L *et al*, *Altern Ther Health Med* 1999; 5: 57–65.

Children with cystic fibrosis benefit from massage therapy, Hernandez-Reif M *et al*, *J Pediatr Psychol* 1999; 24: 175–81.

Deep transverse friction: its analgesic effect, de Bruijn R, *Int J Sports Med* 1984; 5 (Suppl): 35–6.

Effectiveness of a physical therapy regimen in the treatment of tension-type headache, Hammill JM *et al*, *Headache* 1996; 36: 149–53.

Effects of massage & use of oil on growth, blood flow & sleep pattern in infants, Agarwal KN *et al*, *Indian J Med Res* 2000; 112: 212–17.

Effects of slow stroke back massage on relaxation in hospice clients, Meek SS, *Image J Nurs Sch* 1993; 25: 17–21.

Expanding the nursing repertoire: the effect of massage on post-operative pain, Nixon M *et al*, *Austral J Adv Nurs* 1997; 14: 21–6.

Infant massage compared with crib vibrator in the treatment of colicky infants, Huhtala V *et al*, *Pediatrics* 2000; 105: E84.

Infant massage improves mother-infant interaction for mothers with postnatal depression, Onozawa K *et al*, *J Affect Disord* 2001; 63: 201–7.

Influence of reflex zone therapy of the feet on intestinal blood flow measured by color Doppler sonography, Mur E *et al*, *Forsch Komp Med Klass Naturheilkd* 2001; 8: 86–9.

Massage for low back pain, Furlan AD *et al*, Cochrane Database Syst Rev 2000; (4): CD001929.

Massage for promoting growth and development of preterm and/or low birth-weight infants, Vickers A *et al*, Cochrane Database Syst Rev 2000; (2): CD000390.

Massage reduces anxiety in child and adolescent psychiatric patients, Field T *et al*, *J Am Acad Child Adolesc Psychiatry* 1992; 31: 125–31.

Massage therapy is associated with enhancement of the immune system's cytotoxic capacity, Ironson G *et al*, *Int J Neurosci* 1996; 84: 205–17.

Psychophysiological effects of back massage on elderly institutionalized patients, Fraser J and Kerr JR, *J Adv Nurs* 1993; 18: 238–45.

Randomized controlled study of premenstrual symptoms treated with ear, hand and foot reflexology, Oleson T and Flocco W, *Ob Gyn* 1993; 82: 906–11.

Randomized trial comparing traditional Chinese medical acupuncture, therapeutic massage, and self-care education for chronic low back pain, Cherkin DC *et al*, *Arch Intern Med* 2001; 161: 1081–8.

Reflexology and bronchial asthma, Petersen LN *et al*, *Ugeskrift Laeger* 1992; 154: 2065–8.

Respiratory function and the rheological status of bronchial secretions collected by spontaneous expectoration after physiotherapy, Pham QT *et al*, *Bulletin d'Physio-pathologie Respiratoire* 1973; 9: 292–311.

Sensing an improvement: an experimental study to evaluate the use of aromatherapy, massage and periods of rest in an intensive care unit, Dunn C *et al*, *J Adv Nurs* 1995; 21: 34–40.

Slow stroke back massage for cancer patients, Sims S, *Nurs Times* 1986; 83: 19–25.

The effect of massage on pain in cancer patients, Weinrich SP and Weinrich MC, *Nurs Res* 1990; 3: 140–5.

The effect of muscle relaxation, imagery and relaxing music intervention and a back massage on the sleep and psychophysiological arousal of elderly males hospitalized in the critical care environment [dissertation], Richards KC, Austin, Tex: University of Texas; 1993.

The effects of massage in patients with chronic tension headache, Puustjarvi K *et al*, *Acupunct Electrother Res* 1990; 15: 159–62.

The use of therapeutic massage as a nursing intervention to modify anxiety and the perception of cancer pain, Ferrell-Torry AT and Glick OJ, *Cancer Nurs* 1993; 16: 93–101.

The psychophysiological effects of aromatherapy massage following cardiac surgery, Stevensen C, *Comp Ther Med* 1994; 2: 27–35.

Chapter 14. Meditation

A physiological and subjective evaluation of meditation, hypnosis, and relaxation, Morse DR *et al*, *Psychosom Med* 1977; 39: 304–24.

A randomised controlled trial of stress reduction for hypertension in older African Americans, Schneider RH *et al*, *Hypertension* 1995; 26: 820–7.

A relaxation technique in the management of hypercholesterolemia, Cooper MJ and Aygen MM, *J Human Stress* 1979; 5: 24–7.

Acute effects of transcendental meditation on hemodynamic functioning in middle-aged adults, Barnes VA *et al*, *Psychosom Med* 1999; 61: 525–31.

Adrenocortical activity during meditation, Jevning R *et al*, *Horm Behav* 1978; 10: 54–60.

Adverse effects of meditation: a preliminary investigation of long-term meditators, Shapiro DHJ, *Int J Psychosom* 1992; 39: 62–7.

Altered responses of cortisol, GH, TSH, and testosterone to acute stress after four months' practice of transcendental meditation (TM), MacLean CR *et al*, *Ann NY Acad Sci* 1994; 746: 381–4.

Breath suspension during the transcendental meditation technique, Farrow JT and Herbert R, *Psychosom Med* 1982; 44: 133–53.

Can lifestyle changes reverse atherosclerosis?, Ornish D *et al*, *Lancet* 1990; 336: 129–33.

Catecholamine levels in practitioners of the transcendental meditation technique, Infante JR *et al*, *Physiol Behav* 2001; 72: 141–6.

Changed pattern of regional glucose metabolism during yoga meditative relaxation, Herzog H *et al*, *Neuropsychobiol* 1990–91; 23: 182–7.

Changes in myocardial perfusion abnormalities by positron emission tomography after long-term, intense risk factor modification, Gould KL *et al*, *JAMA* 1995; 27: 894–901.

Cognitive behavioral techniques for hypertension: are they effective?, Eisenberg DM, *et al*, *Ann Intern Med* 1993; 1118: 964–72.

Depersonalization and meditation, Castillo RBJ, *Psychiatry* 1990; 53: 158–68.

Differential effects of relaxation techniques on trait anxiety: a meta-analysis, Eppley KR *et al*, *J Clin Psychol* 1989; 45: 957–74.

Effect of transcendental meditation on breathing and respiratory control, Wolkove N *et al*, *J Appl Physiol* 1984; 56: 607–12.

Effect of Buddhist meditation on serum cortisol and total protein levels, blood pressure, pulse rate, lung volume and reaction time, Sudsuang R *et al*, *Physiol Behav* 1991; 50: 543–8.

Effectiveness of transcendental meditation program in preventing and treating substance misuse: a review, Gelderloos P *et al*, *Int J Addict* 1991; 26: 293–325.

Effects of a behavioral stress-management program on anxiety, mood, self-esteem and T-cell count in HIV positive men, Taylor DN, *Psychol Rep* 1995; 76: 451–7.

Effects of stress reduction on cartoid atherosclerosis in hypertensive African Americans, Castillo-Richmond A *et al*, *Stroke* 2000; 31: 568–73.

Electrophysiologic characteristics of respiratory suspension periods occurring during the practice of the transcendental meditation program, Badawi K *et al*, *Psychosom Med* 1984; 46: 267–76.

Elevated serum dehydroepiandrosterone sulfate levels in practitioners of the transcendental meditation (TM) and TM-Sidhi programs, Glaser JL *et al*, *J Behav Med* 1992; 15: 327–41.

Evaluation of transcendental meditation as a method of reducing stress, Michaels RR *et al*, *Science* 1976; 192: 1242–4.

Improved stenosis geometry by quantitative coronary arteriography after vigorous risk factor modification, Gould KL *et al*, *Am J Cardiol* 1992; 69; 845–53.

Lower lipid peroxide levels in practitioners of the transcendental meditation program, Schneider RH *et al*, *Psychosom Med* 1998; 60: 38–41.

Management of hypertension by reduction in sympathetic activity, Mathias CJ, *Hypertension* 1991; 17: 69–74.

Medical care utilization and the transcendental meditation program, Orme-Johnson D, *Psychosom Med* 1987; 49: 493–507.

Non-pharmacological treatment of hypertension, Silverberg DS *et al*, *J Hypertens* 1990; (Suppl 8): S21–S26.

Physiological responses during meditation and rest, Delmonte MM, *Biofeedback Self Regul* 1984; 9: 181–200.

Precipitation of acute psychotic episodes by intensive meditation in individuals with a history of schizophrenia, Walsh, R and Roche L, *Am J Psychiatry* 1979; 136: 1085–6.

Spontaneous Remission, O'Regan B, Sausalito, California: Institutes of Noetic Sciences 1993.

The effects of the transcendental meditation and TM-Sidhi program on the aging process, Wallace RK *et al*, *Int J Neurosci* 1982; 16: 53–8.

The impact of a meditation-based stress reduction program on fibromyalgia, Kaplan KH *et al*, *Gen Hosp Psychiatry* 1993; 15: 284–9.

The impact of the transcendental meditation program on government payments to physicians in Quebec, Herron RE *et al*, *Am J Health Promot* 1996; 10: 208–16.

Three case reports of the metabolic and electroencephalographic changes during advanced Buddhist meditation techniques, Benson H *et al*, *Behav Med* 1990; 16: 90–5.

Transcendental meditation, mindfulness, and longevity: an experimental study with the elderly, Alexander CN *et al*, *J Pers Soc Psychol* 1989; 57: 950–64.

Treating and preventing alcohol, nicotine, and drug abuse through transcendental meditation: A review and statistical meta-analysis, Alexander C N *et al*, *Alcoholism Treatment Quarterly* 1994; 11: 13–87.

Trial of stress reduction for hypertension in older African Americans II: sex and subgroup analysis, Alexander CN *et al*, *Hypertension* 1996; 28: 228–37.

Usefulness of the transcendental meditation program in the treatment of patients with coronary artery disease, Zamarra JW *et al*, *Am J Cardiol* 1996; 77: 867–70.

Chapter 15. Naturopathy

A dietary management of severe childhood migraine, Carter CM *et al*, *Hum Nutri Appl Nutri* 1985; 39A: 294–303.

A prospective study of alcohol, diet, and other lifestyle factors in relation to obstructive uropathy, Chyou PH *et al*, *Prostate* 1993; 22: 253–64.

A review and analysis of the health and cost effective outcome of comprehensive health promotion and disease promotion at the worksite: 1991–1993 update, Pelletier KR, *Am J Health Promotion* 1993; 8: 50–61.

Co-enzyme Q10 as an adjunctive treatment of congestive heart failure, Hofman-Bang C *et al*, *J Am Coll Cardiol* 1992; 9: 216A.

Effect of coenzyme Q10 in patients with congestive heart failure: a long-term multicenter randomized study, Morisco C *et al*, *Clin Invest* 1993; 71 (Suppl 8): S134–6.

Effect of zinc on androgen metabolism in the human hyperplastic prostate, Wallae AM and Grant JK, *Biochem Soc Trans* 1975; 3: 540–2.

Electromyographical ischemic test and intracellular and extracellular magnesium concentrations in migraine and tension type headache patients, Mazotta G *et al*, *Headache* 1996; 36: 357–61.

Food allergy and adult migraine: double-blind and mediator confirmation of an allergic etiology, Mansfield LE *et al*, *Ann Allergy* 1985; 55: 1126–9.

Food allergy in migraine, Monro J *et al*, *Lancet* 1980; 2: 1–4.

Is migraine a food allergy? Eger J *et al*, *Lancet* 1983; 2: 865–9.

Is there a role for thiamine supplementation in the management of heart failure? Leslie D and Gheorghiade M, *Am Heart J* 1996; 131: 1248–50.

L-Carnitine – a preliminary review of its pharmacokinetics, and its therapeutic use in ischemic cardiac disease and primary and secondary carnitine deficiencies in relationship to its role in fatty acid metabolism, Goa KL and Brogden RN, *Drugs* 1987; 34: 1–24.

Magnesium in the prophylaxis of migraine – a double-blind placebo-controlled study, Pfaffenrath V *et al*, *Cephalalgia* 1996; 16: 436–40.

Migraine and magnesium: eleven neglected connections, Swanson DR, *Perspect Biol Med* 1988; 31: 526–57.

Naturotherapist told diabetic to stop using insulin, NCRHI Newsletter: The National Council for Reliable Health Information, 30 June 2000: 1.

Prophylaxis of migraine with oral magnesium: results from a prospective multi-center, placebo-controlled and double-blind randomised study, Peikert A *et al*, *Cephalalgia* 1996; 16: 257–63.

Prostatic hypertrophy as part of a generalized metabolic disease, evidence of the presence of lipopenia, Boyd EM and Berry NE, *J Urol* 1939; 41: 406–11.

Results of a decade of naturopathic treatment for environmental illness: a review of clinical records, *J Naturopathic Med* 1997; 7: 21–7.

The lipids of the prostatic fluid, seminal plasma and enlarged prostate gland of man, Scott WW, 1945; 53: 712–18.

Unconventional approaches to nutritional medicine, Vickers A and Zollman C, *BMJ* 1999; 319; 1419–22.

Vegetarian diets. Is avoiding meat good for everyone? Thomas, P, *What Doctors Don't Tell You* 1998; 9(8): 1–4.

What is better? An investigation into the use and satisfaction with complementary and official medicine in the Netherlands, Oojendijk WT, Netherlands Institute of Preventative Medicine and Technical Industrial Organization, 1980.

Zinc treatment for the reduction of hyperplasia of the prostate, Fahim M *et al*, *Fed Proc* 1976; 35: 361.

Chapter 16. Osteopathy & Chiropractic

A comparison of osteopathic spinal manipulation with standard care with low back pain, Andersson GBJ *et al*, *N Eng J Med* 1999; 341: 1426–31.

A controlled trial of cervical manipulation of migraine, Parker GB, *Aust NZ J Med* 1978; 8: 589–93.

Attention deficit disorder. The hyperactive child, Agresti LM, *Osteopathic Annals* 1989; 14: 6–16.

Benefits of osteopathic manipulative treatment for hospitalized elderly patients with pneumonia, Noll DR *et al*, *J Am Osteopath Assoc* 2000; 100: 776–82.

Chiropractic management of primary nocturnal enuresis, Reed WR *et al*, *J Manip Physiol Ther* 1994; 17: 596–600.

Chronic asthma and chiropractic spinal manipulation: a randomised clinical trial, Neilsen NH *et al*, *Clin Exp Allergy* 1995; 25: 80–8.

Effect of osteopathic medical management on neurologic development in children, Frymann V *et al*, *J Am Osteopath Assoc* 1992; 92: 729–44.

Effectiveness of spinal manipulative therapy in treatment of primary dysmenorrhea: a pilot study, Thomason PR *et al*, *J Manip Physiol Ther*, 1979; 2: 140–5.

Infantile colic treated by chiropractors: a prospective study of 316 cases, Klougart N *et al*, *J Manip Physiol Ther* 1989; 12: 281–8.

Inpatient osteopathic manipulative treatment: impact on length of stay, Cantieri MS, *J Manip Physiol Ther* 1998; 21: 435–6.

Lasting changes in passive range motion after spinal manipulation: a randomized, blind, controlled trial, Nillsson N, *J Manip Physiol Ther* 1996; 19: 165–8.

Learning difficulties of children viewed in the light of the osteopathic concept, Frymann V *et al*, *J Am Osteopath Assoc* 1976; 76: 46–61.

Low back pain of mechanical origin: randomised comparison of chiropractic and hospital outpatient treatment, Meade TW *et al*, *BMJ* 1990, 300: 1431–7.

Managing back pain in general practice – is osteopathy the new paradigm?, Williams N, *Br J Gen Pract* 1997; 47: 653–5.

Manipulation and mobilization of the cervical spine. A systematic review of the literature, Hurwitz EL, *Spine* 1996; 21: 1746–59; 1759–60.

Manipulative therapy of upper respiratory infections in children, Purse FM, *J Am Osteopathic Assoc* 1966; 65: 964–72.

Misuse of the literature by medical authors in discussing spinal manipulative therapy injury, Terrett AG, *J Manip Physiol Ther* 1995; 18: 203–10.

Practical Osteopathic Procedures, Magoun H Sr, Belen, NM/Kirskville, MO: Journal Printing Co, 72–3.

Randomised comparison of chiropractic and hospital outpatient management for low back pain: results from extended follow up, Meade TW *et al*, *BMJ* 1995; 311: 349–51.

Spinal manipulation for low back pain. An updated systematic review of randomized clinical trials, Koes BW *et al*, *Spine* 1996; 21: 2860–71.

Spinal manipulation vs. amitriptyline for the treatment of chronic tension-type headaches: a randomized clinical trial, Boline PD *et al*, *J Manip Physiol Ther*, 1995; 18: 148–54.

The effect of manipulation (toggle recoil technique) for headaches with upper cervical joint dysfunction: a pilot study, Whittingham W, *J Manip Physiol Ther* 1994; 17: 369–75.

The effect of spinal manipulation in the treatment of cervicogenic headache, Nillsson N, *J Manip Physiol Ther* 1997; 20: 326–30.

The effects of spinal manipulation on prostaglandin levels in women with primary dysmenorrhea, Kokjohn K *et al*, *J Manip Pysiol Ther* 1992; 15: 279–85.

The immediate effect of activator vs. meric adjustment on acute low back pain: a randomized controlled trial, Gemmell HA and Jacobson BH, *J Manip Physiol Ther* 1995; 18: 453–6.

The short-term effect of a spinal manipulation on pain/pressure threshold in patients with chronic mechanical low back pain, Cote P *et al*, *J Manip Physiol Ther* 1994; 17: 364–8.

Chapter 17. Placebo

A controlled trial of transcutaneous electrical nerve stimulation (TENS) and exercise for chronic low back pain, Deyo RA *et al*, *N Engl J Med* 1990; 322: 1627–34.

A telephone support service to reduce medical care use among the elderly, Infante-Rivard C *et al*, *J Am Geriatr Soc* 1988; 36: 306–11.

Address to American Psychological Association's Annual Convention, 1996, Sapirstein G, APA News Release, 9 August 1996.

An investigation of drug expectancy as a function of capsule color and size and preparation form, Buckalew LW and Coffield KE, *J Clin Psychopharmacol* 1982; 2: 245–8.

Angina pectoris and the placebo effect, Benson H and McCalle DP, *N Eng J Med* 1979; 300: 1424–9.

Anticipation of analgesia. A placebo effect, Laska E and Sunshine A, *Headache* 1973; 13: 1–11.

Can the provision of information to patients with osteoarthritis improve functional status? A randomized, controlled trial, Weinberger M *et al*, *Arthritis Rheum* 1989; 32: 1577–83.

Caring effects, Tudor Hart J and Dieppe P, *Lancet* 1996; 347: 1606–8.

Continuous emotional support during labor in a US hospital. A randomized controlled trial, Kennell J *et al*, *JAMA* 1991; 265: 2197–201.

Cultural variations in the placebo effect: ulcers, anxiety and blood pressure, Moerman DE, *Med Anthropol Quarterly* 2000; 14: 51–72.

Demonstration to medical students of placebo responses and non-drug factors, Blackwell B *et al*, *Lancet* 1972; 1: 1279–82.

Doctors, Patients and Placebos, Spiro HM, Conn: Yale University Press 1986.

Effect of colour of drugs: systematic review of perceived effects of drugs and of their effectiveness, de Craen AJ *et al*, *BMJ* 1996; 313: 1624–6.

Eight Weeks to Optimum Health, Weil A, New York: Knopf 1997.

General medical effectiveness and human biology: placebo effects in the treatment of ulcer disease, Moerman DE, *Med Anthropol Quarterly* 1983; 14: 13–16.

Harnessing the power of the placebo effect and renaming it 'remembered wellness', Benson H and Friedman R, *Annu Rev Med* 1996; 47: 193–9.

Healing and the Mind, Bill Moyers, London: Thorsons 1993.

Knowledge and use of placebos by house officers and nurses, Goodwin JS *et al, Ann Intern Med* 1979; 91: 106–10.

Listening to Prozac but hearing placebo: A meta-analysis of antidepressant medication, Kirsch I and Sapirstein G, *Prevention & Treatment* 1998; 1: 0002a. Available online at:
http://journals.apa.org/prevention/volume1/pre0010002a.html.

Meaning and Medicine, Dossey L, New York: Bantam 1992.

Narcotic receptor blockade and its effects on the analgesic response to placebo and ibuprofen after oral surgery, Hersch EV *et al, Oral Surg Oral Med Oral Pathol* 1993; 75: 539–46.

Non-blind placebo trial: an exploration of neurotic patients' responses to placebo when its first inert content is disclosed, Park L and Covi L, *Arch Gen Psychiatry* 1965; 12: 336–45.

Patient outcomes after lumbar spinal fusions, Turner JA *et al, JAMA* 1992; 268: 907–11.

Placebo – efficacy and adverse effects in controlled clinical trials, Weihrauch TR and Gauler TC, *Arzneim Forsch* 1999; 49: 385–93.

Placebo effect in double-blind clinical trials: a review of interactions with medications, Kleinen J *et al, Lancet* 1994; 344: 1347–9.

Pleasing the Patient, Watts G, London: Faber & Faber 1992.

Power Healing, Galland L, New York: Random House 1997.

Predictors of outcome in headache patients presenting to family physicians – one year prospective study, The Headache Study Group of the University of Western Ontario, *Headache* 1986; 26: 285–94.

Reduction of postoperative pain by encouragement and instruction of patients: a study of doctor-patient rapport, Egbert LD *et al, N Eng J Med* 1964; 270: 825–7.

Response expectancies in placebo analgesia and their clinical relevance, Pollo A *et al, Pain* 2001; 93: 77–84.

Surgery as placebo, Johnson AG, *Lancet* 1994; 344: 1440–2.

Surgery for lumbar spinal stenosis. Attempted meta-analysis of the literature, Turner JA *et al, Spine* 1992; 17: 1–8.

Symptom reduction and suicide risk in patients treated with placebo in antidepressant clinical trials: an analysis of the Food and Drug Administration database, *Arch Gen Psychiatry* 2000; 57: 311–17.

Telephone care as a substitute for routine clinic follow-up, Wasson J *et al, JAMA* 1992; 267: 1788–93.

The lie that heals: the ethics of giving placebos, Brody H, *Ann Intern Med* 1992; 97: 112–18.

The lumbar disc herniation. A computer-aided analysis of 2,504 operations, Spangfort EV, *Acta Orthop Scand Suppl* 1972; 142: 1–95.

The power of nonspecific effects in healing: implications for psychosocial and biological treatments, Roberts HA, *Clin Psychol Rev* 1993; 13: 375–91.

The power of the sugar pill, Evans JF, *Psychol Today,* April 1974.

Response of patients with myofascial pain-dysfunction syndrome to mock equilibrium, Goodman P *et al, J Am Dent Assoc* 1976; 92: 755–8.

Chapter 18. Spiritual Healing

A randomized controlled trial of the effects of remote, intercessory prayer on outcomes in patients admitted to the coronary care unit, Harris WS *et al, Arch Int Med* 1999; 159: 2273–8.

An experimental study of the effects of distance, intercessory prayer on self-esteem, anxiety and depression, O'Laoire S, *Altern Ther Health Med* 1997; 3: 38–53.

Attendance at religious services, interleukin-6, and other biological indicators of immune function in older adults, Koenig HG *et al*, *Int J Psychiatry Med* 1997; 23: 233–50.

Beyond the Relaxation Response, Benson H, New York: New York Times Books 1984.

Church attendance and health, Comstock GW and Partridge KB, *J Chronic Dis* 1972; 25: 665–72.

Does religious observance promote health? Mortality in secular versus religious kibbutzim in Israel, Kark JD *et al*, *Am J Public Health* 1996; 86: 341–6.

Effects of intercessory prayer on patients with rheumatoid arthritis, Matthews DA *et al*, *South J Med* 2000; 93: 1177–86.

Frequent attendance at religious services and mortality over 28 years, Strawbridge WJ *et al*, *Am J Pub Health* 1997; 87: 957–61.

General and comparative study of the psychokinetic effect on a fungus culture, Barry J, *J Parapsychol* 1968; 32; 237–43.

Healing as a therapy for human disease: a systematic review, Abbott NC, *J Altern Comp Med* 2000; 6: 159–69.

Intercessory prayer for ill health: a systematic review, Roberts L *et al*, *Forsch Komp Med* 1998; 5 (Suppl S1): 82–6.

Intercessory prayer for the alleviation of ill health, Roberts L *et al*, Cochrane Database Syst Rev 2000; (2): CD000368.

Intercessory prayer in the treatment of alcohol abuse and dependence: a pilot study, Walker SR *et al*, *Altern Ther Health Med* 1997; 3: 79–86.

Perceived religiousness is protective for colorectal cancer: data from the Melbourne Colorectal Cancer Study, Kune GA *et al*, *J Royal Soc Med* 1993; 86: 645–7.

Stress-induced immunosuppression and therapeutic touch, Olson M *et al*, *Altern Ther Health Med* 1997; 3: 68–74.

Positive therapeutic effects of intercessory prayer in a coronary care unit population, Byrd RC, *South J Med* 1988; 81: 826–9.

Prayer is Good Medicine: How to Reap the Healing Benefits of Prayer, Dossey L, New York: HarperCollins 1996.

Psychological recovery from coronary artery bypass graft surgery: the use of complementary therapies, Ai AL *et al*, *J Altern Comp Med* 1997; 3: 343–53.

Reed, D, Religion and mortality among the community-dwelling elderly, Oman D, *Am J Public Health* 1998; 88: 1469–75.

Religion and health: is there an association, is it valid, is it causal?, Levin JS, *Soc Sci Med* 1994; 38: 1475–82.

Religion and subjective well being in adulthood: a quantitative synthesis, Witter RA *et al*, *Rev Religious Res* 1985; 26: 332–42.

Religion, spirituality and medicine, Sloan RP *et al*, *Lancet* 1999; 353: 664–7.

Religious coping and depression among elderley, hospitalized medically ill men, Koenig HG *et al*, *Am J Psychiatry* 1992; 149: 1693–700.

Religious involvement and mortality: a meta-analytic review, McCullough ME *et al*, *Health Psychol* 2000; 19: 211–22.

Religious involvement and US adult mortality, Hummer RA *et al*, *Demography* 1999; 36: 273–85.

Religious research in gerontology, Levin JS, 1980–94, *J Religious Gerontol* 1997; 10: 3–31.

Religious struggle as a predictor of mortality among medically ill elderly patients: a 2-year longitudinal study, Pargament K *et al*, *Ann Intern Med* 2001; 161: 1881–5.

Some biological effects of laying on of hands – a review of experiments with animals and plants, Grad B, *J Am Soc Psychical Res* 1965; 59: 95–126.

Systematic analysis of research on religious variables in four major psychiatric journals, 1978–82, Larson DB *et al*, *Am J Psychiatry* 1986; 143: 329–34.

The effects of therapeutic touch on patients with osteoarthritis of the knee, Gordon A *et al*, *J Fam Pract* 1998; 47: 271–7.

The efficacy of 'distant healing': a systematic review of randomized trials, Atin, JA *et al*, *Ann Intern Med* 2000; 132: 903–10.

The Field – the Quest for the Secret Force of the Universe, McTaggart L, London: Thorsons 2001.

The Healing Power of Faith – Science Explores Medicine's Last Great Frontier, Koenig H, New York: Simon & Schuster 1999.

The Medium, Mystic and the Physicist: Toward a General Theory of the Paranormal, LeShan L, New York: Penguin 1995.

The relationship between religious activities and cigarette smoking in older adults, Koenig HG *et al*, *J Gerontol A Biol Sci Med Sci* 1998; 53: 6.

The significance of belief and expectancy within the spiritual healing encounter, Wirth DP, *Soc Sci Med* 1995; 41: 249–60.

Timeless Healing: the Power and Biology of Belief, Benson H, New York: Scribner 1996.

Use of health services by hospitalized medically ill depressed elderly patients, Koenig HG *et al*, *Am J Psychiatry* 1998; 155: 536–42.

Why experimenters upset results, Manning M, *Alpha*, November 1979: 11.

Chapter 19. Traditional Chinese Medicine

A controlled trial of traditional Chinese medicinal plants in widespread non-exudative atopic eczema, Sheehan MP and Atherton DJ, *Br J Dermatol* 1992; 126: 179–84.

A trial of artemether or quinine in children with cerebral malaria, Van Hensbroek MB *et al*, *N Eng J Med* 1996; 335: 69–75.

Anti-tumor effects of PC-SPES, an herbal formulation in prostate cancer, Tiwari RK *et al*, *Int J Oncol* 1999; 14: 713–19.

Chinese medicinal herbs for asymptomatic carriers of hepatitis B virus infection, Liu JP *et al*, Cochrane Database Syst Rev 2001; 2: CD002231.

Chinese medicinal herbs for chronic hepatitis B, Liu JP *et al*, Cochrane Database Syst Rev, 2001; 1: CD001940.

Clinical and biologic activity of an estrogenic herbal combination (PC-SPES) in prostate cancer, DiPaola RS *et al*, *N Eng J Med* 1998; 339: 785–91.

Comparison of artemether and chloroquine for severe malaria in Gambian children, White NJ *et al*, *Lancet* 1992; 339: 317–21

Complications resulting from the use of Chinese herbal medications containing undeclared prescription drugs, Gertner E *et al*, *Arthrits, Rheum* 1995; 38: 614–17.

Do certain countries produce only positive results? A systematic review of controlled trials, Vickers A *et al*, Control Clin Trials 1998; 19: 159–66.

Does dong quai have estrogenic effects in postmenopausal women?: a double-blind placebo-controlled trial, Hirata JD, *Fertil Steril* 1997; 68: 981–6.

Dong quai, Zhu DP, *Am J Chin Med* 1987; 15: 117–25.

Drug overdose and other poisoning in Hong Kong – the Prince of Wales Hospital (Sharin) experience, Chan TYK *et al*, *Hum Exp Toxicol* 1993; 13: 512–15.

Efficacy of traditional Chinese herbal therapy in adult atopic dermatitis, Sheehan MP *et al*, *Lancet* 1992; 340: 13–17.

Herbal therapy PC-SPES: in vitro effects and evaluation of its efficacy in 69 patients with prostate cancer, de la Taille A *et al*, *J Urol* 2000; 164: 1229–34.

Ma-huang strikes again: ephedrine nephrolithiasis, Powell T *et al*, *Am J Kidney Dis* 1998; 32: 153–9.

Oestrogen-like effect of ginseng, Punnonen R and Lukola A, *BMJ* 1980; 281: 1110.

One-year follow up of children treated with Chinese medicinal herbs for atopic eczema, Sheehan MP and Atherton DJ, *Br J Dermatol* 1994; 130: 488–93.

PC-SPES: a unique inhibitor of proliferation of prostate cancer cells in vitro and in vivo, Khubota T *et al*, *Prostate* 2000; 42: 163–71.

Qinghaosu, Hein TT and White NJ, *Lancet* 1993; 341: 603–8.

Rediscovering wormwood: qinghaosu for malaria, [No author listed], *Lancet* 1992; 339: 649–51.

Risks associated with the practice of traditional Chinese medicine: an Australian study, Bensoussan A *et al*, *Arch Fam Pract* 2000; 9: 1071–8.

Treatment of irritable bowel syndrome with Chinese herbal medicine: a randomized controlled trial, Bensoussan A *et al*, *JAMA* 1998; 280: 1585–9.

Treatment of severe malaria with artemisinin derivatives: a systematic review of randomised controlled trials, McIntosh HM and Olliaro P, *Med Trop (Mars)* 1998; 58 (3 Suppl): 61–2.

Chapter 20. Urine Therapy

Effects of urea treatment in combination with curretage in extensive periopthalmic malignancies, Danopoulos ED and Danopoulou IE, *Opthalmologica* 1979; 179: 52–61.

Effects of urea treatment in malignancies of the conjuntiva and cornea, Danopoulos ED *et al*, *Opthalmologica* 1979; 178: 198–203.

Eleven years' experience of oral urea treatment in liver malignancies, Danopoulos ED and Danopoulou IE, *Clin Oncol* 1981; 7: 281–9.

Melatonin supplementation from early morning auto-urine drinking, Mills MH and Faunce TA, *Med Hypotheses* 1991; 36: 195–9.

The results of urea treatment in liver malignancies, Danopoulos ED and Danopoulou IE, *Clin Oncol* 1975; 1: 341–50.

The Water of Life: the Golden Fountain; the Complete Guide to Urine Therapy, Coen van der Kroon 1993. English translation by Merilee Dranow, Oxford: Amethyst Books 1996.

Your Own Perfect Medicine, Christy MM, Self Healing Press 1994.

Chapter 21. Yoga

A new physiological approach to control essential hypertension, Selvamurthy W *et al*, *Ind J Physiol Pharmacol* 42: 205–13.

A study of response pattern of non-insulin-dependent diabetics to yoga therapy, Jain SC *et al*, *Diabetes Res Clin Pract* 1993; 19: 69–74.

An integrated approach to yoga therapy for bronchial asthma: a 3–54 month prospective study, Nagendra HR and Nagarathna R, *J Asthma* 1986; 23: 123–37.

Clinical study of yoga techniques in university students with asthma: a controlled study, Vedantham PK *et al*, *Allergy Asthma Proc* 1998; 19: 3–9.

EEG changes during forced alternate nostril breathing, Stancak A Jr and Kuna M, *Int J Psychophysiol* 1994; 18: 75–9.

Effect of yoga breathing exercises (pranayama) on airway reactivity in subjects with asthma, Singh V *et al*, *Lancet* 1990; 355; 1381–3.

Effect of yoga training on exercise tolerance in adolescents with childhood asthma, Jain SC *et al*, *J Asthma* 1991; 28: 437–42.

Evaluation of a yoga based regimen for treatment of osteoarthritis of the hands, Garfinkel M *et al, J Rheumatol* 1994; 21: 2341–3.

Improvement in static motor performance following yogic training of school children, Telles S *et al, Perceptual and Motor Skills* 1993; 76: 1264–6.

Kapalabhati – yogic cleansing exercise. II. EEG topography analysis, Stancak A Jr *et al, Homeost Health Dis* 1991; 33: 182–9.

Lipid profile of coronary risk subjects following yogic lifestyle interventions, Mahajan AS *et al, Indian Heart J* 1999; 51: 37–40.

Mind-body fitness: encouraging prospects for primary and secondary prevention, La Forge R, *J Cardiovasc Nurs* 1997; 11: 53–65.

Mood change and perceptions of vitality: a comparison of the effects of relaxation, visualization and yoga, Wood C, *J Royal Soc Med* 1993; 86: 254–8.

Nasal airflow asymmetries and human performance, Klein R *et al, Biological Psychol* 1986; 23: 127–37.

Oxygen consumption during pranayamic type of very slow rate breathing, Telles S and Desiraju T, *Ind J Med Res* 1991; 94: 357–63.

Pain management and yoga, Nespor K, *Int J Psychosom* 1991; 38: 76–81.

Physiological changes in sports teachers following 3 months of training in yoga, Telles S *et al, Indian J Med Sci* 1993; 47: 235–8.

Randomised controlled trial of yoga and bio-feedback in management of hypertension, Patel C and North WR, *Lancet* 1975; 2: 93–5.

Selective hemispheric stimulation by unilateral forced nostril breathing, Werntz DA *et al, Human Neurobiol* 1987; 6: 165–71.

The effect of yogic lifestyle on hypertension, Sachdeva U, *Homeost Health Dis* 1994; 35: 264.

The effects of unilateral forced nostril breathing on cognition, Shanahoff-Khalsa DS *et al, Int J Neurosci*, 1991; 57: 239–49.

The integrated approach of yoga: a therapeutic tool for mentally retarded children: a one year controlled study, Uma K *et al, J Mental Deficiency Res* 1989; 33: 415–21.

Treatment of essential hypertension with yoga relaxation therapy in a USAF aviator: a case report, Brownstein A, *Aviat Space Environ Sci* 1989; 60: 684–7.

Yoga and bio-feedback in the management of hypertension, Patel C, *Lancet* 1973; 10: 1053–5.

Yoga based intervention for carpal tunnel syndrome: a randomised trial, Garfinkel M *et al, JAMA* 1998; 280: 1601–3.

Yoga for bronchial asthma: a controlled study, Nagarathna R and Nagendra R, *BMJ* 1985; 291: 1077–9.

Yoga for epilepsy, Ramaratnam S and Sridharan K, *Cochrane Database Syst Rev* 2000; 3: CD001524.

Yoga therapy for NIDDM, Monro R *et al, Comp Med Res* 1992; 6: 66–8.

Yoga, Garfinkel M and Schumacher HR Jr, *Rheum Dis Clin North Am* 2000; 26: 125–32.

329

Index